Instrument-assisted Myofascial Therapy

of related interest

Mobilizing the Myofascial System
A Clinical Guide to Assessment and Treatment of Myofascial Dysfunctions
Doreen Killens
Forewords by Diane Lee, Thomas W. Myers and BetsyAnn Baron
ISBN 978 1 90914 190 2
eISBN 978 1 90914 191 9

The Myofascial System in Form and Movement
Laurie Nemetz
ISBN 978 1 91208 579 8
eISBN 978 1 91208 580 4

Fascial Dysfunction, Second Edition
Manual Therapy Approaches
Leon Chaitow
ISBN 978 1 90914 194 0
eISBN 978 1 90914 195 7

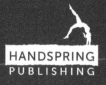

HANDSPRING
PUBLISHING

Instrument-assisted Myofascial Therapy

Principles and Clinical Applications

Edited by

Jürgen Förster ◆ Phillip Page

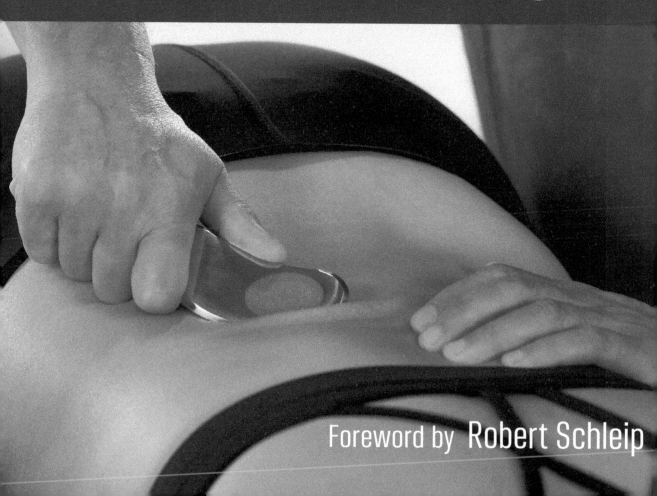

Foreword by Robert Schleip

First published in Great Britain in 2023 by Handspring Publishing, an imprint of Jessica Kingsley Publishers
An imprint of Hodder & Stoughton Ltd
An Hachette UK Company

1

A CIP catalogue record for this title is available from the British Library and the Library of Congress

ISBN 978 1 9134 2645 3
eISBN 978 1 9134 2646 0

Printed and bound in Great Britain by Ashford Colour Press Limited

Jessica Kingsley Publishers' policy is to use papers that are natural, renewable, and recyclable products and made from wood grown in sustainable forests. The logging and manufacturing processes are expected to conform to the environmental regulations of the country of origin.

Handspring Publishing
Carmelite House
50 Victoria Embankment
London EC4Y 0DZ

www.handspringpublishing.com

DEDICATION

To Gella, Mikka and Nathalie – *JF*

To Angela, Andrew, Hannah, Caitlin, and Madison – *PP*

CONTENTS

CONTENTS *continued*

ABOUT THE EDITORS

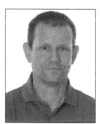

Jürgen Förster PT MA is a physiotherapist from the German-speaking community of Belgium. He first studied physiotherapy and education in Belgium (Brussels and Liège), and then undertook further studies in Germany in the management of health and social care institutions. He has managed several physical therapy schools in his career, including the one at the University Hospital RWTH Aachen. Jürgen has a long track record as lecturer in the physical therapy program at Aachen University and the University of Applied Sciences Aachen. Jürgen received his doctorate in theoretical medical science. He has been an international speaker in the field of musculoskeletal therapy for many years, and for more than ten years he has been intensively involved in the development of the Myofascial Connected System and Instrument-assisted Myofascial Therapy (IAMT). He is the author of several articles and wrote the first German-language book on this subject.

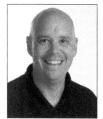

Phillip Page PhD PT ATC LAT CSCS FACSM is an Associate Professor and research director at Franciscan University Physical Therapy program, Baton Rouge, Louisiana. He is a licensed physical therapist and certified athletic trainer. He has a Master's degree in Exercise Physiology and a PhD in Kinesiology from Louisiana State University (LSU). Dr Page is a Fellow of the American College of Sports Medicine, as well as recipient of the Lifetime Excellence in Education award from the American Academy of Sports Physical Therapy section of the American Physical Therapy Association. He has presented over 200 international lectures and workshops on exercise and rehabilitation topics and has written over 100 publications, including three books. His research interests include electromyography and pathokinematic analysis, as well as the use of technology in rehabilitation. He has worked with the athletic programs at LSU, Tulane, and the NFL New Orleans Saints and Seattle Seahawks, as well as the United States Olympic Track and Field Trials.

ABOUT THE CONTRIBUTORS

Shawn Burger PT, DPT, CSCS operates Burger Physical Therapy, California, providing outpatient, acute, and long-term care rehabilitation services. He currently lectures internationally on various topics related to manual therapy, rehabilitation, and business management solutions.

Ashley M. Campbell PT, DPT, SCS is Director of Rehabilitation at the Nashville Hip Institute, Tennessee Orthopaedic Alliance, and Managing Editor of the *International Journal of Sports Physical Therapy*.

Gregory H. Doerr DC, CCSP is the co-developer of FAKTR and developer of Functional Soft Tissue. He is the owner and Clinical Director of Bergen Chiropractic and Sports Rehabilitation Center, New Jersey.

Sue Falsone PT, DPT, MS, SCS, ATC, CSCS, COMT is the owner of Structure and Function Education, and Associate Professor of Athletic Training Programs at A.T. Still University, Arizona.

Arndt Fengler qualified as a physiotherapist in 1996 and as an osteopath in 2004. Arndt has also worked as an alternative practitioner since 2010, and is based in Koppigen, Switzerland.

Brian V. Hortz PhD, ATC, SFDN is Director of Research and Education at Structure and Function Education, Columbus, Ohio.

Ute Imhof is a specialist in pediatric physiotherapy and teaches internationally in the field of child treatment. She is the owner of Barnasfysioterapeut Clinic, Rasta-Lørenskog, Norway.

Markus Rossman is a movement and body therapist, international lecturer, certified physical education teacher, and Rolfer™. He is a member of the ARTZT Fazer expert team, and fascial expert at Kirinus Alpenpark Klinik, Bad Wiessee, Germany.

Bodo von Unruh is a physiotherapist, sports physiotherapist, member of the ARTZT Fazer expert team, and teacher for taping, myofascial therapy and athletic training based in Stuttgart, Germany.

James Wagner OTD, OTR/L, CHT, CPAM, CSCS is an occupational therapist and certified hand therapist. He is currently the team leader of the Guthrie Hand Center and is an adjunct professor of occupational therapy programs at both Keuka College and Ithaca College in New York state.

FOREWORD by Robert Schleip

If you have already learned the art of using your hands as tools of love, as soft-surgery instruments, as musical instruments, as temperature sensors, as finely tuned craft tools, as listening touch devices, and as extensions of your heart, then this book is a gift for you.

Like the two editors of this book, Jürgen Förster and Phillip Page, I continue to touch most of my clients with my bare hands. This sets us apart from mainstream Western orthopedic medicine, which tends to align its values with the slogan "high tech and low touch." In contrast, most myofascial therapy practitioners are more deeply inspired by the values of complementary medicine, which could be described as "low tech and high touch." To then consider augmenting the use of our hands with the additional usage of hand-held tools requires the uttermost care and consideration. The intention of this book is not to replace the skillful touch of your hands, but to enhance their functioning in particular times and special circumstances. Imagine working with your fingers or knuckles on the heel pad or the lower back of a very tall and strong client, wishing you could continue working with an even stronger melting force for a few more minutes, without losing the sensitivity in your compressed fingers. This is where the specific tool usage recommendations of this excellent book may be useful.

The use of small hand-held devices has been developed in many cultures for a long time. Modern research has additionally revealed that our human brains are specially gifted in incorporating the sensory information from prosthetic tools into our own body schema and perceptual organization. For example, some blind people are specially gifted in sensing subtle vibrations of the ground with their walking stick; yet, this perceptual extension demands an intimate coupling process of the sensing person with the specific tool in their hands. I therefore advise you to choose your tools very wisely. Apply a similar degree of appreciative attention that you would devote to choosing a long-term prosthesis for your body or selecting a musical instrument. My personal advice, based on several decades of working with such tools in addition to regular myofascial release work, is to always start and end your session with your bare hands and then consciously choose to temporarily augment their precision with one of the tools shown here. The book will inspire you on how to enrich your technical expertise in a myriad of manners, with the use of different instruments in many different situations. In fact, seeing the impressive line-up of contributing authors, I can attest to you that this book covers the largest context of related therapeutic applications that I have ever seen for instrument-assisted manual work.

In addition to the specific technical presentations in this book, I find the step-by-step approach particularly significant. This systematic approach through evaluation and treatment recognizes the myofascial connected system and the application of specific instrumented techniques to address common myofascial impairments. This new approach will certainly enrich the treatment of myofascial disorders.

Let me finish by sharing one of my favorite situations in which I deeply enjoy working with a hand-held therapeutic tool. When addressing very dense scar tissues, such as around the greater trochanter after a hip surgery, I try to apply a hypnotically slow sliding speed of my fingertips across the scar. When working this way, I can elicit a deeper rehydration and softening effect compared with more rapid manual strokes. In fact, my intention is to find the slowest possible continuous sliding speed that does not yet fall apart into several "and go" motions. With my bare hands, plus possibly the use of some non-slippery cream, I can go as slowly as 1 cm (½ inch) in a few seconds, but not slower. With the right tool held with both of my touching hands, I can now slide across several times slower while sensing through that tool into the slowly flattening scar underneath. Yes, this requires some mindful and curious experimentation to find the right tool for your hands and for your favorite tissue challenges. Let this book inspire you, giving yourself a valuable gift when working with your educated hands within the context of soft tissue work. Your hands and your clients will applaud you for venturing in this new and enriching direction.

Robert Schleip PhD
Professor of Human Biology
Director, Fascia Research Group
Technical University of Munich and Ulm University
Germany
Vice-President, Fascia Research Society
April 2022

PREFACE

This book is the result of more than ten years of development of a fascinating and very helpful therapeutic technique. For this very reason, it was important to us to share this result with the dear reader. Knowing well that the presented technique of IAMT is not and will not be everyone's cup of tea (and it certainly does not have to be!), we wish that by publishing this work we can make a small contribution to the effective treatment of a certain number of patients. We sincerely hope that the experienced therapists for whom this book is intended will be able to restore range of motion and relieve pain in some of their patients through the judicious use of IAMT. In short, they will be able to improve the quality of life of their patients. If this happens, we will have achieved our most important goal.

The fact that we even came up with the idea of writing the book is thanks to several people who encouraged us to do so. First and foremost, Robert Schleip, who asked us in January 2020 – seemingly casually, at a symposium – why we hadn't already written a book about our experiences with the IAMT. We were initially speechless and a little frightened at the mere thought of taking on this challenge. This put a lot of pressure on us, but also got the ball rolling. This book is our belated answer, so to speak. Thank you (not only) for that! During the editing of the book, we have received important support from numerous colleagues, both in professional and human terms. We would like to thank them all sincerely; to list them all would go beyond the scope of this article, but we are sure that the right ones felt addressed. The same applies, of course, to the employees and co-workers of the publishing house: many thanks for the great care and support. A very special thanks goes to our co-authors, who were all immediately willing to collaborate on the book. The quality of the chapters fully confirms our selection. And a very heartfelt thank you to our families who have always supported us and thus made the realization of this book possible. Last but not least, we would like to thank posthumously Ludwig Artzt. It was he who brought us together in 2000 at a congress in Krakow, Poland. Without him we would not know each other as such friends. He and his idealistic ideas paved the way for this book. Rest in peace dear Ludwig. We will not forget you.

The transatlantic cooperation between the tranquil Eupen, the (secret) capital of the German-speaking community of Belgium, and Baton Rouge, the capital of the US state of Louisiana, worked out very well and was a great pleasure. We hope that the result will reflect this. As mentioned earlier, the book is a structured rendering of the IAMT experience. The therapy results achieved daily in patients encourage us to continue on the path we have chosen and to further develop the concept presented here. We would be very pleased to receive your suggestions. We would also – and especially – be pleased if the path towards scientific research into the effectiveness of IAMT would continue to develop. Any contribution will be very welcome.

Jürgen Förster and Phillip Page
Eupen and Baton Rouge
April 2022

Of course, the editors would be very pleased if readers "devoured" this whole book attentively and with interest, but this is probably only the case with an exciting and captivating novel; in any case, it isn't necessary with the text that is in front of you or in your hands right now. The book is based on the practical experience of using instruments in the treatment of myofascial lesions. It is neither a theoretical foundation nor a scientific treatise, but is intended as a guide to the use of instruments in daily practice. The use of instruments – and therefore also this book – should create added value for the practitioner. Therapists should be able to integrate the devices into their daily practice, immediately after reading these chapters and without any further effort. The book should enable them to use the instruments profitably, both for the well-being of the patient, in terms of higher effectiveness and efficiency of the therapy, and for the well-being of the therapist, in terms of protecting their own joints! The text is designed in such a way that it is possible for therapists (!) to carry out the procedures in complete safety without any problems. Thus, users can gain their own experience and further improve their skills.

The book aims to be a kind of introductory guide to the topic – not a directive. On the one hand, the techniques and therapy protocols presented have proven themselves in practice; on the other hand, they are intended only as a basis on which therapists can build as reflective practitioners. Thus, there are no restrictions – apart from valid medical contraindications, of course – on the handling of the devices. The techniques are suggestions for use; they have been tested in a variety of ways and are constantly being developed further.

These chapters are the fruit of years of professional use. The therapy results we have achieved have been continuously evaluated over this time and treatment has been adapted accordingly. Nevertheless, therapists should let their own experience flow into the use of the instruments – and perhaps share it with the community. In this way, Instrument-assisted Myofascial Therapy (IAMT) could constantly develop and improve. The concept of IAMT does not pretend to be evidence-based but has the ambition to evolve towards it. It is, however, based on scientific knowledge and has been developed in close collaboration with leading scientists and practitioners in the field of myofascial lesions – so it is an evidence-*informed* and *theory*-based approach to practice. After reading the book, therapists should therefore integrate the devices into their therapy plan – which they have drawn up on the basis of their findings or diagnosis – and be creative.

To ensure that they can do this in complete safety and that the therapy results are correspondingly good – because that, in essence, is what it is all about – the handling is described in this book in a highly standardized and precise manner: embedded in a frequently encountered lesion, a treatment protocol is first presented for one particular structure. An exact description is given of which instrument is to be used and in which starting position the therapy is carried out. The progressions in the therapy are then listed, as well as the possible treatment options within the entire myofascial system. Starting from the structure treated initially, the so-called "myofascial junctions" are presented: first regionally in a distal to proximal direction and finally within a functional myofascial chain. We call this the Myofascial Connected System (MCS). The use of this system greatly simplifies the way this book may be employed, and is explained below. It is an essential point to grasp and is presented in a short but important chapter (see Chapter 1).

In order to round off the entire treatment and to place it in the real-life context of a modern physiotherapeutic treatment, preparatory and follow-up techniques are described. Although the results of the therapy are not scientifically evaluated (this is by no means our claim) practical tests are presented which guide therapists safely in their work. The book is richly

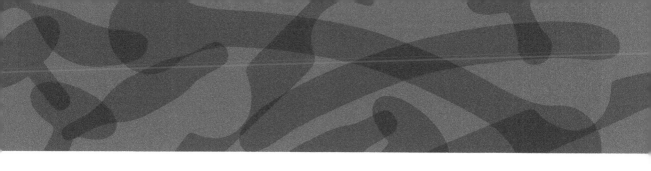

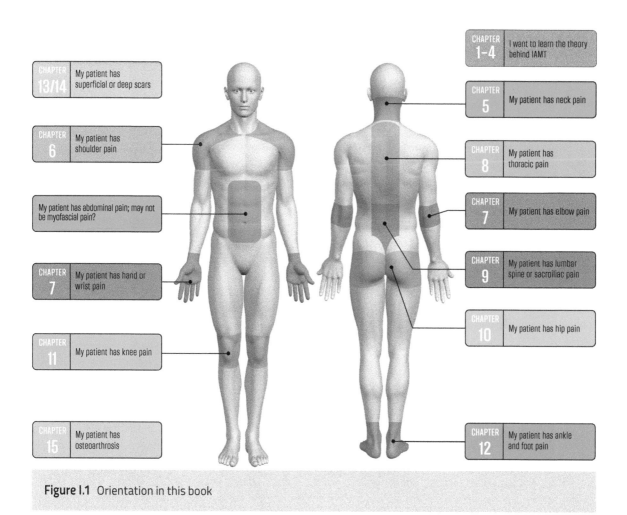

Figure I.1 Orientation in this book

CHAPTER 13/14	My patient has superficial or deep scars
CHAPTER 6	My patient has shoulder pain
	My patient has abdominal pain; may not be myofascial pain?
CHAPTER 7	My patient has hand or wrist pain
CHAPTER 11	My patient has knee pain
CHAPTER 15	My patient has osteoarthrosis

CHAPTER 1-4	I want to learn the theory behind IAMT
CHAPTER 5	My patient has neck pain
CHAPTER 8	My patient has thoracic pain
CHAPTER 7	My patient has elbow pain
CHAPTER 9	My patient has lumbar spine or sacroiliac pain
CHAPTER 10	My patient has hip pain
CHAPTER 12	My patient has ankle and foot pain

illustrated and has numerous tables also. The text has been consciously reduced to the minimum. In summary, it can be said that the book has been written from the practice for the practice and is a manual for daily use in physiotherapy. In order to optimize its use, Figure I.1 gives readers a quick orientation.

The scheme provides readers with a quick-start guide. First, they find the page on which the structure

they want to treat is presented. From this starting point, therapists can, if they wish, use the MCS to find the treatment of structures connected to the injured one. This connected body-wide network of myofascial structures is represented by honeycombs (Figure I.2). On each side of these hexagons are structures which are directly related, both anatomically and functionally, to the structure to be treated. The parts of the MCS influence each other in the sense of forming an inseparably connected and interrelated system without beginning or end. There are no one-way streets nor directions – only connections, which serve a common goal as an ingenious network: moving! The therapy becomes more effective and efficient by treating these connections. Each structure is assigned a certain (arbitrarily selected) number, which should make the system easier for the reader to handle. The structure keeps the same number throughout the book, guiding the reader easily and quickly through an incredibly complex web of myofascial structures. Once therapists are familiar with the system, they will discover completely new therapy methods and possibilities. Doc. MUDr. František Véle, CSc., of the Charles University in Prague, once compared it to a mountain hike. In the valley you see a mountain; if you climb it, you see another mountain range; and at the top of this range, you see a completely new landscape, which you could not see from the valley. The MCS serves as a reliable guide for the therapist during this hike.

Here's an example of how the MCS works: let's take the painful structure of the Achilles tendon. The therapist treats this first; then – depending on the findings, of course – they continue with the treatment of the connected structures, such as the iliotibial tract (IT band). From this new starting point, the treatment continues: for example, via the gluteus maximus muscle to the fascia thoracolumbalis and so on. The therapist thus receives the theory-based legitimation to treat the whole body if necessary: to use the words of therapist and educator David Butler, the license to look at the whole body.

The treatments here are always related to anatomical structures. The presentation of the treatment of individual diagnoses or clinical pictures on the International Classification of Functioning, Disability and Health (ICF) structural level is, however, didactic in nature. Of course, the treatment must always be seen in the context of the activity and participation level. The treatment presented for these structures can be easily applied by the experienced therapist to other

1 Achilles tendon
2 Plantar aponeurosis
3 Peroneus longus
4 Gastrocnemius
5 Tibialis posterior
6 Flexor digitorum brevis
7 Iliotibial tract
8 Biceps femoris
9 Flexor hallucis longus

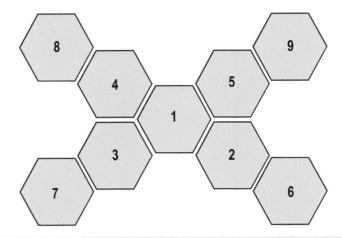

Figure I.2 Representation of the Myofascial Connected System

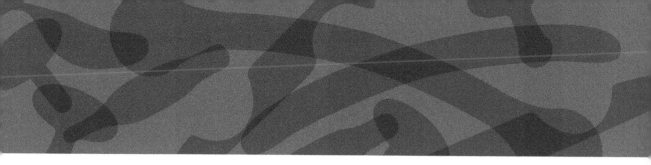

diagnoses relating to the same structures. Thus, the diagnoses can be described as truly exemplary.

Finally, the editors would like to return briefly to the first sentence of these remarks. This book is written to enable the practitioner to immediately apply the techniques safely and profitably for the patient. No one needs to read the book as a whole in order to integrate the techniques into their therapy. Thus, the reader may very well tackle a single chapter and begin treatment straight away. While the editors attach great importance to this practicability, we would like be clear that this decisive advantage for the reader has meant that we sometimes repeat various statements several times throughout the book. This is the only way to ensure that readers can integrate the techniques into their daily therapeutic routine as quickly as possible. These repetitions thus have a practical and didactic background and are as sensible as they are indispensable; in no way do they serve to artificially increase the length of the book. We will, of course, be pleased if every reader "devours" the book in its entirety, but at the same time we would like to apologize to our colleagues for these redundancies.

We hope you enjoy exploring or delving into the fascinating world of IAMT, and sincerely hope that it becomes an integral part of your therapy and of physical therapy worldwide.

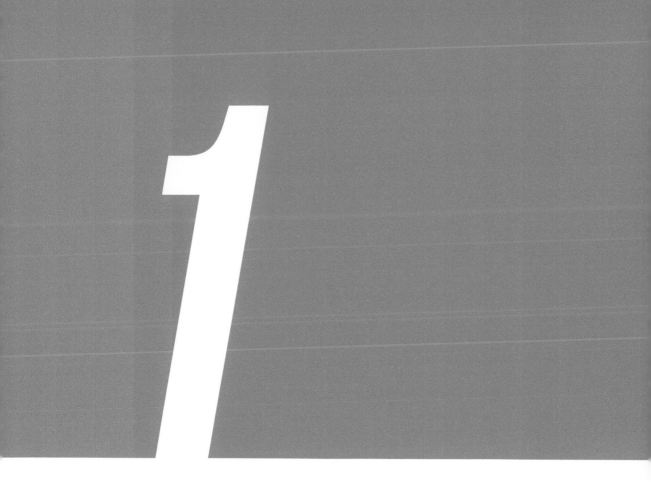

1

Evidence-based Practice

The first part of this book deals with the theoretical background to IAMT. Some or all of this information may already be familiar to readers; however, everyone should be able to follow the techniques presented in later sections. This seems to the authors to be the prerequisite for the successful and sustainable integration of the techniques into our colleagues' daily therapeutic routine. We have chosen a comprehensible structure that makes this possible. Therefore, the structures that will be treated later are described first: the myofascial system. This is not approached classically in the sense of descriptive anatomy, but rather from the authors' own point of view, so that "only" the essential information is passed on; the book should not be unnecessarily overloaded. The same principle is applied in the next chapter, where the theory of IAMT is presented appropriately, in just enough detail, and in a clearly structured way. Unnecessary explanations have been deliberately omitted in favor of easy readability, but we consider it important to briefly describe the history of IAMT, as well as the various instruments available on the market. This clearly serves a better understanding of the therapy. The current literature on IAMT is also described in this chapter. The evidence is presented transparently and readers are provided with the information they need to evaluate the therapy for themselves. The concept described here is not evidence-based but is understood to be evidence-*informed*. Chapter 3 then describes the application techniques in detail, so that the reader will be better able to understand their individual use later on. Finally, and logically, integration into the therapeutic routine is described. Here the indications, contraindications, and limitations are presented, along with complementary and preparatory techniques and clinical decision-making.

Evidence-based Practice

There are several excellent books on the myofascial system, authored by experts in the field of anatomy. Several of these are referenced in this book; therefore, a detailed anatomical description of the structures treated has been considered beyond the scope of this text. It is not our aim to impart anatomical knowledge; rather, the objective is to share and disseminate our knowledge of Instrument-assisted Myofascial Therapy (IAMT), and especially our practical experience of it. It is more of a question of why we use the instrument as opposed to the structural anatomy, and so we propose a more functional viewpoint: the Myofascial Connected System.

Functional Anatomy of the Myofascial System

When we talk about fascia, we first need to put these structures in the right context. Fascia is a type of connective tissue; however, the term "connective tissues" is often used as a synonym for fascia. Connective tissue comes in several different forms, including fatty tissue, cartilage, bone, and the three-dimensional network that forms the framework of all organs (except the glia cells in the central nervous system, CNS). Fascia can be thought of as the tissue connecting muscles and bones. Fascial structures include tendons, ligaments, joint capsules, muscle connective tissue, and even organ capsules. Fascial structures can be classified as loose or tight tissue, or as reticular tissue (see page 6).

Fascia plays another supporting part in movement by providing for the absorption, conduction, processing, and excretion of vital nutrients. It also serves an important role during hemodynamic and biochemical processes, especially during the recovery process in tissue after injuries. Therefore, viewing this system as a purely fascial one (that is, as a mere connecting and supporting system for organs, vessels, and nerves) does not do justice to the current state of knowledge. This system, integrated with a contractile component, becomes extremely versatile and important for the human being: this is the myofascial system, essential for survival because it makes both structure and function possible in human beings. The myofascial system, as a completely interconnected and body-spanning system, is destined for that which ensures human life: movement. Thus, we will call it the Myofascial Connected System (MCS), consisting of various individual structures working together that serve the common goal of supporting human movement.

In the literal sense, the word "fascia" means something that holds structures together. The first International Fascia Research Congress (Findley and Schleip 2007) described the fascia as a rough or coarse membrane, or as "soft tissue components of the tissue which run through the whole body as a wrapping and connecting tension network. These include all collagen containing fiber-like tissues, in particular joint and organ capsules, aponeurosis, muscle septa, ligaments, tendons, retinacula" (Findley and Schleip 2007). These elastic structures build a so-called "body-wide network" or a "body-wide web." This connected web is built to hold all the structures of the human body together in the right place; this is called "structural integrity." In addition to this structural integrity, various authors speak of a so-called "tensegrity," a term that integrates tension and integrity. In the human body, it describes a network responsible for the correct tension in the entire myofascial system: in every part of the system, at every time, and in every situation. This "bio-tensegrity" is the key to purposeful, effective, and efficient functioning of the system. Myofascial tensegrity generally consists of two components:

- transmission of force (or of power) from one structure to the other throughout the myofascial system

- the resulting movement (or stabilization) of the trunk and extremities.

As in any system, the system is only as strong as the weakest link in the (myokinetic) chain. Often, therapists look for the weakest link and treat it to restore kinetic chain function.

The myofascial system functions in its entirety and should be considered in this way both diagnostically and therapeutically. Many muscles have so-called myofascial "expansions" that provide for the optimal transmission of forces. These expansions essentially spread the muscle insertion across a broader area beyond the individual tendon insertion. An isolated tendon insertion cannot do this; the myofascial expansions make this optimal transmission possible. The origins and attachments of muscles discussed in descriptive anatomy are merely insertions of individual muscle fibers, the proportion of which can also vary.

The human body is designed for movement. The structural components of movement (namely, bones, joints, and muscles) are innately connected and supported by the myofascial system.

One must also consider the neurological components of human movement, which control the muscles that move bones and joints. This neurological control begins in the CNS but also must interact with the peripheral nervous system. In addition to supporting movement, the myofascial system forms a matrix for intercellular communication.

The MCS serves an important feedback role in human movement. Afferent stimuli (extero- and interoceptive) are received by receptors and transmitted to the CNS. Many of these afferent sensors (proprioceptors) are found in the fascia: Pacinian corpuscles (sensors for vibration and acceleration), Ruffini corpuscles (sensors for vibration and pressure), Meissner corpuscles (sensors for vibration), Merkel corpuscles (sensors for light touch), Golgi tendon organ (sensor for tissue tension), and the muscle spindle (sensor for tissue length). The afferent information from these fascial receptors leads to efferent responses of the muscular system in controlling movement; thus, the MCS can be considered a sensorimotor system.

In addition to proprioceptors, the MCS contains nociceptors (free nerve endings); it may therefore be considered a "nocimotor" system as well as a sensorimotor system (perhaps this is why some speak of fascia as the sixth sense organ!). Accordingly, fascia plays a major role in the development of pain. Since the causes of myofascial pain lie in the fasciae and are poorly identified with current imaging techniques, they often remain unrecognized or are underestimated. Because the myofascial system is linked throughout the body, myofascial pain tends to be more global than regional, leading to pain being felt throughout the body.

The general structure of human tissue layers can be roughly represented as follows, from superficial to deep: dermis, epidermis, superficial fat layer, superficial fascia, intermediate fat layer, deep fascia, muscle, then bone. The myofascial system can be layered in a superficial and a profound part, and an intramuscular and a visceral part.

The superficial part is subcutaneous and envelops organs, glands, and neurovascular channels; it plays the role of a force transducer and shock absorber, and stores water and fat. As a side note, traction on the veins passing through these fascial elements could be an explanation of the muscular pump action on these vessels, rather than compression by the muscles (Stecco 2017).

The deep or profound fascial layers (fascia proper, aponeurosis, retinacula, ligaments, tendons) consist of dense, fiber-rich tissue that is organized in the form of layers and strands. The direction of the fibers runs parallel within a layer; however, this direction changes in each layer. This creates a three-dimensional structure which, in its entirety, can transmit forces in three planes of movement without restricting mobility. This also demonstrates how important it is that the individual layers maintain their mobility while interacting with other layers. If there is insufficient or no mobility within the individual layers, the system loses its unique effect; individual parts are overloaded while others are underloaded. This again demonstrates the value of physiological stimuli through movement and the specificity of the structures. In the lower limb, the fascial structures are less elastic than in the upper limb because they support human gait and the upright stance. The strong retinacula of the lower limb are also important for proprioception; it is likely that this is why we find them where joints tend to need stability, such as at the ankle and knee. However, in the upper limb, range of motion and mobility are more important. The upper extremity fascial structures are more elastic: the arms are made to move and to manipulate the environment, and we use them to feed ourselves.

Due to the anatomy, the transmission of mechanical forces occurs primarily in the deep fasciae due to their high viscoelastic strength; the superficial fasciae are less suitable for this purpose because of their high mobility. Similar to the superficial fascia, the deep fascia protects and supports movement, but also transmits power. The deep fascia penetrates and surrounds muscles, bones, nerves, and blood vessels.

Microscopically, the major components of fascia are the extracellular matrix (ECM) and cells in relatively small numbers (granulocytes, lymphocytes, plasma cells, and fibroblasts). The lymphocytes and the granulocytes play a role in immunological defense. Plasma is the fluid that contains these components, while fibroblasts are a specific type of cell of the connective tissue that produce mainly collagen fibers. The fact that there are fewer cells in fascia compared to other tissues creates correspondingly larger spacing in this extracellular space. The ECM consists of the basic substance (water, proteins, nutrients, hormones,

electrolytes, and adhesive molecules like heparin, fibronectin, and hyaluronan), as well as fibers (collagen, elastin, and reticulin). The mixture of basic substance and fibers is variable, depending on the function or type of tissue. The basic substance of the ECM consists of approximately 68 percent water; 50 percent of that water in the basic substance is in a bound state (liquid crystal). This composition is mainly responsible for its viscoelasticity (VE). VE represents tissue internal mobility and is mainly dependent on the water content of the tissue (Schleip et al. 2012). If water content decreases, the VE deteriorates (that is, tissues stiffen) and the mechanical transfer of forces between tissues is reduced.

In addition to traditional angular movements of bones around joints in the body (osteokinematics), translational movements occur within the joints (arthrokinematics). Translational movements occur where two or more structures move against each other, as seen in joints, and also between muscle bundles and the different layers of tissue. This movement is referred to as "gliding" and exists in the superficial tissue layers, the tenoperiosteal transitions, and the courses of the tendons and ligaments. Adjacent tissues must be able to glide and slide against each other; if not, hypomobilities can occur that may require mobilization.

Between fascial layers, one may consider translational movement as something like a "fascial joint." These movements make the MCS a gliding system. This tissue gliding is enhanced by hyaluronic acid, produced by "fasciacytes" (fibroblast-like cells) (Stecco et al. 2018) between the layers of fascia.

Tendons are an important component of the myofascial system and the MCS. In the MCS, there are two types of tendon at the functional level: gliding tendons and transmission tendons. While the latter primarily transmit forces (such as the Achilles tendons) and thus must have a high stiffness, the former are primarily responsible for the redirection of forces (such as the peroneal tendons). These gliding tendons change their structure at the deflection points in order to withstand the high loads created by the muscles that are focused on one point of insertion.

Under ideal conditions, with sufficient intra- and inter-tissue mobility and VE, the MCS can develop one of its most important properties: the ability to store kinetic energy. This is also known as the "catapult effect." For example, during the lunging motion of a thrower, structures are stretched to length and corresponding energy is stored, which is then discharged during the throw. Another example comes from the animal world: the leverage of the hip of the red kangaroo is not decisive for its jumping power. Instead, the length of the corresponding tendons and thus the extreme ability to store kinetic energy provide the power needed (Kram and Dawson 1998).

The MCS is thus essential for economic human movement. However, this advantage of the sparing use of energy brings with it some requirements for the structures. These must combine multiple, sometimes contradictory properties (elasticity and stiffness), in order to exhibit low plasticity with high tensile strength. This is accomplished by various tissue types, including collagen, elastin, and reticulin. Collagen is a protein that forms fiber bundles as a structural protein. Of the twenty-eight different types of collagen, type Ia is the most common, and is prevalent in fascia.

Collagen has a high tensile strength; in fact, the body creates collagen in response to tension. In tendons and ligaments, the collagen fiber orientation is parallel; in joint capsules and other ligaments, it is rather inconsistent; and in skin, it is completely inconsistent. The turnover rate (half-life: that is, renewal of half of all cells) of collagen is 300–500 days.

The elastic fibers (elastin) also have high tensile strength but an undulating course. When tissue is stretched, elastin fibers are the first ones to be "stretched" (before the collagen fibers).

The reticular fibers are essentially a thinner form of collagen and have high bending elasticity and low tensile elasticity. Their role is primarily to support the organs, forming a lattice or net of support. This fiber distribution is responsible for both tissue quality and function.

Pathology of the Myofascial System

If the myofascial system is not appropriately challenged and the formation stimuli diminish, such as during immobilization, the ECM changes: degradation of proteoglycans leads to a reduction in water binding and thus to a decrease in the load-bearing capacity of these structures. This lack of movement (gliding) leads over time to adhesions; this in turn goes hand in hand with other consequences, such as a decrease in performance and coordination skills, a tendency for athletes (and non-athletes) to become prone to injuries, an increase in pain sensitivity, and a decrease of body self-perception.

Of course, too many stimuli can also lead to problems; therefore, the dose–response for myofascial structures must be in balance. The stimuli for building and maintaining the MCS are somewhat different for the various components. Concentric and eccentric contractions are important for the contractile components, while traction is the main stimulus for the fascial component. Together, the transmission of the contractions through the fasciae to the bones brings movement in all forms (rotatory and translatory) to all tissue levels (macroscopic and microscopic). Human movement is therefore the all-important formation stimulus for the MCS. But movement is not only important for prevention of injuries; it can be "anti-inflammatory" as well.

If this balance between loading and unloading tissue no longer holds, problems occur in a variety of areas. Muscles atrophy (hypotrophy), fat infiltrates muscle, and collagen synthesis increases with weakening of muscle strength. At the neuromuscular level there is reflex inhibition, hyperalgesia due to chronic inflammation (cytokines), and an increase in the sensitivity of the nociceptors. Overall, deconditioning of the MCS occurs over time and sets off a vicious cycle. Lack of sufficient load leads to a tendency toward adhesion, which, in turn, inhibits movement due to an improper recruitment of muscles fibers. Too much stress, on the other hand, leads to tissue proliferation, which also has an inhibitory effect. Both in turn result in limited mobility and the cycle continues indefinitely. In the early stages, the changes are functional and reversible. Over the course of time, this functional restriction becomes an anatomical problem with permanent restrictions due to remodeling mechanisms. These, in turn, can lead to new problems and cause a progression of deconditioning while the load-bearing capacity decreases and the susceptibility to injury increases.

For the therapist, this mixture of causes and consequences is, at some point, almost impossible to see through. This is because the protective reaction of the body is almost always an increase in tone (tension zone); however, this also occurs due to an overload (overload zone). It is often the case that the location of pain is not always – or is even rarely – identical with the location of lesion. The best way to determine this is through very precise examination.

For example, injuries to the transmission tendons often occur at the tenoperiosteal junction or at the myotendinous junction, whereas injuries to the gliding tendons tend to occur at the deflection point. In both, the symptoms (local pain, local hypertonus in the muscle belly, and hypomobility of the painful areas) are similar. Both injuries are tendinopathies in principle. This inflammatory reaction is the natural response to tissue overload. Even the treatment is the same – only the order differs. Generally, the therapist tries to treat the

cause first, then the consequence. Functional tests are then used to assess the efficacy of the treatment; these tests are presented in each chapter, dealing with each area in turn.

Functional Examples of the MCS

Often, the classical kinesiological approach of addressing human movement is a very mechanistic and structural one. It is characterized by the representation of individual structures and the corresponding assignment of analytical functions. This concept sees the bones as the framework of the body, which are moved by the muscles. Each muscle has at least two bony insertions (origin and insertion); the muscle uses force at origin and insertion that can easily be calculated through biomechanical analysis. However, in our approach to human movement we note that about 30 percent of the muscle fibers have fascial rather than bony attachments. Thus, a complete and body-wide continuous myofascial network is formed. The bones give this system the necessary stability and load-bearing capacity; they are moved around a multitude of joints by this system. In this way of thinking, each body structure is a cogwheel; if you turn one cogwheel, all the others move as well. There is an unconditional mutual influence and dependence.

Let's take the biceps brachii muscle, which is known as an elbow flexor and supinator. In addition, it is active in the shoulder joint as flexor and discrete abductor, and it fixes the humeral head in the glenoid cavity. But the biceps forms fascial connections with surrounding structures too: coracobrachialis, brachialis, supinator, and across the septa into the triceps brachii. It also forms close connections with other structures such as the pectoralis minor and supraspinatus muscles proximally, and distally to the antebrachial fascia, the interosseous membrane, and the finger flexors. All these structures and their relationship to the biceps brachii muscle influence its function; however, when the muscle is considered in its entirety and in the functional context of movements, the structure takes on a much more global significance. For example, during gait, the biceps facilitates the arm swing to counterbalance the contralateral leg swing. The long biceps tendon stores kinetic energy as the shoulder retracts during contralateral stance and releases it in the following gait phase. The biceps influences the gait pattern of the associated structures – and vice versa. Thus, a very comprehensive view of an all-functional network emerges: the MCS.

Summary

Besides its protective, supporting, nutritional, and immunological functions, the MCS performs primarily motor and sensory tasks. In the sensorimotor system, the contractile part (the muscle) produces force, and the fasciae transmit these forces and redirect them if necessary. Within these functions, due to their VE, they can store large amounts of energy and return it at the appropriate time. The MCS is considered the sixth sense: it contains the vast majority of the body's proprioceptors. This makes this system an essential part of the movement system. Its integrity is the basis for coordinated and purposeful movements. In the nocimotor system, on the other hand, due to the high proportion of free nerve endings it contains (nociceptors), it is an equally important component of the protective role. Based on damage signals from the nociceptors, muscle tone is adjusted accordingly for protection. The MCS thus shows its full value for the body, and its homeostasis makes the MCS a system that, on the one hand, protects against injuries and, on the other hand, increases performance.

Because of its vital role in mobility, strength, and pain, it can be argued that the overall health and well-being of the MCS is of the utmost importance to human movement. Thus, IAMT is intended to directly treat the structures of the MCS with the following goals:

- improvement of the maintenance of appropriate tissue hydration regarding water content and transport
- pain reduction
- improvement of tissue mobility
- regulation of muscle tone.

Of course, these goals can be addressed by other therapy options; therefore, we describe additional and complementary modalities in Part 6 of this book. In our experience, IAMT has provided excellent clinical benefits in patients with tendinitis (peroneal tendons, Achilles tendons, rotator cuff, and wrist tendons), joint sprains (finger and ankle joints), De Quervain's stenosis, carpal tunnel syndrome, epicondylitis (medial and lateral), adhesive capsulitis in the shoulder, patellofemoral pain syndrome, plantar fasciitis, various pain syndromes of the spine (cervical and lumbar spine syndromes), muscle strains, scars, and fibromyalgia.

IAMT is not meant to be a "stand-alone" therapy, but part of an integrated approach to treating the MCS. The therapist integrates treatment with the devices into their daily routine. This is the reason why additional pre- and post-treatment techniques are presented in this book. This integrative approach is perhaps best summed up by Warren Hammer (2005): "IASTM [Instrument-assisted Soft Tissue Mobilization; see Chapter 2] is an important adjunct to existing treatment techniques for musculoskeletal conditions."

References

Findley TW, Schleip R (2007) Fascia Research: Basic Science and Implications for Conventional and Complementary Health Care. Munich: Elsevier/ Urban & Fischer.

Hammer W (2005) The benefits of instrument-assisted soft-tissue mobilization. American Chiropractor, August 1. Available: https://theamericanchiropractor. com/article/2005/8/1/the-benefits-of-instrument-assisted-soft-tissue-mobilization [March 17, 2022].

Kram R, Dawson TJ (1998) Energetics and biomechanics of locomotion by red kangaroos (*Macropus rufus*). Comp Biochem Physiol B Biochem Mol Biol 120(1):41–49.

Schleip R, Duerselen L, Vleeming A et al. (2012) Strain hardening of fascia: static stretching of dense fibrous connective tissues can induce a temporary stiffness increase accompanied by enhanced matrix hydration. J Bodyw Mov Ther 16(1):94e100.

Stecco A (2017) Personal communication, Connect 2017 Connective Tissues in Sports Medicine 2nd International Congress, Ulm University, Germany, March 16–19, 2017. March 16 Pre-conference workshop: Antonio Stecco: Fascial Manipulation.

Stecco C, Fede C, Macchi V et al. (2018) The fasciacytes: a new cell devoted to fascial gliding regulation. Clin Anat 31(5):667–676. doi:10.1002/ca.23072.

History

The history of Instrument-assisted Soft Tissue Mobilization (IASTM) is long and yet short at the same time: long because the technique has existed for over 2,000 years, short as it has only recently become popular in physiotherapy. Traditionally, IASTM was used personally to relieve pain and improve function. It was a very long time before these everyday devices began to be employed for medical purposes as well. In the beginning, the devices were naturally made of materials that were commonly found and affordable. It was not unusual for them to be household items such as porcelain spoons or combs, or even coins or stones (such as jade), as well as animal (buffalo) horn. Manufactured instruments, such as the so-called "strigilis" or "racloir," were handmade scrapers in iron or bronze. They were specifically made for the treatment of athletes or healthy people, and used after sports or bathing, probably for cleansing or regeneration. It is curious that some of these instruments, in addition to fitting the curves of the body, were created with a channel for collecting liquids. Apparently, sweat from famous athletes and gladiators was collected into vessels in this way and may have been offered for sale to fans. Contemporary authors such as Travell and Simons (Simons et al. 1989) also describe a very similar application – even if the goal is a therapeutic one. They write of the use of oil on the skin while slowly gliding the fingers along the length of the muscle to "milk out" the muscle fluid content.

Far Eastern medicine uses these "scraping" devices extensively. Their names vary according to their individual country of origin: in China they are called "Gua Sha," in Indonesia "Kerik," in Vietnam "Cao Gio," in Laos "Khoud Lam," and in Cambodia "Kos Khyol." In these regions, however, we find a different mode of action: with

Gua Sha ("Gua" meaning scraping, "Sha" skin reddening), for example, a visible skin discoloration is produced, probably to stimulate the body's own defense mechanisms or to eliminate toxins. In Western culture, these subcutaneous hematomas could be problematic, and might even have legal consequences as a form of bodily injury. Interestingly, there was even a movie made called *The Guasha Treatment*, whose main purpose was to educate people about this form of therapy in traditional Chinese medicine. However, in Gua Sha, tissue is not only rubbed or scraped, but also beaten (in the sense of clapping, called "Pak Sha") and pinched (in the sense of pressing, "Tsien Sha").

The spread of this type of therapy beyond the East happened very late. It was introduced, probably in the 1970s, to the USA by acupuncturist Arya Nielsen, and also to Europe, where the Swedish physiotherapist Kurt Ekman developed a device-based therapy that he called "Crochetage" or "Fibrolysis." In Germany, the technique was given the name "Gentle Myofascial Tacking Technique" and was developed as a form of relief for the hands of therapists performing transverse friction. Ekman was an early student of James Cyriax, who performs cross-frictions with fingers shaped like a hook; therefore, the instruments are also hook-shaped to loosen the so-called "cross-links" in the treated tissue (van den Berg 1999). (For websites, see the References at the end of this chapter.)

Today, this type of device use is usually referred to by the collective term "Instrument-assisted Soft Tissue Mobilization" (IASTM). The devices are made of very different materials, such as steel, aluminum, and various plastics, although wood and even jade and buffalo horn are still in service today. A lubricant is also often employed to reduce the occurrence of skin irritation (Gautschi 2013).

The concept of IASTM emerged from these techniques. It was developed in 2010, and since then has been refined through the close collaboration of an international team of experts to which the authors belong, as well as there being numerous course participants in Europe and Asia. On the one hand, then, IASTM sees itself as a part of a large group of soft tissue treatment techniques, while on the other hand, from what the authors know, IASTM is somewhat unique and novel in its approach: based on human anatomy, structures are treated specifically – albeit indirectly. The authors expect the targeted treatment of anatomical structures to be more effective and thus more efficient. Experience has shown that it also gives therapists greater security to know which structures they are treating – and why. The modes of action are both mechanical and neurophysiological, following an easy understandable logic.

A second important point in the development of IASTM is the view of the myofascial system as a body-wide network: the Myofascial Connected System (MCS). Thus, IASTM is not limited to local treatments, but may be extended to regional and even global therapy. One exception in the IASTM approach is "Sound-assisted Soft Tissue Mobilization" (SASTM). This particular modality is designed to differentiate physiological and pathological tissue qualities, and is a special case in that it can be used both therapeutically and diagnostically (for website, see end of chapter).

IASTM and IAMT

With the assistance of Robert Schleip, Instrument-assisted Myofascial Therapy (IAMT) has been developed in Europe after the foundations were established by traditional IASTM. Rather than focusing on instruments and techniques, IAMT is a more holistic approach to myofascial therapy utilizing instruments. IAMT incorporates the techniques of IASTM but goes beyond an instrument-based approach. It integrates the physiological benefits of instruments within the context of

the myofascial and sensorimotor systems. The mechanical benefits of IASTM are recognized at a cellular level as a stimulator of fibroblast production and facilitator of collagen alignment. The mechanical effects are thought to potentially break down and remodel fascial adhesions arising from collagen cross-bridging within and between fascial layers. While it is commonly thought that IASTM stimulates an inflammatory response to facilitate this realignment, this remains to be proven. These mechanical changes with IASTM are ultimately thought to improve tissue and joint mobility.

As mentioned previously, the neurophysiological aspects of mechanical stimulation of fascia may also be involved in proprioception and the management of nociception. Reducing pain during motion can improve movement patterns. The IAMT approach combines the mechanical and neurophysiological effects with the concepts of myofascial tensegrity and motor control to provide both local and global effects.

The techniques of IAMT differ from those of IASTM; thus, whether the mode of action and efficacy differ is unclear to date. In the literature for IASTM, an action at the cellular level is often stated as the mechanism of action: most often, the mode of action is connective tissue remodeling by stimulating the action of fibroblasts, with an effect on the quality/functionality of unwanted tissue (scar tissue and adhesions, for example) or regeneration of physiological connective tissue with regained functionality (toughness and stiffness). This mechanism is often presented as triggering a healing response. This may possibly apply to IAMT, since, to begin with, the stimuli are mechanically similar: namely, pressure, and traction on the structures. The way of thinking in IAMT is somewhat different and is characterized by considerations that are both local – mechanical (improvement of joint mobility by improving the displaceability of the tissue layers) – and central – neurophysiological (regulation of tone, mostly in the sense of lowering). These hypotheses are possible explanations for the very frequent direct response of the body to treatment. This will be discussed in more detail in the next chapter.

In summary, the authors believe that the functional benefit appears to be principally an improvement in range of motion (ROM) and thus a clinical improvement in use of the treated area. Other claims, however, such as pain relief with a reduction in medication use, faster rehabilitation, and improvement of blood and lymph circulation, seem to be supported by experience. IAMT focuses mainly on functional changes (ICF: activity level) and less on setting healing processes in motion. It is the application of techniques to anatomical structures (ICF: structural level) that may have a relevant connection with the patient's condition.

Types and Features of IASTM Instruments

Many devices are offered for self-treatment, mostly intended to apply pressure to the tissues to induce relaxation. This is often referred to as "Self-(Myo)Fascial Release." Increasingly, various devices are used in sports, and bear at least some relation to those described here. So-called "foam rollers" are a good example. They are now widely used and available in many variants, including options for vibration and heating.

IASTM tools and techniques seem very popular in today's culture. A simple search using one of the well-known search engines and the term "Instrument-assisted Soft Tissue Mobilization tool" yields about 630,000 hits (May 14, 2021). Searching for videos on a well-known platform with the same search term yields an almost infinite number of results.

As we have seen, in addition to there being different techniques, different materials are also used to make the instruments, including wood, jade, plastics, and metals. Questions immediately arise as to why these various materials are used and whether the material plays a role. The first question cannot be answered easily. There may be many reasons for choosing one material over another: perhaps because of a personal preference for a certain material, or for economic reasons, or simply due to its availability. The role of the material itself is somewhat easier to address. The authors do not see any therapeutic effect in the choice of material other than the benefit for the therapist.

Perhaps a therapist is very close to a certain company that manufactures or distributes devices. The authors themselves were involved in the development of devices with one particular company but would like to state clearly that they have no financial involvement in the sale of the devices and never have had. Their advisory activity was limited exclusively to development of the devices: selection of material and specific design. The devices were designed and manufactured according to the authors' requirements.

Be that as it may, the most important job the material has to do is relieve the therapist's hands. Also, the authors expect an increase in the effectiveness of the therapy through greater precision in application. To achieve these goals, it is necessary to "extend" the therapist's hand. Although the human hand, as a sensory and motor part of the body, does not seem to be replaceable, the device should be able to transmit information from the treated tissue to the therapist's hand through a logical choice of material. In order to perceive this order of resonance, the material needs to be of a high density. This requirement is fulfilled in particular by high-quality stainless steel materials that are also used in surgery; these devices are correspondingly rustproof and corrosion-resistant. In addition, stainless steel meets the highest standards of hygiene: it can easily be cleaned, disinfected, and even sterilized (like a surgeon's instruments). It is durable and therefore sustainable.

The therapist can easily cool or warm the stainless steel if desired or necessary. Due to its heavy weight, stainless steel fits well in the hand; in the best-case scenario the device becomes integrated into the therapist's body scheme after a period of use. The weight of a steel instrument also seems to reduce the pressure that has to be provided by the therapist, thus reducing their effort.

Having addressed the issue of the material, we can move on to the shape of the devices: both the size, type, and purpose of the corners and edges (bevels and angles) and the overall shape (convex and concave areas). The devices should be adapted as well as possible to the requirements of IASTM, with each area of the instrument having a specific purpose. The mechanical actions that the therapist wants to achieve with the instrument should be well described. For example, the device should lend itself to being placed both vertically (perpendicular to the skin) and horizontally (parallel to the skin) on many different parts of the body. Because every human body is differently proportioned, the device should have a concave area that adapts to the curves of the body and a convex area that adapts to the concavities of the body. The shape of the edges can affect the "intensity" of application: a rounded edge is smoother and less intense, while a single bevel at a 45-degree angle can be quite intense. The size of these areas on the instrument should be different to reach all parts of the body safely. In order to achieve the desired strength of the effect through the device, these areas should be partly rounded and partly beveled. There should also be some kind of tip for application of pressure. Depending on the area treated, the tip should be a different size in diameter and length. Finally, it should be possible to "hook" it on to various structures (muscle bellies, tendons and so on).

It is clear that no one device can have all these features. That is why the authors took the opportunity to help develop treatment instruments and training with various companies. Sometimes, we described to manufacturers what qualities and characteristics the instruments should have and were given the opportunity to help develop their "optimal" instruments. For example, the devices described below were developed under the guidance of an international expert in the research and treatment of the myofascial system: Dr Robert Schleip. However, the reader can rest assured that all the techniques described in this text can be performed regardless of the choice of equipment.

The devices were initially named "Fazer" by Dr Schleip, based on the term "fascia." The initial "F" and the number of the instrument within the five-part set were chosen as shorthand. To complete the naming and for uniform communication among all users, the authors have assigned names to the instruments based on their shape (Figure 2.1):

- F1, called "whale"
- F2, called "boomerang"
- F3, called "finger"
- F4, called "thumb"
- F5, called "cone."

The F1, or "whale," is designed to have one end shaped as a hook and a mid-shaft convexity. The hook is rounded at its end and has an edge that is about 2 cm wide and beveled at a 45-degree angle. Due to its shape, the end can be used for hooking as well as for scraping and pushing. With its small size, it can also be chosen for work in relatively small or hard-to-reach areas (such as retromalleolar). The mid-portion is primarily suitable for scraping. In order to adapt to the contours of the body, it has an indentation with a rounded edge and a corresponding convexity with truncated edges. The other end is rounded with a beveled edge, mainly used for mobilization. To optimize handling, two finger recesses are incorporated.

The F2, or "boomerang," was designed to facilitate superficial blood circulation; one edge (the

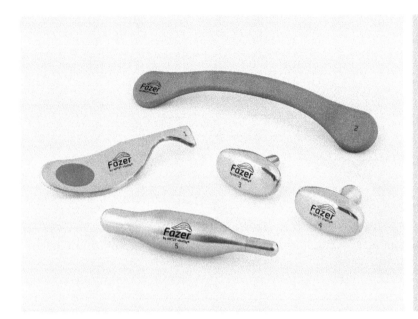

Figure 2.1 Fazer five-instrument set from Artzt Vitality®

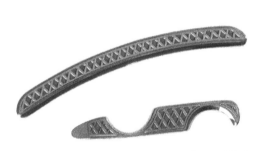

Figure 2.2 HawkGrips two-instrument set

manufacturers available around the world; sometimes, manufacturers make tools that appear very similar at different price levels. Some tools combine the features of other instruments: for example, the HawkGrips Boomerang (Figure 2.2), Scanner, and Dual Edge instruments are similar to the F2 from Artzt. It can sometimes be confusing for clinicians when they have to decide which instrument is best for a particular application.

To give the reader a neutral view of the instruments available, the authors have tried to summarize their most important characteristics in the list below and Table 2.1. The aim here is only to present, as objectively as possible, the ways in which the instruments are similar against the background of their apparent differences. In this way, the reader will be better able to choose the appropriate instrument for a specific technique. It is not about presenting the advantages or disadvantages of individual instruments. The table is therefore intended as a "generic" schematic of the specific characteristics of instruments across the spectrum.

convexity) is rounded, while the other (concavity) is beveled at 45 degrees. Other applications include large-scale scraping or pushing, or use as a kind of lever: for example, to mobilize larger structures.

The F3 ("finger"), F4 ("thumb"), and F5 ("cone") share a similar structure but have different diameters. These instruments are mainly used to apply pressure in vertical and horizontal directions.

Throughout this book, the authors explain the clinical techniques for use with various IASTM tools. Obviously, there are many different instruments and

Table 2.1 A comparison of some of the instruments available

Tool	Category			
	Straight elongated instruments	Straight short instruments	Curved instruments	Combination curve instruments
Artzt F1				x
Artzt F2			x	
Artzt F3, 4, 5		x		
HG Pro Multi Tool				x
HG Handlebars			x	
HG Multi Curve				x
HG Scanner	x			
HG Boomerang			x	
HG Tongue Depressor		x		
Edge Mobility Tool, Star				x
GT1			x	
GT2				x
GT3		x		
GT4	x			
GT5			x	
GT6				x
FAKTR1, 3, 4				x
FAKTR2	x			
STM1, 2, 5				x
STM3			x	
STM4	x			

F: Fazer; FAKTR: Functional and Kinetic Treatment with Rehabilitation; GT: Graston Technique; HG: HawkGrips; STM: SMART tools.

- Straight elongated instruments:
  - with beveled and/or rounded edges
  - straight and curved treatment edges
  - for scanning, scraping, and shoving
- Straight short instruments:
  - with thin- or thicker-end treatment edges
  - for pushing and pinning
- Curved instruments:
  - bilateral concave and/or convex curvature treatment edge

- ○ with beveled and/or rounded edges
- ○ for scraping and shoving
- Combined curve instruments:
  - ○ with concave and/or convex curvatures in different diameters; the concavity can be so pronounced that the instrument is almost hook-shaped
  - ○ for scraping, shoving, and hooking

IASTM Lubricants

When equipment is used for therapeutic purposes, human skin is exposed to stress. Depending on the technique and the pressure applied, as well as the duration and frequency of the treatment, this stress varies. The sensitivity of the patient also plays a role. Of course, the main goals of any treatment are not to harm the patient and, if possible, to make the treatment pleasant. For this reason, therapists performing IASTM often use a lubricant. As with the different types of instrument, there are various lubricant products on the market. The aim of these products is to reduce the sliding friction of the instrument on the skin, thus lowering the impact on the skin. This can be accomplished through the use of specific emollients (oil or water-based), shea butter, synthetic or natural beeswax, natural oil (olive, almond, or jojoba), or mineral oils. Some therapists simply use massage lotion or massage oil.

In addition to this mechanical action, some products claim to have an additional therapeutic effect due to their ingredients. For example, the addition of arnica is said to provide an anti-inflammatory benefit. This effect could certainly be useful when there is an inflammatory reaction in the treated tissue; however, it has yet to be proven that these ingredients are truly beneficial in IASTM. Other ingredients may be added to emollients to improve the blood circulation, such as cayenne pepper (capsaicin).

A reasonable lubricant should have the following properties:

- It should ensure harmonious sliding of the instruments on the skin.
- It should not be absorbed too quickly.
- It should not cause allergic reactions.
- It should be as neutral as possible; this also applies to olfactory ingredients (such as lavender and rosemary).
- An additional pharmacological effect can be useful but may not be necessary or proven.

For these reasons, the authors usually use a neutral lubricant in an amount that is both necessary and purposeful.

Lubricants should be applied with caution; a reduction of sliding friction can both reduce the mechanical effectiveness of the therapy and make the use of certain techniques almost impossible. This is the case with a technique that will be described in detail later: mobilization. Here it is essential that there is no sliding between the instrument and the skin.

IASTM Research

As an emerging therapeutic intervention, IASTM research is developing. Most current clinical applications are based on anecdotal and empirical evidence. The current scientific evidence (as of May 2021) may be described in two areas: mechanisms of action and outcomes.

To the authors' knowledge, there are currently no studies on the different materials or techniques. Metal devices have been studied most frequently; this may be related to the prevalence of this material in IASTM. Applicability of the results to other materials is therefore unclear. In fact, one approach (Astym®) insists on claiming that the research and outcomes related to it should not be considered the same as those relating to IASTM in general. Unfortunately, the quantity of studies on IASTM is limited at present, though the quality of the studies is certainly a more important factor in assessing the current effectiveness of a therapy. In a systematic review, Cheatham and colleagues conclude that:

The literature measuring the effects of IASTM is still emerging. The current research has indicated insignificant results which challenges the efficacy of IASTM as a treatment for common musculoskeletal pathology, which may be due to the methodological variability among studies. There appears to be some evidence supporting its ability to increase short term joint ROM. (Cheatham et al. 2016)

However, not only are further high-quality studies necessary if this type of therapy is to be practiced profitably and safely, but equally qualitative and standardized training is also needed.

In order to maintain consistent quality and standard of IASTM treatment, it is recommended that clinicians utilizing IASTM receive training in the application and administration of the treatment, and specialized training should be at the discretion of the clinician or the clinician's employer. (Moore et al. 2020)

These measures should allow efficacy studies in the future.

In the experience of the authors, the lack of evidence is criticized when a new form of therapy is established, often despite the fact that older or established forms of therapy have also failed to provide proof of efficacy. The longer history of application or the level of popular awareness seems to compensate for the lack of proof of effectiveness. From this perspective, IASTM might be expected to help support the positive experiences therapists have had with using the devices in recent years, as well as the consistently positive feedback patients have given despite the lack of evidence.

Disclaimer

The authors declare that they have no financial interest in the sale of these instruments; however, a certain portion of the Artzt company's sales generated with the IASTM tools flows directly into fascia research at the Fascia Research Group of the University of Munich (http://www.fascia research.de).

References

Cheatham SW, Lee M, Cain M et al. (2016) The efficacy of instrument assisted soft tissue mobilization: a systematic review. J Can Chiropr Assoc 60(3):200–211.

Gautschi R (2013) Manuelle Triggerpunkt-Therapie: Myofasziale Schmerzen und Funktionsstörungen erkennen, verstehen und behandeln. Stuttgart and New York: Georg Thieme.

Moore MG, Daley AR, Winkelmann ZK (2020) An evidence-to-practice review on the efficacy of instrument assisted soft tissue mobilization. Clin Pract Athl Train 3(3):4–11. Available: https://doi.org/10.31622/2020.0003.3.2 [March 28, 2022].

Simons DG, Travell JG, Simons LS (1989) Travell & Simons' Myofascial Pain and Dysfunction: The Trigger Point Manual, 2nd edn. Baltimore: Williams & Wilkins.

van den Berg F (1999) Angewandte Physiologie 1: Das Bindegewebe des Bewegungsapparates verstehen und beeinflussen. Stuttgart and New York: Georg Thieme.

Websites

Guasha: history (n.d.) Guasha Therapy. Available: https://guashatherapie.nl/history/?lang=en [Accessed Apr 23, 2022].

Guasha – Therapie gegen den Schmerz (Dec 21, 2012) Welt/Gesundheit. Available: https://www.welt.de/gesundheit/medizin-ratgeber/article157721869/Gua-Sha-Therapie-gegen-den-Schmerz.html [Accessed Apr 23, 2022].

Less damage. More healing (2012) SASTM. Available: https://www.sastm.com [Accessed Apr 23, 2022].

From the anatomical and physiological aspects of the myofascial system and its function reviewed in Chapter 1, the following may be considered objectives of myofascial therapy:

- pain reduction
- improvement in tissue fluid content and transport (rehydration)
- improvement of mobility
- regulation of muscle tone.

From these, the authors have developed five goal-specific techniques:

- Rehydration Technique (ReT)
- Pain Relief Technique (PRT)
- Regulation of Tone Technique (RoT)
- Mobilization Technique (MoT)
- Metabolization Technique (MeT).

These techniques were first explained by describing the handling of the IAMT devices according to the actions that the therapist performs: shoving, rolling, scraping, pressing, and rubbing. Then, several assumptions behind IAMT were applied to the techniques, as listed in Table 3.1.

Note that a clear distinction between the techniques is not always possible; nor is it absolutely necessary. The techniques' objectives will overlap somewhat: rubbing the skin naturally has a certain mechanical and metabolic effect on the underlying structures, for instance. The name given to each technique therefore corresponds to the technique's main objective.

Technique 1: Rehydration Technique (ReT)

The technique consists of a superficial shoving ("gliding") or a deep shoving ("rolling"). The IAMT device is continuously pushed with pressure (like the bow of a boat through a wave), working away from the therapist, while the return to the starting point is pressure-free; thus, fluid should be forced ahead of the device as it moves. The pressure depends on the location of the structure to be treated: the deeper the structure, the greater the pressure. Continuous pressure should be applied in all directions since tissues are not always organized in parallel structures. However, if swelling or edema is visible, a retrograde (proximal/cranial) direction seems more prudent. The treatment

	Table 3.1 Assumptions behind IAMT techniques	
	Assumption	**IAMT Technique**
1	The myofascial structures are dehydrated and must be rehydrated	Rehydration technique: ReT
2	The patient is in pain and needs pain relief	Pain Relief Technique: PRT
3	Muscle tone is increased from overuse (primary hypertonus) or reflexive protection (secondary hypertonus); this tone must be reduced and normalized	Regulation of Tone: RoT
4	Hypomobility results from both disuse (lack of movement) and overuse (chronic or recurrent inflammation); tissue mobility must be increased	Mobilization Technique: MoT
5	Circulating blood is a transport system, carrying fresh oxygen and nutrients to an area while removing waste substances and metabolites; local blood circulation must be improved	Metabolization Technique: MeT

area is rather large, while the depth of treatment is superficial or deep, depending on the location of the structure. The speed is low and continuity of movement is important to maintain fluid movement. This technique could be executed with different tools. Rather larger devices with a wide, rounded surface are best suited. The use of a lubricant is often necessary. The continuous pressure should first push fluid out of the tissue (reduction of fluid content), as if squeezing a sponge, resulting in reciprocal fluid absorption. This effect should occur at the cellular level, and by altering fluid absorption and release, the extracellular matrix should rehydrate and improve the quality of the tissue. This technique has a local site of action. Its therapeutic approach is direct and reflexive; due to its gentleness it is usually very well tolerated and painless; therefore, it is recommended as an initial therapy.

Technique 2: Pain Relief Technique (PRT)

The technique consists of a quick scraping, meaning a friction in the sense of scraping; pressure is maintained on both the outward and return paths. The direction of scraping is irrelevant; it may be that starting in a direction parallel to the treated structure is more comfortable for the patient. There are some variants: with or without rotation of the instrument. Working without rotation, the therapist induces the sliding of the instrument by a whip-like movement of the whole arm; the wrist is relaxed and moves loosely along. Working with rotation, the therapist induces the sliding of the device by a movement with the forearms in pronation and supination; thus the device rotates around its own axis. The treatment area is a maximum of 10–15 cm (medium-sized area). The treatment depth is shallow, while the speed is high; through brisk movements the therapist achieves a high input in a short time. Small or larger devices with rounded or sharp areas are best suited. The use of a lubricant is often recommended. The principle of action is based on the Gate Control Theory of Melzak and Wall (1965). Scraping produces an increased proprioceptive input, which is thought to lower nociceptive perception in return. This phenomenon is explained by a faster conduction of mechanoreceptive afferents compared to nociceptive conduction due to the increased myelination of the afferent sensory fibers. The technique also has a local effect on the treated tissue; the blood circulation in this area is increased as well as the perception. While these effects are positive, they are not the primary goal of therapy. Therefore the site of action is not the treated area, but goes via the central nervous system (CNS). The therapeutic approach is symptomatic, indirect, and reflexive therapy.

Technique 3: Regulation of Tone (RoT)

The technique consists of applying pressure with the instrument on the underlying structures. The therapist places the instrument at the desired point and applies vertical pressure to the tissue until they perceive an initial "end feel." The pressure is held until the tone noticeably decreases. The technique can then be repeated on a new "end feel." A variant is the so-called "melting" technique, in which the vertical pressure is supplemented by even small lateral or circular movements of the instrument. Sometimes the therapist finds not only one point in a structure, but a whole row, or a strand of continuous tissue. This can be treated individually or as a whole. When the whole strand is being treated, the instrument is pushed without releasing the pressure over the imaginary line that seems to connect the individual points. The treatment area is small and localized. The depth of treatment depends on the depth of the treated structure: superficial or deep – mostly rather deep.

The speed of the pressure is very low and progressive. The most suitable instruments are those with an elongated extremity, rounded at the end; the appearance of these devices is often reminiscent of a mushroom. The diameter of the round tip of the extremity is very small because the technique is very local and needs to reach specific structures: it should be between 0.5 and 1 cm.

The use of a lubricant is not recommended. The presumed principle of action is based on the action of the sensorimotor system. The nociceptive afference (the pressure by the instrument) is responded to with a localized relaxing efference through a multi-synaptic circuit in the CNS. This is also known as diffuse noxious inhibitory control (Patel and Dickenson 2020). The site of action is therefore the CNS. The therapeutic approach is indirect and reflexive therapy; due to the pressure, the therapy is sometimes painful. It produces a pain of a certain characteristic; this is usually in contrast to the actual pain of the patient. The pain is only temporary and rather radiates around the area. It is quite a "feel-good" type of pain that quickly subsides when the pressure is removed and does not linger. Of course, the technique also has a local effect on the treated tissue. The blood circulation in this area is increased by releasing the hypertonus (which occludes blood flow), as well as the perception. While these effects are positive, they are not the primary goal of therapy.

Technique 4: Mobilization Technique (MoT)

The technique resembles Cyriax's transverse friction massage or Ekmann's "Crochetage" in its modalities of execution. It restores mobility by "releasing" reversible myofascial lesions, also known as "restrictions." The technique consists of a rubbing or a frictioning or a hooking. First, the instrument is applied to the restriction to be treated; then it is moved with pressure in the direction of the restriction until the displaceability of the tissue is at a maximum. Now, either the instrument is returned to the starting position without pressure (but also without loss of contact) or the final position is held for some time (approximately 20 seconds) before it is returned. The instrument does not slide over the skin at all, but moves in solidarity with the mobilized structure; therefore, the use of a lubricant is not necessary. Sometimes this can even be counterproductive: namely, when the instrument slides over the skin unintentionally due to the lubricant.

The technique is actually a transverse friction in the sense of being an intermittent displacement of tissue layers in a perpendicular direction to the direction of the fibers. The deep fasciae are arranged in at least three fiber layers. Within each layer, the fibers are parallel, but the fibers of the individual layers are not; this seems to allow transmission of forces in all directions. Therefore, the technique should always be performed in different directions. The beginning can be parallel to the superficial layer. In the case of superficial fascia, the direction of restriction is decisive, as these fasciae are built in a looser and less structured architecture. The treatment area depends on the extent of the restriction. In the case of large-scale restrictions, the techniques are divided into a corresponding number of smaller sequences. The depth of treatment depends on the depth of the treated structure. The speed of the technique is low.

The most suitable instruments are those with a curved end. This looks like or is a kind of hook. The curvature of the hook can vary; the end should not be pointed, but rounded. This allows targeted and precise therapy and is gentle on the skin. Avoiding the use of a lubricant is strongly recommended. The principle of action consists in a mobilizing of the different tissue layers against each other. In this way, the mobility of these layers can be restored or at least improved.

It remains unclear whether non-physiological fascial "cross-links" between structures or within the same structure are released in the process, so the site of action is direct and local. The therapeutic approach is consequently a direct action on the local fibers with increase of the micro- and macroscopic range of motion.

Technique 5: Metabolization Technique (MeT)

This technique is based on the historic use of "scraping" to increase blood flow as a means of removing toxins (that is, Gua Sha). The technique consists of a quick scraping, similar to the ReT, but pressure is applied in one direction only. The instrument is returned without losing contact with the body. The direction of scraping is not of concern. There are variants in the execution: with or without rotation of the instrument. Working without rotation, the therapist induces the sliding of the instrument by a whip-like movement of the whole arm; the wrist is relaxed and moves loosely along. Working with rotation, the therapist induces the sliding of the device by a movement with the forearms in pronation and supination; thus the device rotates around its own axis. The treatment area is considered to be medium: slightly larger than for the PRT, but smaller than for the ReT and MoT. The depth of treatment is definitely superficial, while the speed is also medium: slightly lower than that of the PRT, but higher than that for the ReT and MoT. Rather flat devices with a rounded surface are best suited. The use of a lubricant is recommended. The principle of action is based on an increase of local superficial blood circulation (microcirculation) in the treated area due to the scraping. A short duration is needed to achieve the desired activation of the metabolism (metabolization), noted through the presence of erythema (reddening of the skin). The site of action is, of course, direct and local. The therapeutic approach also has a direct action on the local superficial blood vessels.

Summary

The different IAMT techniques are summarized in Table 3.2.

Table 3.2 Summary of different IAMT techniques						
Technique	**Action**	**Treatment Area**	**Depth**	**Speed**	**Instrument**	**Lubricant**
Rehydration	Shoving	Large	Superficial or deep	Low	Straight elongated Curved Combination curve	Yes
Pain relief	Scraping	<10–15 cm	Superficial	High	Straight elongated Curved Combination curve	Yes
Regulation of tone	Pressing	Small	Superficial or deep	Low	Straight short	No
Mobilization	Rubbing	Varies	Superficial or deep	Low	Straight elongated Curved Combination curve	No
Metabolization	Scraping	Medium	Superficial	Medium	Straight elongated Curved Combination curve	Yes

Table 3.3 Recommended techniques for specific tissues		
Tissue	**Recommended Techniques**	**Comment**
Superficial fascia	PRT, ReT, RoT, MoT, MeT	Superficial fascia tends to be more accessible; therefore, they are treated with all techniques.
Deep fascia	PRT, ReT, MoT, MeT	Deep fascia is obviously deeper and less accessible; therefore, the MeT is not used.
Muscle	PRT, ReT, RoT, MeT	IAMT is helpful in muscle pathologies to avoid reduction of displacement during scar formation. This is also to prevent recurrences. However, the treatment starts at the earliest after the inflammatory phase.
Tendon	PRT, ReT, RoT, MoT, MeT	Tendons and ligaments tend to be more accessible; therefore, they are treated with all techniques.
Ligament	PRT, ReT, RoT, MoT, MeT	
Scar	ReT, RoT, MoT, MeT	If scars are painful, they can be treated with PRT. However, one should clarify the cause of the pain before treating it with IAMT. Only the degree of restriction of movement (quantity) and, above all, the type of restriction (quality) is decisive: a scar with a fixed stop is more connective tissue-like and the MoT is increased in intensity and held at the end to produce improvement.

MeT: Metabolization Technique; MoT: Mobilization Technique; PRT: Pain Relief Technique; ReT: Rehydration Technique; RoT: Regulation of Tone Technique.

The duration for which each treatment technique should be implemented depends on the therapeutic situation. Most techniques, as individual parts of treatment, last only seconds (indirect, reflexive techniques), or several minutes (direct, local) techniques. Remember, however, that IAMT is not a stand-alone treatment; it serves as an adjunct to enhance other treatments such as joint mobilization or therapeutic exercise such as stretching, strengthening, or sensorimotor training. As with other adjunctive therapies, the amount of time spent should correspond to the severity of the impairment being addressed: the fewer the symptoms, the less IAMT is required.

Different tissues have unique properties that can benefit from the various techniques. Table 3.3 summarizes the authors' suggestions for specific IAMT techniques, depending on the tissue.

The attentive reader may be surprised to learn that the Regulation of Tone technique is used not only in its classic application of muscle. The technique may also be applied to other structures of the myofascial system for two reasons: first, fascia, ligaments, and tendons also have contractile elements; and second, the MCS is a continuum throughout the body (that is, pressure or traction on one element of the system affects the entire system). Thus, a reduction in tone may be felt in the non-contractile areas as well.

This chapter has described five different IAMT techniques with specific therapeutic goals directed at various tissues. Therapists should apply the scientific and theoretical basis of IAMT to implement specific techniques based on the individual patient impairments and goals.

References

Melzack R, Wall PD (1965) Pain mechanisms: a new theory. Science 150(699):971–979.

Patel R, Dickenson AH (2020) A study of cortical and brainstem mechanisms of diffuse noxious inhibitory controls in anaesthetised normal and neuropathic rats. Eur J Neurosci 51(4):952–962.

The indications for using IAMT include restoring or enhancing function in a variety of tissues to address impairments such as pain, decreased mobility, or increased tone. Clinicians should use the three pillars of evidence-based practice to determine whether IAMT would be beneficial and which technique would be best: the best evidence available, the clinical experience of the therapist, and the goals and values of the patient.

According to Pierre Bisschop, a student of James Cyriax MD and co-author of *A System of Orthopaedic Medicine*, Cyriax is said to have stated, "If I don't know whether I am allowed to use the therapy or not, I don't use it! If I don't know whether the therapy helps or not, I try it!" (Bisschop 1993). Thus, the use of the equipment must always serve to improve the patient's condition. The instruments should be employed judiciously, ensuring absolute safety for the patient. A thorough assessment of the patient's condition (including an accurate medical history, regional inspection, functional testing, and careful palpation) should be the basis of any therapeutic action. In particular, "Functional Evaluation Tests" (see page 26) are indispensable for directing treatment.

Based on the authors' clinical experience, the concept of IAMT is designed to be directly and efficiently integrated into readers' daily therapeutic routine. If a therapist had to learn a new, possibly complicated and complex technique, its use in practice might become questionable, thus preventing integration in practice. Furthermore, IAMT consists of a series of techniques that have very specific objectives to address clinical findings. It should be another complementary tool in the therapist's toolbox of adjunct therapies.

As with any adjunctive therapeutic tool, its integration and use depend on the individual therapist. The authors recommend that therapists maintain their current approach to the assessment of patients and utilize IAMT techniques as a tool to reach their therapeutic goals. The use of IAMT should always be conscious and purposeful, targeted to the goals of the patient. Therapists often experience uncertainty and may lack advanced practical skills when integrating new techniques. However, successful experiences will certainly encourage the therapist to use IAMT increasingly to improve the effectiveness and efficiency of therapy.

Two possible approaches are recommended for the smooth and positive integration of IAMT into the therapeutic routine:

- The therapist initially uses the devices to treat known patients for whom therapy has reached a relative plateau; or
- The therapist uses the techniques on new patients as part of the routine treatment of known conditions.

The therapist may find that the results are faster, more comprehensive, or more permanent compared to their traditional approach (or the opposite!). Either way, both approaches are intended to make the integration of IAMT safe, easy, and thus more beneficial. It is important for clinicians to understand when to use the instruments, as well as when not to use them.

The prerequisites for clinical integration are, among other things, knowledge of the indications and contraindications of IAMT, and of its limits, as well as observation of certain precautions. Based on their years of experience, the authors present a recommended protocol for each treatment in the following chapters, despite a lack of direct evidence. These protocols have no claim to validity and generalizability but are intended to provide therapists with an initial introduction to IAMT. As with any protocol, they should be considered as a "starting point" for clinicians to adapt and apply to individual patients. These protocols are by no means intended to be followed word for word.

To address the highly individual situations encountered by therapists in different settings (including hospitals, rehabilitation centers, private clinics, and sports teams), the authors have added optional therapy protocols to individualize therapy.

Indications

The indications for IAMT naturally refer to the myofascial system to address painful conditions and functional impairments. While there are many conditions that may be represented through the myofascial system, the authors have decided to list the most common ones that benefit from IAMT to serve as examples:

- plantar fasciitis
- Achilles tendinopathy
- anterior knee pain/patellofemoral pain syndrome
- hamstring strain/tendinopathy
- groin strain/pubalgia
- mechanical/chronic lower back pain
- sacroiliac joint dysfunction
- chronic neck pain/whiplash-associated disorder
- cervicogenic headache
- subacromial impingement syndrome
- biceps tendinopathy
- elbow epicondylopathy (tennis elbow/golfer's elbow)
- carpal tunnel syndrome
- Dupuytren's contracture
- superficial and deep scars
- osteoarthritis (independent of the affected joint).

Contraindications and Precautions

Absolute contraindications include allergy to the type of material the device is made of (metal, plastic and so on) or to the lubricant. The devices preferred by the authors (stainless steel) are hypoallergenic and suitable for nickel allergy sufferers. Obviously, skin diseases and injuries over the site of treatment are contraindications. If the patient suffers from any condition that may cause severe harm from increased blood flow or bleeding (such as hemophilia or metastasized cancer), IAMT should not be used. Similarly, patients taking blood thinners should be treated with caution. Gautschi (2013: 51) recommends only treating those with a Quick value (for prothrombin time) of at least 20; however, IAMT should be applied with less intensity and the Metabolization Technique should be avoided. Some acute soft tissue injuries have been successfully and safely treated immediately after injury (such as a ligament sprain). In this case, the aggressiveness of IAMT must be adjusted (for example, using less pressure and depth for acute injury).

Cheatham and colleagues (2019) provide an extensive list of contraindications including:

- acute injury
- acute infection
- fever
- advanced osteoporosis
- unstable fracture
- myositis ossificans
- peripheral vascular disease
- varicosis.

However, clinicians should apply common sense in determining if IAMT is potentially harmful for the individual patient: any condition or diagnosis that can become worse with skin and soft tissue massage/mobilization should be carefully considered.

Limitations

While IAMT is thought to be most effective on the structure and mechanical aspects of tissue, less is known of its effects on acute or chronic inflammation. Further limitations relate to chronic overloading of the structures: for example, using monotonous postures and movements without appropriate adaptation. Here, the effectiveness of IAMT is decisively reduced, in the experience of the authors, as symptoms cannot be eliminated sufficiently and permanently. Therefore, in these cases the authors combine IAMT with additional measures that combat chronic overload and sustained postures and movements.

Fortunately, IAMT can help in other aspects of chronic overload, specifically addressing compensatory changes in other structures. Thus, it can be used at the beginning of the therapy to create the necessary mechanical conditions for potentially permanent changes in the patient. Following treatment with IAMT, postures and movements are trained accordingly, then "reprogrammed," and finally automated. During this process, IAMT can be used selectively to eliminate the discomfort that often arises during this intense period of change.

These structural change processes are rather prolonged in the fascial tissues, sometimes taking months. In a way, this duration must be considered as a limiting factor. But it is worthwhile considering that – according to the principles of Jean-Baptiste de Lamarck (1744–1829) or Étienne Geoffroy Saint-Hilaire (1772–1844), "C'est la fonction qui forme l'organe," or Horatio Greenough (1805–1852), "Form follows function" – the body needs a certain input (*function*) as a stimulus for its structures (*form*) (Brügger 2000: 52).

Swiss neurologist Alois Brügger MD furthered these ideas and claims by stating, "No organ without a function and no function without an organ" (Brügger 1996). In this case, the "organ" can be considered to be a myofascial structure, such as a muscle, tendon, or ligament: each structure has a specific function, and that function is not possible without that structure. The interaction of structure and function can be applied to both large structures (the biceps femoris muscle) and smaller ones (popliteus); every structure is therefore considered when treating the MCS, regardless of its volume, size, visibility, and so on. The individual components of this system function according to the principle of mechanical gears: the movement of one of these gears influences the other gears in the system.

British neurologist Charles Edward Beevor (1854–1908) noted, "The brain knows no muscles, only movements" (Beevor's Axiom). However, movements result from the coordinated activity of individual muscles; the reader will therefore find that the treatment of smaller and possibly "forgotten" structures is also presented in this text. Because these other structures are often compensating for the primary dysfunction, it is important to inform the patient that such treatment may result in the emergence of "new" complaints.

Clinical Decision-making

Clinical decision-making in IAMT is analogous to that in non-instrument therapy and is based on the therapeutic diagnosis and the experience of the therapist. Thus, each treatment is individually planned, designed, and guided. With experience, therapists treating myofascial problems may note the existence of clinical patterns: that is, certain structures are more frequently affected, often in combination with a lesion of certain other structures. This may be due to the problems having similar causes: specifically, repetitive and monotonous postures and movements. While these postures and movements are individual and characteristic, the basic motor program is the same between individuals, in terms of both neurophysiology (natural processes; sensorimotor system) and neuropathophysiology (pathological processes; nocimotor system).

This assumption is the basis for the following chapters. Treatment protocols are presented by the authors as decision-making aids and suggestions, which, of course, can and must be adapted to the situation and the patient. Therapy usually has to be modified by the therapist several times during the treatment process to suit changing situations using clinical reasoning. In order to do so, therapists should be aware of specific tests to guide progress. These simple clinical tests reflect the influence of the interventions carried out by the therapist. The authors call these Functional Evaluation Tests (FETs). The definition of a FET is a technique for evaluation of a therapeutic technique or a therapy result. These FETs are chosen to be simple in application but are, in principle, systematic and standardized.

Clinical experience shows that, in many unsuccessful cases, the right intervention site has not been identified. In the sense of therapy in kinetic chains, it is sometimes the case that the treated structure is not currently primarily responsible for the symptomatology. This approach is based on the recognition that function is the best guide in therapy. The tests are therefore mostly motor programs known to the patient; these programs are generally executed subconsciously and organized at the subcortical level to minimize the influence of cortical volition.

In the authors' experience, the best FETs are active movements in upright stance because they involve the CNS and require postural control. This type of test also allows an assessment of the willingness to move. Examples include head rotation, (bilateral) rotation or lifting (flexion) of the arms, forward-bend finger–floor distance, and gait patterns. The assessment criteria are movement quality, pain during movement, and quantity (ROM). Of course, the usual scales can be used to evaluate pain: the visual analog scale (VAS) or numeric rating scale (NRS).

If these tests are not feasible or do not allow a conclusion to be drawn, passive tests can also be used: either a passive movement test based on the same criteria as the active tests (with a correspondingly lower relevance), or a pain (symptom) provocation test. Sometimes a combination of active and passive tests is useful. Either way, the improvement in the test result will almost always plateau as the treatments progress. Because improvements are not always linear and there can sometimes be setbacks (usually related to the patient's daily activities), this is usually a clear sign that the therapy progression needs to be readjusted. Experience suggests that implementing the following progressions may be effective:

- tissue tension (from relaxed to contracted)
- initial position (from unloaded to loaded)
- without–with movement (from immobile to mobile)
- without–against resistance (from free movement to resistive movement)
- functionality (use of stability trainers, elastic bands, exercise ball and so on).

The commonly used algorithm "Test–Treat–(Re)Test" is applied here. It is clear that pre- and post-tests are comparable only if the execution is identical. The simplicity not only has the advantage of great practicality in daily practice, but also can lower the error rate. Without the need for exact scientific quantification, patients can respond to the test after treatment as "better, worse, or same," similar to a traffic light system. Above all, the interpretation is unambiguous: if the test result is better (positive), the intervention seems to be beneficial. The intervention location, timing, and intensity appear to have been adequate; consequently, the therapy is continued. If the test result is worse (negative), the intervention does not seem to be beneficial. As a consequence, the therapy is adjusted, as the intervention location, timing, or intensity does not appear to have been adequate. The therapist must then decide, according to an updated therapeutic diagnosis, which parameter(s) (intervention location, timing, or intensity) to adjust.

Complementary Treatments and Pre- and Post-processing Techniques

There are many ways to complement IAMT with pre- and post-treatment techniques. Obviously, the optional use of other treatments and techniques with IAMT should be based on the needs of the patient and the experience of the therapist. Some of these complementary treatments are described in Chapters 23–25 by experts in the fields of cupping, kinesiology taping, and fascial training. The main expectation in implementing these techniques is always the same: namely, a better and lasting therapeutic result. While these interventions are not described in detail in this text, the aim is to show how they can be used in a meaningful and complementary way within the framework of IAMT. Readers are encouraged to learn more about the techniques individually as part of their overall clinical practice. In order to place the application of the techniques in the context of IAMT, the authors have chosen to present them within a classification according to treatment objectives. Of course, all interventions have a common goal of relieving pain or maintaining a pain-free state (PRT; see Chapter 3). Other objectives are the treatment of functional lesions (support of RoT and MoT), an increase in blood and lymph flow (support of ReT and MeT), and the restoration of a healthy posture and healthy movement pattern (support of RoT and MoT).

Treatment of Functional Lesions (Support of RoT and MoT)

The goal of these techniques is to stimulate neuromuscular control mechanisms to compensate for an existing imbalance within a function; both passive and active techniques are available for this purpose. Passive techniques include so-called "Shaking." Fast, shaking movements are used to lower the tone in the treated structures (Dr Brügger Institut 1994). Another passive technique is the "Spontaneous Release by Positioning" or "Strain–Counterstrain" of Lawrence H. Jones (Jones Institute 2022). Here, relaxation is to be achieved via a spontaneous response to slow and precise changes in joint position. There are also a few active techniques for correcting an imbalance, for example: Muscle Energy Techniques (Noto-Bell et al. 2019), Kabat's Proprioceptive Neuromuscular Facilitation (PNF) techniques (that is, Hold–Relax and Contract–Relax; Buck et al. 1996: 35–40), Lewitt's Post-isometric Relaxation Techniques (Noto-Bell et al. 2019), and Agistic Eccentric Contraction Techniques according to Alois Brügger and colleagues (1998).

In order to achieve a lasting effect, the patient can perform movement exercises against external resistance. Here, balance is to be achieved through targeted exercise of the neglected muscle function groups. The authors find elastic resistance training to be the most versatile and effective technique for many patients. Several elastic resistance brands, such as TheraBand® (Akron, Ohio, USA), offer a progressive system of resistance so that appropriate resistance can be given to all muscle groups in virtually every patient throughout the length of the treatment.

Increasing Blood and Lymph Flow (Support of ReT and MeT)

The goal of these interventions is to activate the mechanisms that provide improved tissue metabolism. Here, the lymphatic system in particular is addressed, which drains the extracellular space. The removal of fluid components together with the metabolic waste products they contain should be increased in order to rehydrate the extracellular matrix and support remodeling. Recommended techniques include thermotherapy through a moist heat in the form of a so-called "hot roll" or moist heat pack (as a therapist technique) or foam rolling (as a patient technique). The "hot roll" is applied with one or two terry towels rolled tightly in a funnel shape while very hot water – not boiling – is poured in. In the context of IAMT, foam rolling is used to improve tissue hydration through the mechanical effect of external pressure and subsequent relief rather than to improve ROM or to reduce muscle tone. Therefore, the authors recommend a prolonged and targeted application of foam rolling.

Restoration of a Healthy Posture and Healthy Movement Pattern (Support of RoT and MoT)

The view of the myofascial system as an anatomical entity (continuum) and as a functional entity (tensegrity) supports the use of therapy to maintain posture and movement throughout the entire body. This is to be achieved by correction and training of posture and movement which supports the optimal load of all structures during everyday life. Experience suggests that it is beneficial if the patient can actively participate in the rehabilitation.

Summary

This chapter has described the elements of integrating IAMT into daily clinical practice including indications, contraindications, and precautions. Clinical decision-making and application with complementary therapies were also discussed.

As Cheatham and colleagues wrote in their clinical commentary (2019):

Instrument assisted soft-tissue mobilization (IASTM) has become a popular myofascial intervention for sports medicine professionals. Despite the widespread use and emerging research, a consensus on clinical standards, such as describing the intervention, indications, *precautions, contraindications, tool hygiene, safe treatment, and assessment, does not exist. There is a need to develop best practice standards for IASTM through a universal consensus on these variables. The purpose of this commentary is to discuss proposed clinical standards and to encourage other sports medicine professionals and researchers to contribute their expertise to the development of such guidelines.*

The authors would like to contribute to this discussion with their experience; thus, the integration of IAMT into clinical practice is probably one of the most important chapters in this book. After all, a technique that is difficult to integrate into the therapist's daily routine is unlikely to be adopted and will likely fade from clinical practice. Nevertheless, the results of IAMT are convincing to both the authors and their patients, and our ultimate goal is to share our experiences with interested therapists in order to constantly improve patient care.

References

Bisschop P (1993) Personal communication, advanced training course on orthopaedic medicine according to James Cyriax, Leuven, Belgium, October.

Brügger A (1996) Personal communication, internal training session, Brügger Institute, Zürich.

Brügger AEK, Rock C-M, Petak-Krueger S (1998) Agistisch-exzentrische Kontraktionsmaßnahmen gegen Funktionsstörungen des Bewegungssystems. Zürich: Dr. Bruegger Institut.

Brügger A (2000) Lehrbuch der funktionellen Erkrankungen des Bewegungssystems. Zollikon and Benglen, Switzerland: Brügger-Verlag.

Buck M, Beckers D, Adler S (1996) PNF in der Praxis, 3rd rev edn. Berlin, Heidelberg, and New York: Springer.

Cheatham SW, Baker R, Kreiswirth E (2019) Instrument assisted soft-tissue mobilization: a commentary on clinical practice guidelines for rehabilitation professionals. Int J Sports Phys Ther 14(4):670. doi:10.26603/ijspt20190670.

Dr. Brügger Institut (1994) Course documents. Düsseldorf: Evangelisches Krankenhaus Düsseldorf.

Gautschi R (2013) Manuelle Triggerpunkt-Therapie: Myofasziale Schmerzen und Funktionsstörungen erkennen, verstehen und behandeln. Stuttgart and New York: Georg Thieme.

Jones Institute (2022) What is Counterstrain? [Online] Available: https://www.jicounterstrain.com/counterstrain [27 April 2022].

Noto-Bell L, Vogel BN, Senn DE (2019) Effects of post–isometric relaxation on ankle plantarflexion and timed flutter kick in pediatric competitive swimmers. J Am Osteopath Assoc 119(9):569–577.

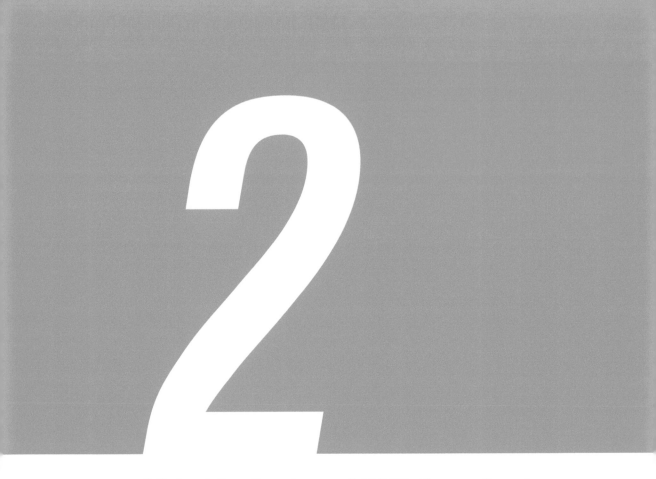

2

Clinical Applications of IAMT: Upper Quarter

The chapters in Parts 2–4 deal with the clinical application of the instruments on the patient: IAMT in daily practice. The structure follows the internationally recognized division of the body into quarters; the upper quarter is described first in Part 2. As we mentioned in the book's Introduction, we are also concerned with good readability and high relevance to everyday practice. It would be unusual to have the opportunity to read the whole book in one go, and so a structure has been chosen that allows the reader to tackle each chapter separately and still be able to apply the corresponding therapy directly.

All the chapters here are developed in the same way: at least two important – and common – diseases have been selected for each area. A detailed description of the treatment is given first, followed by a schematic representation of the treatment with numerous illustrations. The authors hope that this will lead to an immediate and optimal implementation of the therapy in the reader's practice. A treatment protocol is provided, which has proven itself in practice. Of course, it can and should always be adapted to the patient or the condition. Sometimes not all steps are necessary; sometimes a certain part of the treatment must be carried out more intensively. However, especially when the therapist is still gaining experience with IAMT, it is advisable to follow the protocols; they lend a certain structure and often give the therapist a corresponding sense of security. They also increase comparability between patients.

A visual representation of the treatment is also provided, for quick reference. Finally, the authors give information on the possible duration of the therapy, suggest evaluation tests, and present possibilities for progression as well as pre- and post-treatment techniques. In the latter case, reference should always made to Chapter 4 since these techniques are almost always identical.

Clinical Applications of IAMT: Upper Quarter

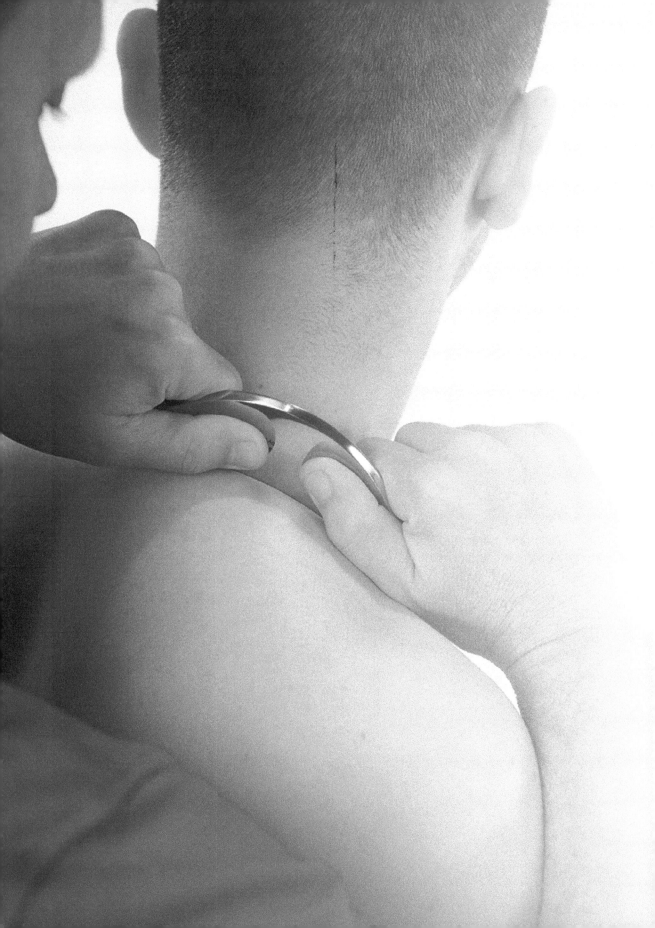

This chapter focuses on the treatment of two frequent and practice-relevant diagnoses for this area: non-specific or mechanical neck pain (cervicalgia) and headache with a myofascial cause (suboccipital headache). These diagnoses are representative of the range of other cervical pathologies; treatment is adapted according to the symptoms and the suspected causes.

Non-specific or Mechanical Neck Pain (Cervicalgia)

Detailed Description of the Treatment

The affected structure is the cervical spine with its myofascial structures:

- Nuchal fascia and ligamentum nuchae.
- Trapezius (descending/upper part and transverse/middle part).
- Serratus posterior superior.
- Levator scapulae.
- Short neck extensor muscles (obliquus capitis inferior and superior, rectus capitis posterior major and minor).

While the specific treatment of the lateral and medial muscular tract is somewhat difficult, attempts are made to specifically treat the suboccipital short neck muscles because of their role in headache symptoms. The treatment of these short neck muscles is described accordingly under the "headache" heading, separately from classical cervicalgia. Experience also shows that non-specific headaches tend to be associated with lower cervical dysfunction and are more likely to be treated functionally with the upper thoracic spine, whereas vertebrogenic headaches tend to originate in the higher cervical segments (C1–3).

In most chapters of this book, a standard treatment (for the so-called "primary structures affected") and an additional treatment (for the so-called "secondary structures affected") are presented. In the cervical spine, two parts of a treatment are described due to the complexity of the area and of the clinical diagnosis being treated. It is not always necessary to perform both parts consecutively. Usually, the therapist starts with treatment of the dorsal structures and then performs a second treatment on the ventral structures. It is also possible to address both areas with one treatment; thus, individual techniques from both parts can be combined. The reader will find a detailed description of the treatment of adjacent structures in corresponding chapters. (Figure I.1 in the Introduction also helps readers quickly find the corresponding structures in this book.) Through the Myofascial Connected System, the reader is also guided through the entire body-wide network of fascial structures. In this way, a holistic treatment of the human body is provided, even for seemingly local problems.

Treatment of the dorsal (posterior) structures of the cervical spine

The patient lies prone (relaxation of the treated structure), with ankles or feet overhanging the edge of the table. The arms should be relaxed next to the body. The patient's head should not be rotated but in neutral. The side lying position is an alternative, although it allows only one-sided treatment. As with the thoracic and lumbar spine, the side lying position is used to treat the ligamentous structures between the vertebrae. The seated position or use of a massage chair may also be an alternative.

The treatment starts with the Rehydration Technique by applying large-area sliding of the entire area of the cervical spine. It is best to use a curved instrument or a combination curve instrument, with its convex side. Starting from the acromion, the instrument is continuously pushed medially and cranially, upwards toward the occiput. The instrument is then placed a little further medially with each repetition so that the entire surface is gradually treated. The pressure is proportional to the thickness of the soft tissue layers. The more tissue under the instrument, the higher the pressure can be; however, uniformity of the pressure is important. Each of these parts is treated several times. Then the painful areas of the cervical spine are treated; there are usually several pain points in the cervical spine area. It is best to use a relatively short part of the instrument for this local treatment.

Sometimes the patient's hair or hairstyle may be problematic. Due to the occipital insertions of muscles and ligaments, the treatment sometimes has to take place in the area of the patient's hair. The therapist should address this problem before treatment and refrain from treating this area if necessary.

The Rehydration Technique can be used on large areas, although some areas are difficult to reach. This is where the value of the equipment and its special properties become apparent, as the therapist may rehydrate these hard-to-reach areas with the narrow part of the instrument. The muscular attachments (tenoperiosteal junctions) on the scapula (the acromion and spine of the scapula for the trapezius muscle, the superior angle for levator scapulae, and the medial border for serratus anterior), along with the occiput (occipital protuberance for the ligamentum nuchae), should be treated as well. Usually, both the affected side of the cervical spine and the apparently unaffected or non-painful side are treated because of the broad ligamentous and muscular attachments across the spine and the role of the cervical spine as an organ of protection, support, and movement. Furthermore, experience shows that non-specific neck pain is often deep, broad-based, and bilateral; usually, one side is more affected than the other.

After the Rehydration Technique, the Pain Relief Technique is usually performed. Of course, it is possible to start with this; however, beginning therapy with the gentle and rather pleasant Rehydration Technique has proven to be very positive in the authors' experience. The technique is, naturally, limited to the painful area(s). Pain localization, discussed above, is often broad-based cervical (between C7 and C3) and bilateral. These painful areas, which the patient is almost always well able to identify, are then treated accordingly. The area may extend along the nuchal fascia and even beyond, into the fascia of the shoulder girdle and the arm.

In order to achieve the greatest pain relief, the painful areas are provided with a high degree of mechanical stimulation through scraping. The technique is performed directly over the painful areas with a progressive pressure (which should not increase the pain already present). The pressure is applied in both treatment directions: away from the treated area and then on the return. If there are several pain points, they are treated consecutively.

The next technique applied is Regulation of Tone. Application is again dependent on the physiotherapeutic findings. The hypertonia is visualized on palpation and immediately treated accordingly. In the area of the cervical spine, hypertonic structures are usually located in its entirety: trapezius (descending and transverse parts), serratus posterior superior, levator scapulae, and the short neck muscles. Other cervical muscles may be hypertonic as well. Once the therapist has located a hypertonic area, they place the (straight short) instrument on the point, apply vertical pressure to the tissue, and maintain this pressure until the tone subsides. The therapist may then feel they can penetrate deeper into the tissue. At the new point of tension, the pressure is held again, and the therapist waits for a new release. The technique can be completed by small movements of the instrument.

In this case, the therapist moves the instrument back and forth on the spot or performs small circular movements. Often, this "melting technique" brings an additional relaxing effect and thus increases the overall benefit.

The next technique applied is the Mobilization Technique. The experienced therapist will have no difficulty locating the hypomobile zones of the cervical spine, particularly those superficial ones involving the nuchal fascia. They are treated according to the protocol already described: first sensed by the superficial displacement test, then treated accordingly. The importance of these superficial hypomobilities is often underestimated, in the authors' view, as their treatment is integral to IAMT.

The deeper hypomobilities are somewhat more difficult to locate; they are mostly in the trapezius muscle and at its insertions at the acromion and spine of the scapula, superior angle, and medial border, as well as the external occipital protuberance, the ligamentum nuchae, and the spinous process of vertebrae C7–T3.

Special attention should be paid to the direction of the tissue mobility limitation. This is not necessarily identical over the entire course of the same structure; moreover, several or even all directions can be affected. The limitation can be determined by a simple test of displaceability using the therapist's hand or the instrument. In our experience, there is seldom a single point, but the loss of mobility usually extends to the entire structure. These characteristics can vary from one patient to another. Depending on the structure, the mobilization is carried out with the hook or the short, flat side of the instrument. It is important that the instrument always remains in contact with the same area. An important technical point is that the instrument is not pushed over the skin, but the anatomical structure is moved in the restricted direction. The return movement is then done without pressure and is described as returning to the starting position.

The tenoperiosteal junctions at the spine (at T3) should always be mobilized and they are often chosen as an entry point for mobilization. This is done either more locally with the end of the instrument, or more regionally with the convex side of the instrument. The therapist then works further cranially along the spine from hypomobility to hypomobility and mobilizes the attachments at the occiput. Next, the tenoperiosteal junctions at the scapula are treated: acromion, superior angle, and medial border. This is also best done with the hook and the edge of the hook of an instrument. The therapist may also find severe hypomobilities at the ventral edge of the descending (upper) trapezius muscle. These can also be mobilized very well with the hook of an instrument.

The following intermuscular septa should be mobilized with the edge of the hook of the instrument: those between trapezius, levator scapulae, and serratus posterior superior muscles.

Finally, the authors would like to point out that the ligamentum nuchae requires treatment. This is best done in the side lying position. The patient's neck is flexed to "open" the dorsal area as much as possible. In the typical neck pain patient, flexion is severely limited and it is often very difficult for the therapist to treat this structure initially; however, after treatment, mobility improves as the pain is reduced. The treatment is best performed with the hook of the instrument.

The last technique recommended in this standard treatment session is the Metabolization Technique. Unlike other treatments, this is considered more of a "finishing" technique to end the therapy and stimulate blood circulation, resulting in a pleasant sensation for the patient. The therapist scrapes with the instrument over the area to be treated, with relatively high pressure that varies according to the volume of the tissue: the greater the volume (that is, the thicker the layer of tissue), the greater the pressure can be. The pressure is applied in one direction only and the speed of

67 Rhomboids
76 Nuchal ligament
77 Trapezius, descending/superior part
78 Trapezius, transverse/middle part
79 Serratus posterior superior
80 Levator scapulae
81 Obliquus capitis inferior
82 Obliquus capitis superior
83 Rectus capitis posterior major
84 Rectus capitis posterior minor

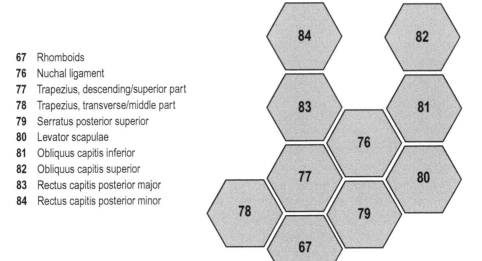

Figure 5.1 Non-specific or mechanical neck pain (cervicalgia): representation of the MCS of the dorsal cervical spine

execution is also relatively high. It is important to note that the pain already present must not increase with this technique.

Myofascial Connected System (MCS) (Figure 5.1)

Schematic Representation of the Treatment of the Dorsal Cervical Spine

Diagnosis
(Non-specific) neck pain.

Primary structures affected (Figure 5.2)
- Nuchal fascia and ligamentum nuchae.
- Trapezius (descending/upper part and transverse/middle part).
- Serratus posterior superior.
- Levator scapulae.
- Short neck muscles (obliquus capitis inferior and superior, rectus capitis posterior major and minor).

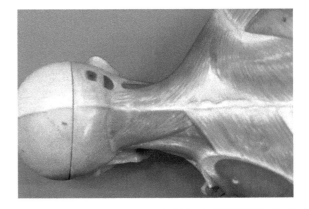

Figure 5.2 Non-specific or mechanical neck pain (dorsal): primary structures affected

Initial position
- Lying prone, with ankles or feet overhanging the table; arms are relaxed next to the body, and the head in neutral.

- Alternatives: side lying or seated on a massage chair.

Material
- Recommended: combination curved, straight short instrument.
- Optional: straight elongated instrument, curved instrument.

Technique
- Recommended: Rehydration, Pain Relief, Regulation of Tone, Mobilization, Metabolization.
- Optional: none.

Recommended treatment protocol (Table 5.1)

Rehydration Technique (ReT)

- Entire area of the cervical spine (nuchal fascia).

Pain Relief Technique (PRT)

- Broad-based cervical (between C7 and C3) and bilateral pain.

Regulation of Tone Technique (RoT)

- Trapezius (descending/superior and transverse/middle parts).
- Serratus posterior superior.
- Levator scapulae.
- Short neck muscles.

Mobilization Technique (MoT)

- Nuchal fascia.
- Trapezius (descending and transverse parts).
- Levator scapulae.
- Serratus posterior superior.
- Ligamentum nuchae.

Metabolization Technique (MeT)

- Broad-based cervical (between C7 and C3) and bilateral.

Table 5.1 Non-specific or mechanical neck pain (cervicalgia): summary of recommended treatment protocol (dorsal structures)

ReT	PRT	RoT	MoT	MeT
Nuchal fascia	Painful area	Trapezius (descending and transverse parts)	Nuchal fascia	Painful area
		Serratus posterior superior	Trapezius (descending and transverse parts)	
		Levator scapulae	Levator scapulae	
		Short neck muscles	Serratus posterior superior	
			Ligamentum nuchae	

Visual Presentation of the Treatment Unit

Recommended treatment protocol

Rehydration Technique (ReT)

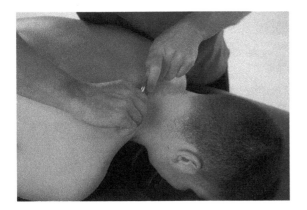

Figure 5.3 Cervical spine: starting position 1

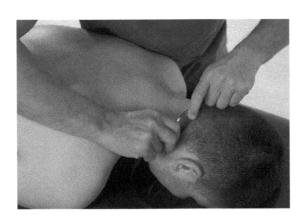

Figure 5.4 Cervical spine: end position 1

Pain Relief Technique (PRT)

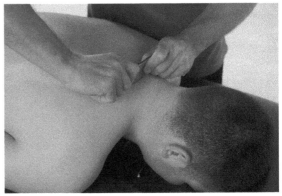

Figure 5.5 Cervical spine: large area

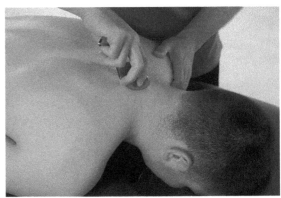

Figure 5.6 Cervical spine: small area

Regulation of Tone Technique (RoT)

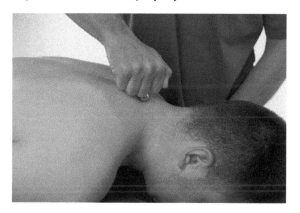

Figure 5.7 Trapezius, descending part

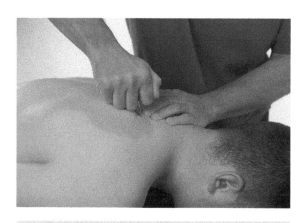

Figure 5.8 Levator scapulae

Mobilization Technique (MoT)

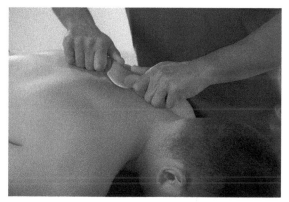

Figure 5.9 Trapezius insertions at the spinous processes of the thoracic spine

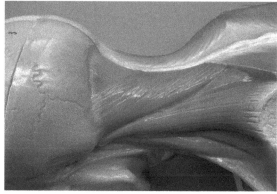

Figure 5.10 Structures involved in the Mobilization Technique: dorsolateral view

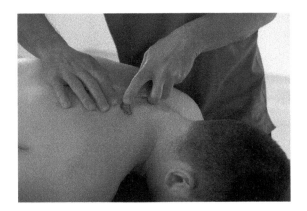

Figure 5.11 Levator scapulae (superior angle of the scapula)

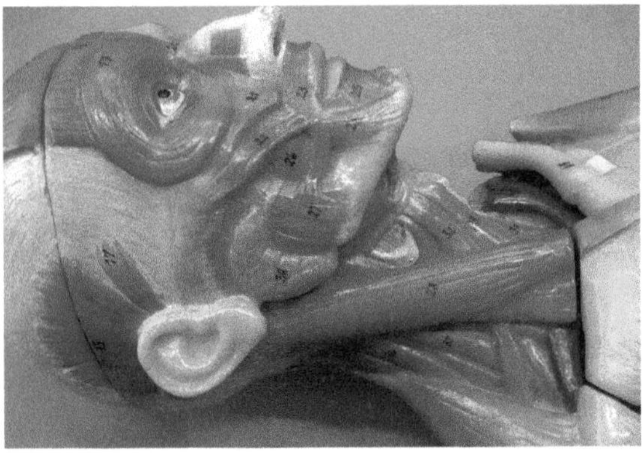

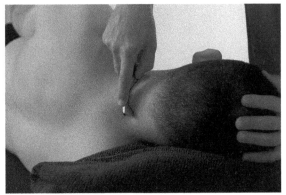

Figure 5.13 Ligamentum nuchae in side lying with hook

Metabolization Technique (MeT)

Figure 5.12 Structures involved in the Mobilization Technique: anterolateral view

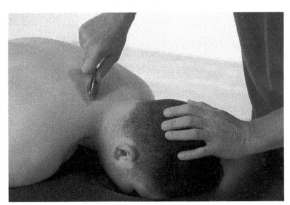

Figure 5.14 Cervical spine

Duration

Approximately 15 minutes.

Evaluation

- Numeric rating scale (NRS).
- Global ROM cervical spine: distance sternum–chin (flexion–extension and rotation); distance ear–acromion (lateral flexion).
- Segmental mobility tests of the cervical spine.

Exercise progression

- Tissue stretch: stretch starting position in flexion (and rotation):
  - Lying on the side in flexion
  - Sitting on the stool in flexion (and rotation)
  - In standing position in flexion (and rotation).

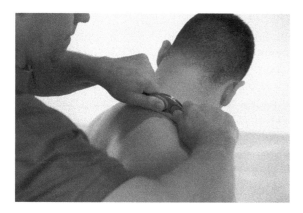

Figure 5.15 Tissue stretch: treatment sitting on the stool in flexion (and rotation)

- Tissue dynamics: active movements of the cervical spine:
  - Lying on the side (flexion)
  - Sitting on the stool (flexion, rotation, lateral flexion)
  - In standing position in flexion (flexion, rotation, lateral flexion).
- Tissue loading: functionality of the starting position:
  - Sitting on the stool
  - In standing position.

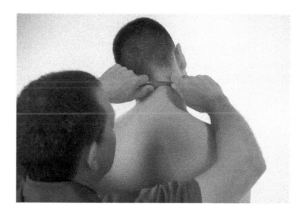

Figure 5.16 Tissue loading: treatment in standing position

Treatment of the ventral (anterior) structures of the cervical spine

The treatment of ventral structures is usually performed unilaterally; if both sides are affected, they are treated one after the other. The authors recommend treatment of the following structures: the sternocleidomastoid muscle; scalenus anterior, medius, and posterior; subclavius; the intercostal muscles; cervical fascia (superficial layer); the platysma muscle; and the ligaments of the sternoclavicular joint and costoclavicular joint. It may seem surprising that the clavicles or their ligaments are discussed at this point, yet experience shows that these short and rather inconspicuous structures have a functional value that should not be underestimated; if we look at the muscular attachments and their spatial distribution, the high value of these structures quickly becomes obvious. Other structures (hyoid musculature and prevertebral cervical muscles, the so-called "deep neck flexors") either are difficult to reach or cannot be differentiated, or they cannot be treated efficiently due to the presence of large vessels and nerves (the carotid artery, jugular vein, and vagus nerve), as well as the larynx and trachea.

The patient lies supine, supporting the knee joints and head to relax the treated structure. In this case it is especially important that the patient's head is stable so that the patient can relax and the therapist can work effectively. The authors recommend the use of pillows that adapt to the structures; these may be molded or filled with materials that conform to the body. The arms should be relaxed next to the body or folded on the abdomen.

The Rehydration Technique starts with rather small and rather superficial sliding of the area at the front and lateral neck. It is essential that the above-mentioned sensitive structures (vessels, nerves, and airways) are left out. Beginning from the lateral side of the clavicle, the instrument (with its concave side) is worked in the direction of the head (towards the mastoid process). Then the instrument is applied further medially to reach all structures. The pressure is proportional to the thickness of the soft tissue layers. The more tissue under the instrument, the higher the pressure can be, while ensuring that it remains uniform; however, the pressure should be kept rather low because the skin in this area is quite thin and sensitive. Each of these parts is treated several times.

The authors recommend the Rehydration Technique for the ligamentous structures of the sternoclavicular and costoclavicular joints. This is best done with the edge of the hook of the instrument. Application of the Rehydration Technique may not be as effective in this region compared to other areas; nevertheless, the authors recommend performing the short and superficial sequence described, if only as preparation of the area for the following techniques.

After the Rehydration Technique, the Pain Relief Technique is usually performed. However, since musculoskeletal pain in the anterior neck region is relatively rare, this treatment may be minimal. If at all, patients occasionally express pain around the sternoclavicular joint, at which point the Pain Relief Technique can be performed (with a small instrument).

The next technique applied is Regulation of Tone. Application is again dependent on the examination findings. The muscular hypertonia is visualized on palpation and immediately treated accordingly. In the area of the anterior neck, sternocleidomastoid, the scalene muscles, subclavius, and the intercostal muscles tend to be hypertonic. The location is mostly the muscle belly; however, it is not uncommon to find several points within sternocleidomastoid. Once the therapist has located a hypertonic point, they place the instrument (straight short instrument) on the point, apply vertical pressure to the tissue, and maintain this pressure until the tone subsides. The therapist can then penetrate deeper into the tissue. At the new point of tension, the pressure is held again and the therapist waits for a new release. The technique can be completed by small movements of the instrument. In this case, the therapist moves the instrument back and forth on the spot or performs small circular movements. Often this "melting technique" brings an additional relaxing effect and thus increases the overall effect.

This technique should also take into account the sensitivity of the area and its structures. Accordingly, the pressure should not be too great. It is advisable to go into the treatment progressions (especially the stretching of the treated structures) at an early stage rather than to increase the pressure and the treatment depth of IAMT.

The next technique applied is the Mobilization Technique. Areas of hypomobility are first addressed; the superficial fascia in particular should be inspected and treated. Deeper hypomobilities are somewhat more difficult to locate; they are mostly in the sternocleidomastoid muscle and at the insertions (tenoperiosteal junction) at the mastoid process, the clavicle, the first ribs, and the sternum. Special attention should be paid to the direction of the limitation, as described earlier. The tenoperiosteal junctions of sternocleidomastoid, the scalene muscles, subclavius, and the intercostal muscles at the clavicle (medial side), the sternum, and the first ribs should be mobilized. As this is a very focused technique, it is best done with the small end of an instrument. The therapist then works along the clavicle, moving laterally with each hypomobility. The tenoperiosteal junction at the first two ribs is treated. Finally, the attachments at the mastoid process should be addressed. This is also best done with the hook and the edge of the hook.

Usually, the last technique applied in this standard treatment session is Metabolization. As already described for the Pain Relief Technique, musculoskeletal pain in the anterior neck region is rare. If the patient does express pain, the Metabolization Technique can theoretically be performed there; however, this is often the exception rather than the rule.

Myofascial Connected System (MCS) (Figure 5.17)

Schematic Representation of the Treatment of the Ventral Cervical Spine

Diagnosis
(Non-specific) neck pain.

Primary structures affected (Figure 5.18)
- Cervical fascia.
- Platysma.
- Sternocleidomastoid.
- Scalenus anterior, medius, and posterior.
- Subclavius.
- Intercostal muscles.
- Ligaments of the sternoclavicular joint and costoclavicular joint (anterior sternoclavicular ligament, interclavicular ligament, costoclavicular ligament).

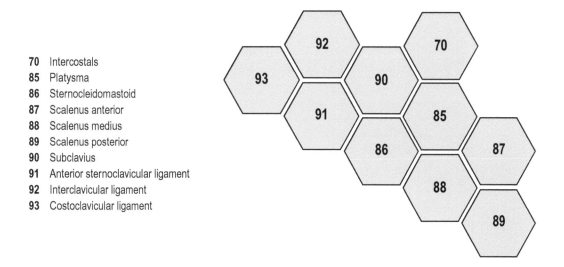

70	Intercostals
85	Platysma
86	Sternocleidomastoid
87	Scalenus anterior
88	Scalenus medius
89	Scalenus posterior
90	Subclavius
91	Anterior sternoclavicular ligament
92	Interclavicular ligament
93	Costoclavicular ligament

Figure 5.17 Non-specific or mechanical neck pain (cervicalgia): representation of the MCS of the ventral cervical spine

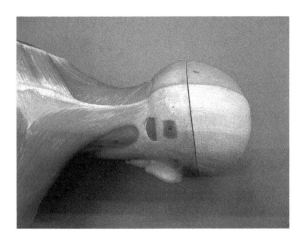

Figure 5.18 Non-specific or mechanical neck pain (ventral): primary structures affected

Initial position

Lying supine, supporting the knee joints and head (relaxation of the treated structure).

Material

- Recommended: combination curved, straight short instrument.
- Optional: straight elongated instrument, curved instrument.

Technique

- Recommended: Rehydration, Regulation of Tone, Mobilization.
- Optional: Pain Relief, Metabolization.

Recommended treatment protocol (Table 5.2)

Rehydration Technique (ReT)

- Front and side neck area.
- Ligaments of the sternoclavicular joint and costoclavicular joint.

Regulation of Tone Technique (RoT)

- Sternocleidomastoid.
- Scalene muscles.
- Subclavius.
- Intercostal muscles.

Mobilization Technique (MoT)

- Cervical fascia.
- Sternocleidomastoid.
- Scalene muscles.
- Subclavius.
- Intercostal muscles.

Table 5.2 Non-specific or mechanical neck pain (cervicalgia): summary of recommended treatment protocol (ventral structures)

ReT	PRT	RoT	MoT	MeT
Front and side of neck area		Sternocleidomastoid	Cervical fascia	
Ligaments of the sternoclavicular joint and costoclavicular joint		Scalene muscles	Sternocleidomastoid	
		Subclavius	Scalene muscles	
		Intercostal muscles	Subclavius	
			Intercostal muscles	

Visual Presentation of the Treatment Unit

Recommended treatment protocol

Rehydration Technique (ReT)

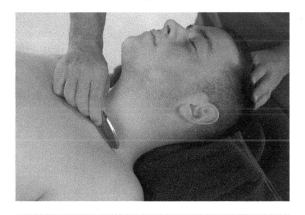

Figure 5.19 Cervical fascia

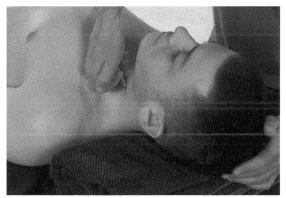

Figure 5.21 Scalene muscles

Regulation of Tone Technique (RoT)

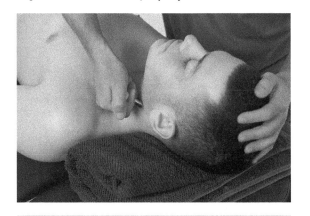

Figure 5.20 Sternocleidomastoid

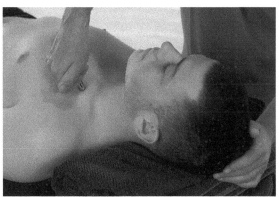

Figure 5.22 Subclavius

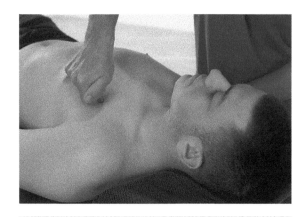

Figure 5.23 Intercostal muscles

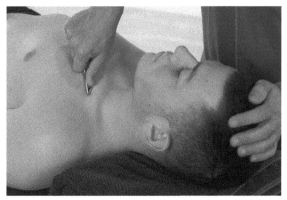

Figure 5.25 Scalene muscles

Mobilization Technique (MoT)

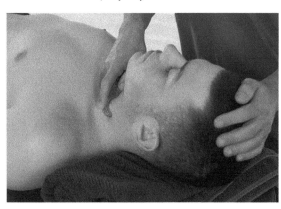

Figure 5.24 Sternocleidomastoid

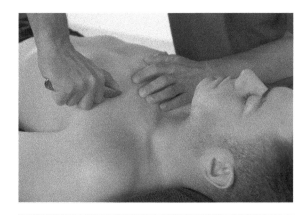

Figure 5.26 Subclavius

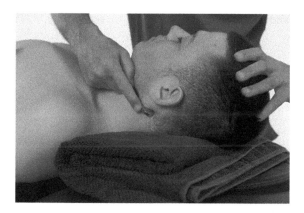

Figure 5.27 Sternocleidomastoid

Duration

Approximately 5 minutes.

Evaluation

- Numeric Rating Scale (NRS).
- Global ROM cervical spine: distance sternum–chin (flexion–extension and rotation); distance ear–acromion (lateral flexion).
- Segmental mobility tests of the cervical spine.

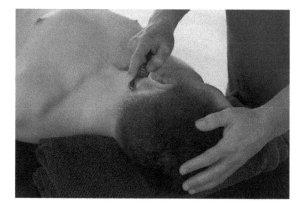

Figure 5.28 Tissue stretch: starting treatment in a stretched position in rotation (lying supine)

Exercise progression

- Tissue stretch: stretch starting position in rotation:
  - Lying supine
  - Sitting on the stool
  - In standing position.
- Tissue dynamics: active movements (rotation) of the cervical spine:
  - Lying supine
  - Sitting on the stool
  - In standing position in flexion.
- Tissue loading: functionality of the starting position:
  - Sitting on the stool
  - In standing position.

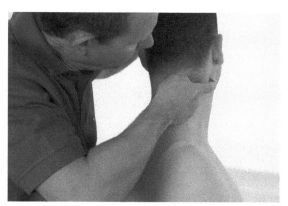

Figure 5.29 Tissue loading: treatment sitting on the stool

Myofascial Headache

Detailed Description of the Treatment

Headaches can result from the short deep cervical extensor muscles. A so-called "myofascial headache" radiates from the occiput into the head via the attachments of the trapezius, sternocleidomastoid, and the erector spinae cervicalis muscles (longissimus capitis and splenius capitis). From there (superior nuchal line), the temporoparietal fascia and the occipitofrontalis and temporoparietalis muscles are mainly responsible for the typical distribution of the pain in the head.

The affected structures are therefore the nuchal fascia and the temporoparietal fascia, the obliquus capitis inferior and superior muscles, rectus capitis posterior major and minor, and the posterior atlanto-occipital membrane, as well as the epicranius muscle group (occipitofrontalis and temporoparietalis muscles with the large epicranial aponeurosis (galea aponeurotica)).

The patient lies prone, with the ankle joints supported (relaxation of the treated structure) or the feet overhanging the table. The arms should be relaxed next to the body. The patient's head should not be rotated. In this case, it is especially important for the patient's neck to be stable so that it can relax and the therapist can work effectively. The seated position on a massage chair may be an alternative.

A problem that should not be underestimated – at least for some patients – is the fact that the treatment almost always takes place or has to take place in the area of the scalp hair, which could be problematic. Treatment of the short neck muscles is not usually problematic after appropriate education by the therapist; however, treatment of the tenoperiosteal transitions at the occiput and of the head muscles sometimes poses a bigger problem for the therapist, although experience has shown that patient education helps here as well. The short neck muscles are treated with all the "classic" techniques of IAMT; on the head, only Regulation of Tone and Mobilization Techniques are used. The other techniques either are not indicated or seem ineffective. In case of doubt, the authors always recommend refraining from the corresponding treatment.

As usual, the therapy starts with the Rehydration Technique, but only with a short, large-area treatment of the neck. Starting from the acromion, the instrument is continuously pushed medially and cranially up to the occiput several times. It is best to use the convex side of the instrument. The affected structures are then directly treated. The area between the spinous process of C2 (axis), the transverse process of C1 (atlas), and the inferior nuchal line is rehydrated from medial to lateral (first one side, then the other) with the instrument, using the edge of the heel. The pressure is increased progressively and very carefully in small steps (due to the vascular–nerve bundle contained in the suboccipital triangle). The aim is to reach the posterior atlanto-occipital membrane that forms the ventral border of this area. Experience has shown that this is successful only when the patient is relaxed.

Then, after rehydration, the Pain Relief Technique is usually performed. Of course, it is also possible to start with this; however, beginning therapy with the gentle and rather pleasant Rehydration Technique has proven to be very positive. The technique is, naturally, limited to the painful area(s). Experience has shown that in the case of myofascial headaches, the patient indicates many pain points that are usually distributed over the entire head area. This makes an exact differentiation of these numerous points nearly impossible. Furthermore, as already mentioned, the Pain Relief Technique is not used in the area of the head due to the problem with hair. In the authors' experience, the possible indirect use of this technique (use of the technique at a distance, usually in the same dermatome) is not very effective. However, the same experience shows that pain relief can be achieved relatively effectively with the Regulation of Tone and Mobilization Techniques.

The next technique applied is the Regulation of Tone. In the case of myofascial headache, hypertonic muscles are usually located in the short neck muscles (obliquus capitis inferior, obliquus capitis superior, rectus capitis posterior major, rectus capitis posterior minor), as well as in the head muscles (epicranius: occipitofrontalis and temporoparietalis). These techniques are used only for the short neck muscles; there the technique is mostly applied with a straight short instrument, which allows precision of application. For the head muscles, due to the anatomical location (under the scalp at the hairline and directly over the skull bones), the technique is performed only once per hypertonic point. The release is also rarely noticeable, since the direct bone contact and the thinness of the musculature do not allow this. Furthermore, it is best for the therapist to use a slightly wider straight short instrument. Patients often describe this as more pleasant than an overly localized pressure with a straight short instrument.

The next technique applied is the Mobilization Technique. The superficial hypomobilities involve the nuchal fascia. They are treated according to the protocol already described.

The experienced therapist will have no difficulty locating the deeper hypomobile zones of the short neck muscles. There is seldom a single point, as the loss of mobility usually extends to the entire structure, particularly if the affected structures are as short as the short neck muscles. Depending on the structure, mobilization is carried out with the hook or the short flat side of the instrument.

The spinous process of C2 (insertion of rectus capitis major and obliquus capitis inferior) is often chosen as an entry point for mobilization. Here one can work with the short side of the instrument or with its hook; sometimes a straight short instrument is an alternative, the advantage being that the therapist can mobilize more selectively and therefore more precisely. The therapist follows the muscles to their cranial insertion, then treats the small area of the arch of the C1 atlas (insertion of the rectus capitis minor muscle) and follows this structure up to the inferior nuchal line. Finally, treat from the arch of the C1 atlas (obliquus capitis superior) and mobilize this muscle, again up to the inferior nuchal line.

Mobilization of the epicranius muscle (which combines the occipitofrontalis muscle with temporoparietalis) begins at the highest nuchal line; from there, the therapist mobilizes, first, the very flat muscle belly of the epicranius muscle and then the epicranial aponeurosis across the entire head, up to the eyebrows. The treatment should always involve both sides (one after the other, of course). For this treatment, the edge of the convexity of the instrument is ideal. Then, the same technique is performed for the temporalis muscle: from the patient's ear (auricular cartilage) to the epicranial aponeurosis. This treatment is also performed successively on both sides.

For the final treatment of the ligamentum nuchae, the patient does not necessarily have to turn onto their side; it is usually sufficient if they pull the chin slightly towards the chest. In the prone position, the cervical spine – at least in the high cervical region – is bent far enough to be able to treat the ligament accordingly due to the opening of the intervertebral area. The treatment is best done with the hook. The patient often has very limited opening of the intervertebral spaces. Nevertheless, experience shows that treatment of these areas is also worthwhile. In the typical neck pain patient, flexion is severely limited and it is often very difficult for the therapist to treat these structures initially.

The Metabolization and Pain Relief Techniques are optional for this region and are less often applied.

Myofascial Connected System (MCS) (Figure 5.30)

Schematic Representation of the Treatment

Diagnosis
Myofascial headache.

Primary structures affected
- Nuchal fascia and temporoparietal fascia.
- Obliquus capitis inferior and superior.
- Rectus capitis posterior major and minor.

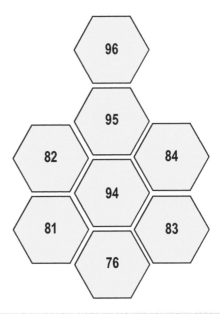

76	Ligamentum nuchae
81	Obliquus capitis inferior
82	Obliquus capitis superior
83	Rectus capitis posterior major
84	Rectus capitis posterior minor
94	Posterior atlanto-occipital membrane
95	Occipitofrontalis
96	Temperoparietalis

Figure 5.30 Myofascial headache: representation of the MCS of the upper cervical region and head

- Posterior atlanto-occipital membrane.
- Epicranius muscle group (epicranial aponeurosis).

Initial position
- Lying prone, with the ankle joints supported (relaxation of the treated structure) or feet overhanging the table, arms relaxed next to the body, head in neutral position.
- Seated on a massage chair (alternative).

Material
- Recommended: combination curved, straight short instrument.
- Optional: straight elongated instrument, curved instrument.

Technique
- Recommended: Rehydration, Regulation of Tone, Mobilization.
- Optional: Pain Relief Technique.

Recommended treatment protocol (Table 5.3)

Rehydration Technique (ReT)
- Neck area.
- Area between the C2 spinous process, the transverse process of C1, and the inferior nuchal line.

Regulation of Tone Technique (RoT)
- Short neck muscles (obliquus capitis inferior, obliquus capitis superior, rectus capitis posterior major, rectus capitis posterior minor).
- Head muscles (epicranius: occipitofrontalis and temporoparietalis).

Mobilization Technique (MoT)
- Nuchal fascia.
- Insertion of rectus capitis major and obliquus capitis inferior at the spinous process of C2 and the inferior nuchal line.

- Insertion of rectus capitis minor (arch of the atlas (posterior tubercle), following this structure up to the inferior nuchal line).
- Insertion of obliquus capitis superior (arch (transverse process) of the atlas and inferior nuchal line).

- Occipitofrontalis: from the highest nuchal line to the eyebrows via the epicranial aponeurosis.
- Temporoparietalis: from the patient's ear (auricular cartilage) to the epicranial aponeurosis.
- Ligamentum nuchae.

Table 5.3 Myofascial headache: summary of recommended treatment protocol				
ReT	**PRT**	**RoT**	**MoT**	**MeT**
Neck area		Short neck muscles	Nuchal fascia	
C2–C1 area and the inferior nuchal line		Head muscles: epicranius	Insertion of rectus capitis major and obliquus capitis inferior at the spinous process of C2 and the inferior nuchal line	
			Insertion of rectus capitis minor (posterior tubercle, following this structure up to the inferior nuchal line)	
			Insertion of obliquus capitis superior (transverse process of the atlas and the inferior nuchal line)	
			Occipitofrontalis: from the highest nuchal line to the eyebrows via the epicranial aponeurosis	
			Temporoparietalis: from the patient's ear (auricular cartilage) to the epicranial aponeurosis	
			Ligamentum nuchae	

Visual Presentation of the Treatment Unit

Recommended treatment protocol

Rehydration Technique (ReT)

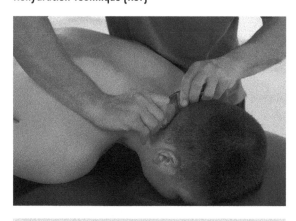

Figure 5.31 Neck and C2–C1 area

Regulation of Tone Technique (RoT)

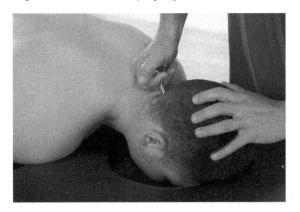

Figure 5.32 Short neck muscles (obliquus capitis inferior, obliquus capitis superior, rectus capitis posterior major, rectus capitis posterior minor)

Mobilization Technique (MoT)

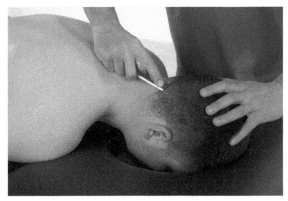

Figure 5.34 Nuchal fascia

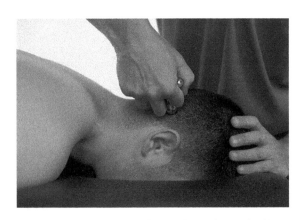

Figure 5.33 Head muscles (epicranius: occipitofrontalis and temporoparietalis)

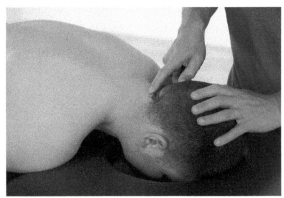

Figure 5.35 Insertion of rectus capitis major and obliquus capitis inferior at the spinous process of C2

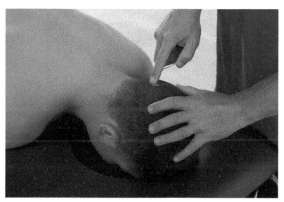

Figure 5.36 Insertion of rectus capitis minor at the inferior nuchal line

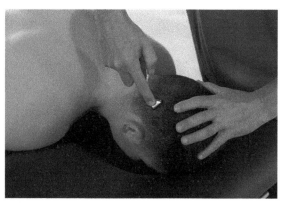

Figure 5.38 Occipitofrontalis: from the highest nuchal line to the eyebrows via epicranial aponeurosis

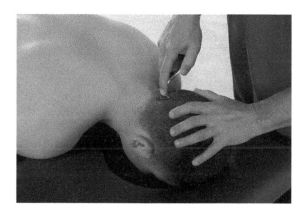

Figure 5.37 Insertion of obliquus capitis superior (arch of the atlas)

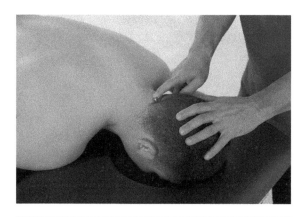

Figure 5.39 Temporoparietalis: from the patient's ear (auricular cartilage) to the epicranial aponeurosis

Duration

Approximately 10 minutes.

Evaluation

- Numeric Rating scale (NRS).
- Global ROM cervical spine: distance sternum–chin (flexion–extension and rotation); distance ear–acromion (lateral flexion).
- Segmental mobility tests of the cervical spine.
- Analysis of head position.

Exercise progression

The exercise progressions are rarely used in this case. Although the causes of the disease are likely to be found in the musculoskeletal system, in the authors' experience they rarely involve truly functional aspects. However, common exercises such as stretching and ROM can be prescribed.

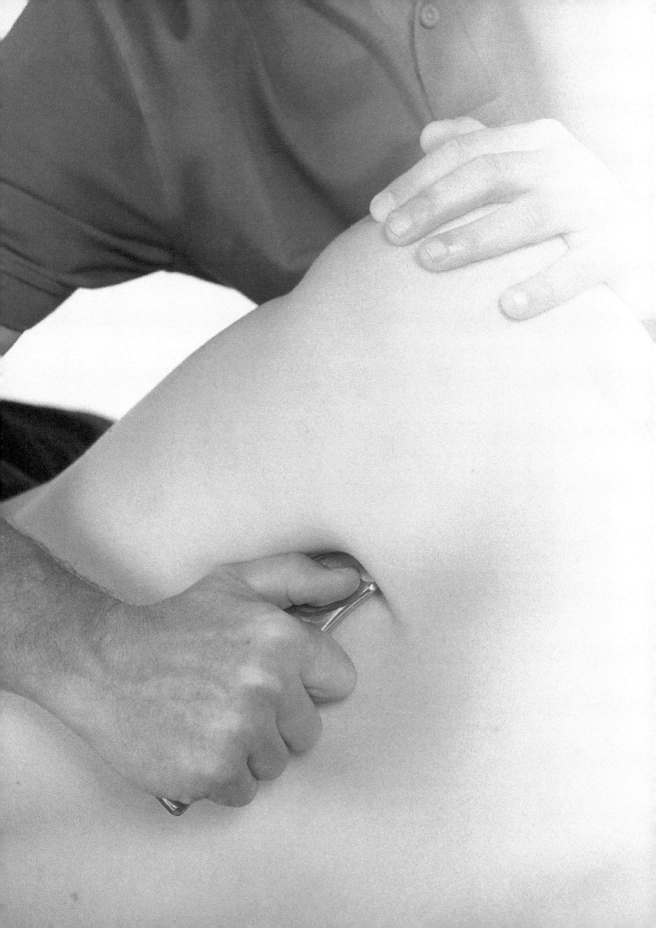

The treatment of two frequent and thus practice-relevant diagnoses have been selected for this area: subacromial impingement syndrome (SIS; also known as impingement syndrome, supraspinatus syndrome, or subacromial pain syndrome) and tendinopathy of the long biceps tendon. As described previously, these diagnoses are representative of the entire range of pathology in the shoulder complex; treatment is adapted according to the symptoms and the suspected causes.

Subacromial Impingement Syndrome

Subacromial impingement syndrome (SIS) cannot be clearly identified as a single diagnosis as far as terminology is concerned; however, it is agreed that SIS particularly affects the rotator cuff, representing a large number of cases seen in practice. It is generally thought to result from faulty positioning of the humeral head in the glenoid fossa of the scapula. For this reason, and because the chapter would otherwise be somewhat confusing, the authors have decided to address the structures that play a major role in the SIS mechanism first. The other structures, particularly the muscles that move the shoulder (such as pectoralis major and so on) are described later in the chapter, in the section on long biceps tendinopathy. Both treatments can be combined in practice, of course. The deltoid muscle occupies a special role: although it does not play a part in all shoulder activities, through its insertions it is involved in almost every shoulder treatment. Accordingly, its treatment is addressed in both sections of this chapter.

In most chapters of this book, a standard treatment (for the so-called "primary structures affected") and an additional treatment (for the so-called "secondary structures affected") are presented at this point. In this case, however, because of the complexity of the area or the clinical diagnosis being treated, the authors have chosen not to offer an optional treatment protocol here.

Detailed Description of the Treatment

Dysfunction of the tissues of the subacromial space (between the acromion and glenoid) are addressed here. The affected structures include the brachial fascia and the muscles of the rotator cuff (supraspinatus, infraspinatus, teres minor, and subscapularis), as well as the adjacent deltoid muscle (acromial part or middle portion, clavicular part or anterior portion, and spinal part or posterior portion). The surrounding scapular muscles are particularly important (rhomboid major and rhomboid minor, serratus posterior superior, serratus anterior and teres major, trapezius and levator scapulae), as are the ventral muscles of the upper thorax that are indirectly involved in the mechanics of the shoulder joint (subclavius and the intercostal muscles) and the coraco-acromio-clavicular ligaments (coracoclavicular, coracoacromial, and acromioclavicular).

For the initial position of the patient there are several alternatives: the classic position is prone. From here, alternation between the prone and supine positions is necessary. The lateral position is also possible, but the arm must be stable and supported so that the patient can relax and the therapist has reasonable access to all structures. Although the lateral position described below is somewhat more complicated, it has the advantage that the patient does not have to change position, which can reduce the time taken up by repositioning. In addition, the therapist can, if necessary, treat dorsal and ventral structures alternately and reach all insertions (including those of serratus anterior at the medial scapular border). Another option is to sit next to the therapy table; the arm to be treated lies relaxed in the plane of the scapula.

We first describe the treatment of the dorsal structures, then that of the ventral structures. As already indicated, the order can be changed if the treatment requires it.

Dorsal structures

The Rehydration Technique starts with large-area sliding of the dorsal side (the area between the inferior angle of the scapula, the deltoid tuberosity, the upper spine, and the humeral head). This is best done with the concave side of a combined curve instrument; a curved instrument is also possible for very large patients. The instrument is attached to the inferior angle of the scapula and pushed to the occiput; from there, the instrument is pushed further, this time in a caudal direction to the acromion. Then, the scapula or the myofascial attachments (tenoperiosteal junctions) are treated. This works well with the hook of the combined curve instrument: the device is attached to the inferior angle of the scapula and pushed to the superior angle. From there, it is pushed along the spine of the scapula to the acromion (supraspinous fossa) and then back along the surface below the spine of the scapula (infraspinous fossa). After the attachments to the lateral scapular border are treated in the same manner, working from the acromion to the inferior angle, the supraspinatus and infraspinatus muscles are finally addressed. The pressure is proportional to the actual thickness of the soft tissue layers. The more tissue under the instrument, the higher the pressure can be – but remember, the uniformity of the pressure is important. Thus, when treating the structures on the scapula, the pressure is naturally reduced somewhat, since the structures lie directly above the bone. In the authors' opinion, it is worth following the tendon of the supraspinatus muscle as far as possible, almost underneath the acromion.

Furthermore, the therapist may place the patient's hand on the patient's back in order to rehydrate the distal insertion on the greater tuberosity; due to the small surface area and the nature of the insertion, the authors prefer to use the edge of the hook of the combined curve instrument here. Finally, the teres major and minor and deltoid (spinal part) muscles are treated, starting from the scapula and working towards the acromion. Each of these parts is treated several times.

After Rehydration, the Pain Relief Technique is usually performed. Of course, it is possible to start with this; however, beginning therapy with the gentle and rather pleasant Rehydration Technique has proven to be very positive in the authors' experience. The Pain Relief Technique is, of course, limited to the painful area(s). Localization of the pain is sometimes difficult, in that the symptoms are partly movement-dependent (such as in abduction during a so-called painful arc). Nevertheless, patients are mostly able to localize the painful area, even at rest. This is usually either fairly centralized in the deltoid muscle between the acromion and the deltoid tuberosity, or in the area of the posterior deltoid between the humerus and the glenoid fossa. The site of pain rarely coincides with the site of the lesion but is nearly always in the same dermatome (C5) or in the region of the axillary nerve. Since the Pain Relief Technique is a reflex technique, it can be performed very well and effectively in the areas indicated by the patient. In the progressions described below, the technique is also performed in the painful positions or movements. In order to achieve the greatest pain relief, the painful areas are provided with a high degree of mechanical stimulation due to the scraping. The technique is performed directly over the painful areas (or, if necessary, at a short distance from them) with a progressive pressure that should not increase the pain that is already present. This pressure is applied in both directions: on the way out and on the way back.

If there are several pain points, they are treated consecutively.

The next technique applied is Regulation of Tone. The application is again dependent on the physiotherapeutic findings. The hypertonia is visualized on palpation and immediately treated accordingly. In the area of the shoulder, hypertonic areas are usually located in the supraspinatus, subscapularis, teres major, and trapezius (descending/upper trapezius and transverse/middle trapezius) muscles, and in levator scapulae. Nevertheless, all the muscles of the shoulder girdle should be examined for local hypertonicity. Once the therapist has located a hypertonic point, they place the short, straight instrument on it, apply vertical pressure to the tissue, and maintain this pressure until the tone subsides. The therapist may then feel that they can penetrate deeper into the tissue. At the new point of tension, the pressure is held again and the therapist waits for a new release. The technique can be completed by small movements of the instrument. In this case, the therapist moves the instrument back and forth on the spot or performs small circular movements. Often, this "melting technique" has an additional relaxing effect and thus increases the overall benefit.

The next technique applied is the Mobilization Technique. The experienced therapist will have no difficulty locating the hypomobile zones of the shoulder. The superficial hypomobilities involve the nuchal fascia and the brachial fascia. They are treated according to the protocol already described: first they are determined by the displacement test, then treated accordingly. The importance of these superficial hypomobilities is often underestimated, but treatment of these disorders is integral to IAMT. Special attention should be paid to the direction of the limitation, which is not necessarily consistent over the entire course of the same structure; moreover, several or even all directions can be affected. The limitation can be determined by a simple test of tissue displaceability using the therapist's hand or the instrument. In our experience, there is seldom a single point, but the loss of mobility usually extends to the entire structure. These characteristics can vary from one patient to another. Depending on the structure, the mobilization is carried out with the hook or the short, flat side of the instrument. It is important for the instrument to always remain in contact with the same area. The instrument is not pushed over the skin but the anatomical structure is moved in the restricted direction. The return movement is then done without pressure and is described as returning to the starting position. The spine of the scapula (tenoperiosteal junction) is often chosen as an entry point for mobilization. Here, the therapist can work along this structure (supraspinatus and infraspinatus) with the short side of the combined curve instrument, the advantage being that mobilization can be more selective and therefore more precise. The therapist then works along the spine of the scapula from hypomobility to hypomobility, trying to mobilize the supraspinatus muscle as much as possible until it disappears under the acromion. It is also necessary to treat the attachments of the serratus anterior muscle at the medial border of the scapula. With the convex side of the combined curve instrument, the therapist penetrates as far as possible under the scapula and mobilizes the structures in a medial to lateral direction. This technique often "frees" the scapula in its mobility. Next, the distal insertions of these muscles on the humerus are mobilized. The tenoperiosteal junction of the supraspinatus tendon is mobilized in the same position (the patient's hand on their back) as described for the Pain Relief Technique. The distal insertions of the infraspinatus and teres minor muscles should be mobilized (at the greater tubercle and lesser tubercle, respectively), as well as the deltoid (at the deltoid tuberosity). The distal insertions of the corresponding muscles on the spine could also be mobilized (the rhomboids, serratus posterior superior, trapezius, and levator scapulae). Two muscular septa are also worth mobilizing: that between the deltoid and teres minor, and that between the infraspinatus and teres minor.

The last technique applied in this standard treatment session is the Metabolization Technique. Unlike other treatment techniques, this is considered more of a "finishing" technique to end the treatment and stimulate blood circulation, resulting in a pleasant sensation for the patient. The therapist scrapes with the instrument over the area to be treated, using relatively high pressure that varies according to the volume of the tissue: the greater the volume (that is, the thicker the layer of tissue), the greater the pressure can be. The pressure is applied in one direction only and the speed of execution is also relatively high. It is important to note that the pain already present must not increase with this technique.

Ventral structures

The Rehydration Technique starts with large-area sliding of the ventral side (the area between the sternoclavicular joint and deltoid tuberosity); this is best done with the concave side of the combined curve instrument. The instrument begins at the mastoid process and is pushed to the acromion; from there, it is pushed further, this time in a medial direction, to the acromioclavicular joint. Then, the ligaments of this joint and the intercostal spaces of ribs 1 to 9 (insertion of the serratus anterior muscle) are treated; this works well with the hook of the combined curve instrument or a short, straight instrument (for the intercostal spaces). Anatomical localization of the anterolateral insertions of serratus anterior and of pectoralis major can lead to potentially difficult situations when treating women, given the existence of the breast. The authors recommend discussing this clearly at the beginning of the patient's treatment. Furthermore, the female breast can be an obstacle

to effective therapy in certain techniques (such as Rehydration, Pain Relief and Metabolization). In this case, the authors recommend refraining from using these techniques. It goes without saying that the female breast is not treated with the instruments in any way. The therapist always adapts the execution of the therapy to the individual situation. The pressure applied is always proportional to the thickness of the soft tissue layers. The more tissue under the instrument, the higher the pressure can be, although uniformity of the pressure is important. Thus, when treating the structures on the clavicle or the ribs, the pressure is naturally reduced because the structures lie directly above the bone. Finally, subclavius and deltoid (clavicular part) are treated. Each of these parts is treated several times.

The Pain Relief Technique is performed on ventral structures similarly to the dorsal structures and will not be reviewed in detail here. It is performed directly over the painful areas or a short distance away, with a progressive pressure that should not increase the pain already present. This pressure is applied in both directions: on the way out and on the way back. If there are several painful points, they are treated consecutively.

The next technique applied is the Regulation of Tone. Application is again dependent on the physiotherapeutic findings. Hypertonic muscles are identified and treated accordingly. In the area of the shoulder, they are usually located in the subclavius and intercostal muscles. Nevertheless, all the muscles of the shoulder girdle should be examined for local tightness. The technique is performed as described above for the dorsal structures and so a detailed description is not given here.

Next comes the Mobilization Technique. The technique is performed in the same way as for the dorsal structures and so a detailed description is not given here. The acromioclavicular joint and its ligaments (coracoclavicular, coracoacromial, and acromioclavicular) are often chosen as an initial point for mobilization. Here, the therapist can work along the clavicle (subclavius muscle) with the short side of the combined curve instrument. Then the therapist mobilizes the intercostal muscles and the insertions of serratus anterior, followed by the distal insertions of the following muscles on the humerus: subscapularis, latissimus dorsi and teres major (at the lesser tubercle), as well as the deltoid (at the deltoid tuberosity).

The last technique applied in this standard treatment session is the Metabolization Technique. This technique is performed in a similar way as for the dorsal structures and does not need to be described in detail again.

Myofascial Connected System (MCS) (Figure 6.1)

Schematic Representation of the Treatment

Diagnosis
Subacromial impingement syndrome (SIS).

Primary structures affected (Figure 6.2)
- Brachial fascia.
- Rotator cuff (supraspinatus, infraspinatus, teres minor, and subscapularis).
- Deltoid muscle (clavicular, acromial, and spinal parts).

66 Trapezius (ascending/lower part)
67 Rhomboids
68 Serratus anterior
70 Intercostals
77 Trapezius (descending/upper part)
78 Trapezius (transverse/middle part)
79 Serratus posterior superior
80 Levator scapulae
90 Subclavius
97 Deltoid (acromial part)
98 Deltoid (clavicular part)

99   Deltoid (spinal part)
100 Supraspinatus
101 Infraspinatus
102 Teres minor
103 Teres major
104 Subscapularis
105 Coracoclavicular ligament
106 Coracoacromial ligament
107 Acromioclavicular ligament

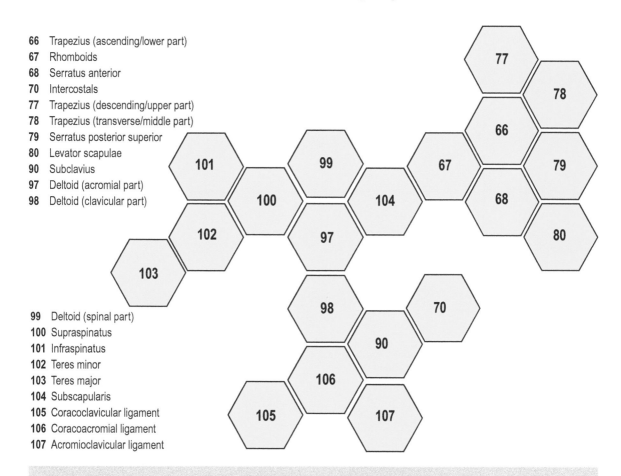

Figure 6.1 Subacromial impingement syndrome: representation of the MCS

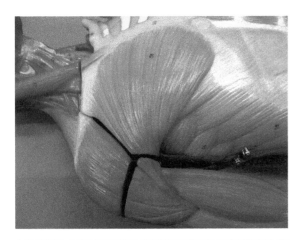

Figure 6.2 Subacromial impingement syndrome: structures affected – anterior part of the shoulder and the arm

- Scapular muscles (rhomboid major and rhomboid minor, serratus posterior superior, serratus anterior, teres major, trapezius, and levator scapulae).
- Subclavius and the intercostal muscles.
- Ligaments of the coraco-acromioclavicular joints (coracoclavicular, coracoacromial, and acromioclavicular).

Initial position
Side lying, arm stable and supported on a cushion.

Material
- Recommended: combination curved, straight short instrument.
- Optional: straight elongated instrument, curved instrument.

Technique
- Recommended: Rehydration, Pain Relief, Regulation of Tone, Mobilization, Metabolization.
- Optional: none.

Recommended treatment protocol: dorsal structures (Table 6.1)

Rehydration Technique (ReT)
- Area between the inferior angle of the scapula, deltoid tuberosity, the spine, and the humeral head (nuchal fascia and brachial fascia).
- Tenoperiosteal junctions around the scapula and at the humerus.

Pain Relief Technique (PRT)
- Painful area:
  ° Centrally in the deltoid muscle between the acromion and the deltoid tuberosity; or
  ° In the area of the spinal part of the deltoid muscle between the humerus and the glenoid fossa.

Regulation of Tone Technique (RoT)
- Supraspinatus.
- Subscapularis.
- Teres major.
- Trapezius (descending and transverse parts).
- Levator scapulae.

Mobilization Technique (MoT)
- Nuchal fascia and brachial fascia.
- Supraspinatus.
- Infraspinatus.
- Serratus anterior.
- Teres minor.
- Deltoid.
- Rhomboid major and rhomboid minor.
- Serratus posterior superior.
- Trapezius.
- Levator scapulae.
- Septa between deltoid and infraspinatus, and deltoid and teres minor.

Metabolization Technique (MeT)
- Centrally, in the deltoid muscle between the acromion and the deltoid tuberosity.

Table 6.1 Subacromial impingement syndrome: summary of recommended treatment protocol (dorsal structures)

ReT	PRT	RoT	MoT	MeT
Area between the inferior angle of the scapula, deltoid tuberosity, spine, and humeral head (nuchal fascia and brachial fascia)	Painful area	Supraspinatus	Nuchal fascia and brachial fascia	Painful area
Tenoperiostal junctions around the scapula and at the humerus	Centrally, in the deltoid between the acromion and deltoid tuberosity	Subscapularis	Supraspinatus	Centrally, in the deltoid between the acromion and deltoid tuberosity
	Area of the posterior deltoid between the humerus and glenoid fossa	Teres major	Infraspinatus	Area of posterior deltoid between humerus and glenoid fossa
		Trapezius (descending and transverse parts)	Serratus anterior	
		Levator scapulae	Teres minor	
			Deltoid	
			Rhomboid major and rhomboid minor	
			Serratus posterior superior	
			Trapezius	
			Levator scapulae	
			Septa between deltoid and infraspinatus, and deltoid and teres minor	

- Area of the spinal part of the deltoid between the humerus and the glenoid fossa.

Recommended treatment protocol: ventral structures (Table 6.2)

Rehydration Technique (ReT)

- Area between the sternoclavicular joint, the deltoid tuberosity, and the humeral head.
- Subclavius and deltoid (clavicular part).

Pain Relief Technique (PRT)

- Painful area: centrally in the deltoid muscle between the acromion and the deltoid tuberosity.

Regulation of Tone Technique (RoT)

- Subclavius.
- Intercostal muscles.

Mobilization Technique (MoT)

- Acromioclavicular joint (and its coracoclavicular, coracoacromial, and acromioclavicular ligaments).

Table 6.2 Subacromial impingement syndrome: summary of recommended treatment protocol (ventral structures)				
ReT	**PRT**	**RoT**	**MoT**	**MeT**
Area between the sternoclavicular joint, deltoid tuberosity, and humeral head	Painful area	Subclavius	Acromioclavicular joint (and its coracoclavicular, coracoacromial, and acromioclavicular ligaments)	Painful area
Subclavius and the anterior deltoid	Centrally in the deltoid muscle between the acromion and the deltoid tuberosity	Intercostal muscles	Subclavius	Posterior area of the deltoid between the humerus and the glenoid fossa
			Intercostal muscles	
			Serratus anterior	
			Distal insertions on the humerus: • subscapularis • latissimus dorsi • teres major • deltoid	

- Subclavius.
- Intercostal muscles.
- Serratus anterior.
- Distal insertions on the humerus:
  - Subscapularis
  - Latissimus dorsi
  - Teres major
  - Deltoid.

Metabolization Technique (MeT)

- Posterior area of the deltoid between the humerus and the glenoid fossa.

Visual Presentation of the Treatment Unit

Recommended treatment protocol: dorsal structures

Rehydration Technique (ReT)

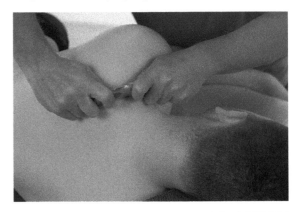

Figure 6.3 Nuchal fascia

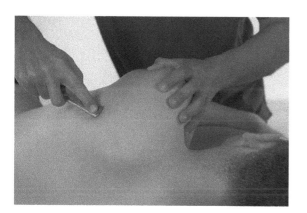

Figure 6.4 Tenoperiosteal junctions around the scapula and at the humerus

Regulation of Tone Technique (RoT)

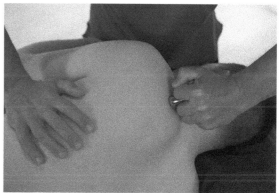

Figure 6.6 Supraspinatus

Pain Relief Technique (PRT)

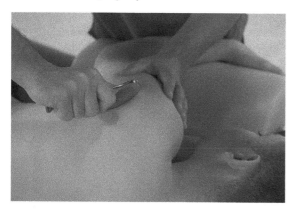

Figure 6.5 Area of the spinal part of deltoid between the humerus and glenoid fossa

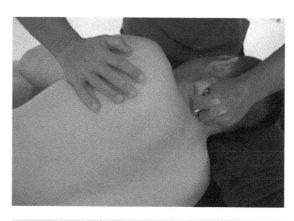

Figure 6.7 Trapezius (descending and transverse parts)

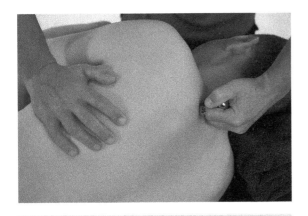

Figure 6.8 Levator scapulae

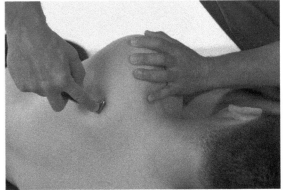

Figure 6.10 Supraspinatus

Mobilization Technique (MoT)

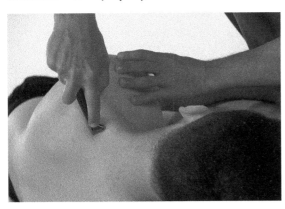

Figure 6.9 Nuchal fascia and brachial fascia

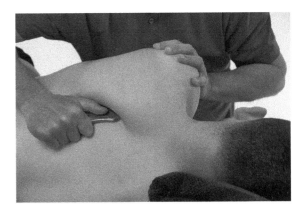

Figure 6.11 Serratus anterior (ventral to the scapula)

Metabolization Technique (MeT)

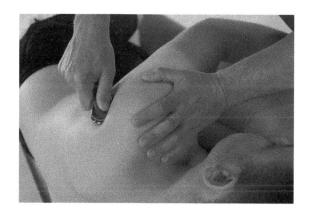

Figure 6.12 Deltoid (convex side of the instrument)

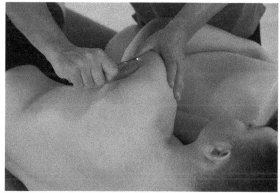

Figure 6.14 Area of the spinal part of deltoid between the humerus and glenoid fossa

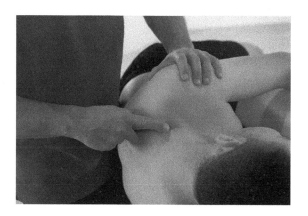

Figure 6.13 Trapezius (hook)

Recommended treatment protocol: ventral structures

Rehydration Technique (ReT)

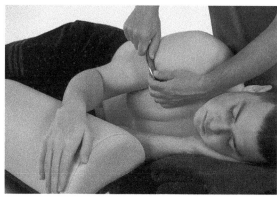

Figure 6.15 Area between the sternoclavicular joint, the deltoid tuberosity, and the head of the humerus

Pain Relief Technique (PRT)

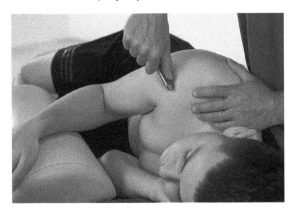

Figure 6.16 Centrally in the deltoid muscle between the acromion and the deltoid tuberosity

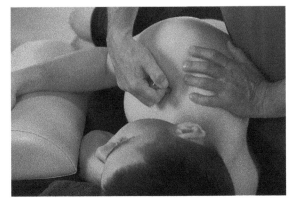

Figure 6.18 Intercostal muscles

Regulation of Tone Technique (RoT)

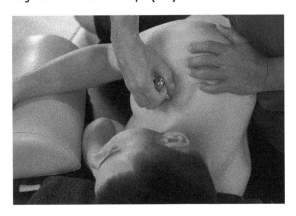

Figure 6.17 Subclavius

Mobilization Technique (MoT)

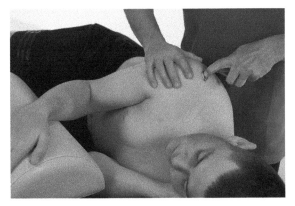

Figure 6.19 Coracoclavicular ligament

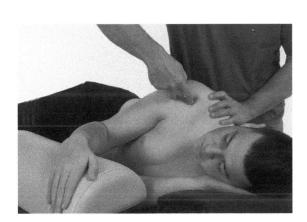

Figure 6.20 Coracoacromial ligament

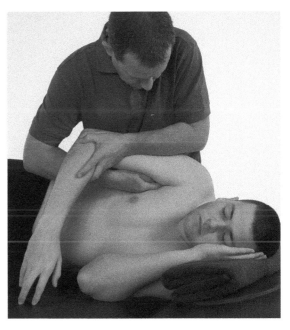

Figure 6.22 Serratus anterior

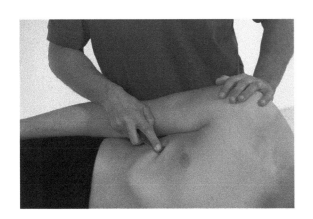

Figure 6.21 Acromioclavicular ligament

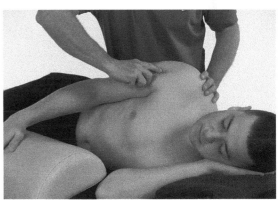

Figure 6.23 Subscapularis (distal insertions on the humerus)

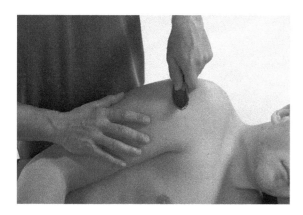

Figure 6.24 Deltoid (distal insertions on the humerus)

Metabolization Technique (MeT)

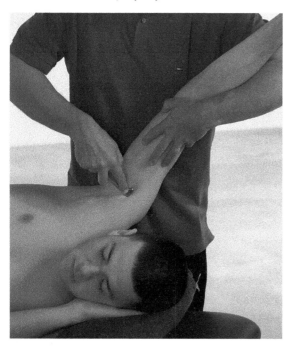

Figure 6.25 Centrally in the deltoid muscle between the acromion and the deltoid tuberosity

Duration

Approximately 20 minutes.

Evaluation

- Numeric rating scale (NRS).
- Provocation tests (Hawkins–Kennedy, Neer, painful arc, empty can, external rotation resistance, cross-body adduction test, drop arm sign).
- ROM glenohumeral joint.
- End-feel flexion, abduction, and external rotation.
- Analysis of standing position with scapula setting.
- Scapula dynamics.

Exercise progression

- Tissue stretch: stretch starting position:
  - Dorsal structures in extension, adduction, and internal rotation
  - Ventral structures in flexion, abduction, and external rotation.
- Tissue dynamics: active movements of the shoulder: flexion–extension and/or abduction–adduction and/or external–internal rotation.

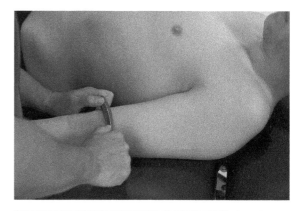

Figure 6.26 Tissue stretch: treatment in stretched position

- Tissue dynamics+: resistive movement against elastic resistance.
- Tissue loading: functionality of the starting position (e.g. sitting or standing).
- Tissue loading+: use of tools, e.g. bands, oscillating bar (FlexBar® or Bioswing®) and so on.

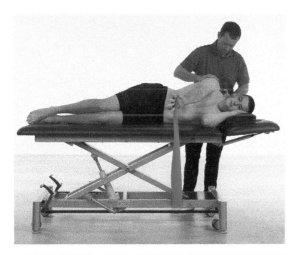

Figure 6.27 Tissue dynamics+: treatment with resistive movement against elastic resistance

Tendinopathy of the Long Biceps Tendon

Detailed Description of the Treatment

Tendinopathy of the long biceps tendon affects the brachial fascia and the biceps brachii muscle (long and short head, as well as the transverse humeral ligament), and the adjacent structures: coracobrachialis, brachialis, pectoralis major and pectoralis minor, and deltoid muscles (clavicular and acromial parts), as well as the antagonist of the biceps brachii muscle: triceps brachii.

For the initial patient position there are several alternatives. The classic one is the supine position, with the arm lying relaxed on a cushion. The shoulder must be turned in maximum internal rotation; if this is not possible, change to the prone lying position for treatment of the triceps muscle. The lateral position and seated position next to the therapy table, with the arm to be treated relaxed on this couch (in the plane of the scapula), are alternatives. Treatment in the supine lying position is described here.

The Rehydration Technique starts with large-area sliding of the ventral area of the whole arm. This is best done with the concave side of the combined curve instrument; the curved instrument is also a possible choice for very large patients. Starting from the caudal location, the technique is performed in a cranial direction up to the humeral head. The pressure is proportional to the thickness of the soft tissue layers; the more tissue under the instrument, the higher the pressure can be. However, uniformity of the pressure is important. It is recommended that the arm is treated in two or three parts, depending on the instrument and the circumference of the arm. Each of these parts is treated several times, and then the painful area of the tendon is treated from the deltoid tuberosity (cranial myotendinous transition), cranially as far as possible. Although the pressure in this area should be low because the tendon runs directly on the bone, it is best to use a relatively short part of the combined curve instrument. The authors recommend that the therapist works with one hand and stabilizes the patient's arm with the other hand. During the treatment, the transverse humeral ligament is rehydrated separately, as this is often the most painful or problematic area. After that, the insertion of the short tendon at the coracoid process and the caudal insertion at the radial tuberosity are addressed, as well as the radiation into the antebrachial fascia; this treatment is best done with the edge of the hook of the combined curve instrument. Finally, the shoulder is turned in internal rotation to treat the dorsal side of the arm in the same way.

After Rehydration, the Pain Relief Technique is usually performed. Of course, it is possible to start with this; however, beginning therapy with the gentle and rather pleasant Rehydration Technique has proven to be very positive in the authors' experience. In order to achieve the greatest pain relief, the painful areas are addressed with a high degree of mechanical stimulation due to the scraping. The pressure is applied in both directions: on the way out and on the way back. If there are several pain points, they are treated one after the other.

The next technique applied is the Regulation of Tone. The application is again dependent on the physiotherapeutic findings. Hypertonic muscles are identified and treated accordingly. In the area of the shoulder, they are usually located in the two heads (long and short) of the biceps brachii muscle, coracobrachialis, brachialis, pectoralis major and pectoralis minor, deltoid (clavicular and acromial parts), and triceps brachii. All the muscles of the shoulder girdle (especially those of the rotator cuff) should be examined for local tightness. Once the therapist has located a hypertonic muscle, they place the short, straight instrument on the point, apply vertical pressure to the tissue, and maintain this pressure until the tone subsides. The therapist will then have the impression that they can penetrate deeper into the tissue. At the new point of tension, the pressure is held again and the therapist waits for a new release. The technique can be completed by small movements of the instrument. In this case, the therapist moves the instrument back and forth on the spot or performs small circular movements. Often, this "melting technique" has an additional relaxing effect and thus increases the overall benefit.

The next technique applied is the Mobilization Technique. The experienced therapist will have no difficulty locating the hypomobile zones. The superficial hypomobilities involve the brachial fascia. They are dealt with according to the protocol previously described: first they are identified by

the displacement test and then treated accordingly. The importance of these superficial hypomobilities is often underestimated but the treatment of these disorders is integral to IAMT. Special attention should be paid to the direction of the limitation. This is not necessarily identical over the entire course of the same structure; moreover, several or even all directions can be affected. The limitation can be determined by a simple test of displaceability using the therapist's hand or the instrument. In the authors' experience, there is seldom a single point; rather, the loss of mobility extends to the entire structure. The characteristics vary from one patient to another.

Depending on the structure, the mobilization is carried out with the hook or the short, flat side of the instrument. It is important that the instrument is always in contact with the same area. The instrument is not pushed over the skin, but the anatomical structure is moved in the restricted direction. The return movement is then done without pressure and is described as returning to the starting position. The caudal insertion at the radial tuberosity (tenoperiosteal junction) is often chosen as an entry point for mobilization. The therapist can work along the biceps with the short side of the combined curve instrument, the advantage being that mobilization can be a little more selective and therefore more precise. At the extremities, the mobilization of muscle septa is of great importance in the view of the authors. In the area of the arm, these are numerous; however, experience suggests that it is worthwhile investing time in mobilization to achieve complete and lasting therapeutic results. The muscular septa between these structures should be mobilized:

- both heads of biceps brachii
- biceps brachii (short head) and coracobrachialis
- biceps brachii and brachialis
- biceps brachii and pectoralis major.

The septa between the adjacent structures should also be mobilized:

- long and lateral heads of triceps brachii
- triceps brachii and teres major, and triceps brachii and teres minor
- triceps brachii and brachialis
- triceps brachii and biceps brachii
- deltoid and triceps brachii
- deltoid and pectoralis major
- pectoralis major and pectoralis minor.

Then, the tendons of the biceps brachii muscle are mobilized from the myotendinous junction to the coracoid process for the short head and as far as possible cranially for the long head. Finally, the insertions of the following muscles at the humerus and the scapula are mobilized: triceps brachii (including anconeus) and pectoralis major and pectoralis minor, as well as latissimus dorsi and teres major. For all these tendons, mobilization

with the hook of the combined curve instrument is an ideal option. It may also be useful to mobilize the muscular septa of adjacent structures:

- long and lateral heads of triceps brachii
- triceps brachii and teres major, and triceps brachii and teres minor
- triceps brachii and brachialis
- triceps brachii and biceps brachii
- deltoid and triceps brachii
- deltoid and pectoralis major
- pectoralis major and minor.

The last technique applied in this standard treatment session is the Metabolization Technique. The therapist scrapes with the instrument over the area to be treated (the myotendinous transition of biceps brachii and the long tendon, as well as the long tendon of biceps brachii) using relatively high pressure that varies according to the volume of the tissue: the greater the volume (that is, the thicker

48 Latissimus dorsi
73 Pectoralis major
74 Pectoralis minor
97 Deltoid (acromial part)
98 Deltoid (clavicular part)
99 Deltoid (spinal part)
102 Teres minor
103 Teres major
108 Biceps brachii
109 Coracobrachialis
110 Brachialis
111 Triceps brachii
112 Anconeus

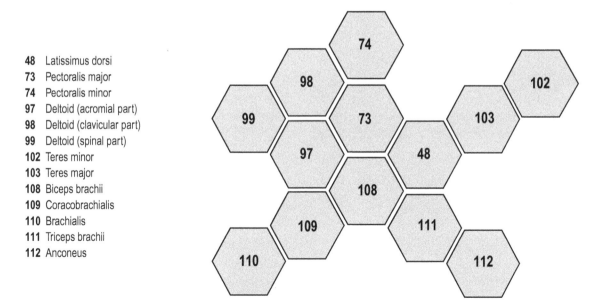

Figure 6.28 Tendinopathy of the long biceps tendon: representation of the MCS

the layer of tissue), the greater the pressure can be. The pressure is applied in one direction only and the speed of execution is also relatively high. The pain already present must not be increased.

Myofascial Connected System (MCS) (Figure 6.28)

Schematic Representation of the Treatment

Diagnosis

Tendinopathy of the long biceps tendon.

Primary structures affected (Figure 6.29)

- Brachial fascia.
- Biceps brachii (long and short heads, transverse humeral ligament).

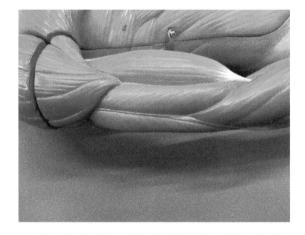

Figure 6.30 Tendinopathy of the long biceps tendon: secondary structures affected

Initial position

Lying supine, arm relaxed on a cushion.

Material

- Recommended: combination curved, straight short instrument.
- Optional: straight elongated instrument, curved instrument.

Technique

- Recommended: Rehydration, Pain Relief, Regulation of Tone, Mobilization, Metabolization.
- Optional: none.

Recommended treatment protocol (Table 6.3)

Rehydration Technique (ReT)

- Brachial fascia: medial, dorsal, and lateral side of the arm (and the forearm).
- Long tendon of biceps brachii.

Pain Relief Technique (PRT)

- Myotendinous transition of biceps brachii and the long tendon.
- Long tendon of biceps brachii.

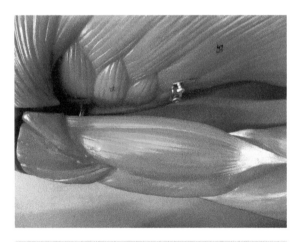

Figure 6.29 Tendinopathy of the long biceps tendon: primary structures affected

Secondary structures frequently affected (Figure 6.30)

- Coracobrachialis.
- Brachialis.
- Pectoralis major and pectoralis minor.
- Deltoid (clavicular and acromial parts).
- Triceps brachii.

Table 6.3 Tendinopathy of the long biceps tendon: summary of recommended treatment protocol

ReT	PRT	RoT	MoT	MeT
Brachial fascia: medial, dorsal, and lateral side of the arm (and forearm)	Painful area	Biceps brachii (long and short heads)	Biceps brachii (tenoperiosteal and myotendinous junctions)	Painful area
Long head of biceps brachii			Long head of biceps brachii	
			Septa between: • both heads of biceps brachii • biceps brachii (short head) and coracobrachialis • biceps brachii and brachialis • biceps brachii and pectoralis major	

Regulation of Tone Technique (RoT)

- Biceps brachii (long and short heads).
- Coracobrachialis.
- Brachialis.
- Pectoralis major and pectoralis minor.
- Deltoid (clavicular and acromial parts).
- Triceps brachii.

Mobilization Technique (MoT)

- Biceps brachii (tenoperiosteal and myotendinous junctions).
- Long head of biceps brachii.
- Muscular septa between:
  - both heads of biceps brachii
  - biceps brachii (short head) and coracobrachialis
  - biceps brachii and brachialis
  - biceps brachii and pectoralis major.

Metabolization Technique (MeT)

- Myotendinous transition of biceps brachii and the long tendon.
- Long tendon of biceps brachii.

Optional treatment protocol (Table 6.4)

Regulation of Tone Technique (RoT)

- Coracobrachialis.
- Brachialis.

Table 6.4 Tendinopathy of the long biceps tendon: summary of optional treatment protocol

RoT	MoT
Coracobrachialis	Coracobrachialis
Brachialis	Brachialis
Pectoralis major and pectoralis minor	Pectoralis major and minor
Deltoid (clavicular and acromial parts)	Deltoid (clavicular and acromial parts)
Triceps brachii	Triceps brachii (including anconeus)
	Latissimus dorsi
	Teres major
	Muscular septa between: • long and lateral heads of triceps brachii • triceps brachii and teres major, and triceps brachii and teres minor • triceps brachii and brachialis • triceps brachii and biceps brachii • deltoid and triceps brachii • deltoid and pectoralis major • pectoralis major and pectoralis minor

- Pectoralis major and pectoralis minor.
- Deltoid (clavicular and acromial parts).
- Triceps brachii.

Mobilization Technique (MoT)

- Insertions of the following muscles at the humerus and the scapula:
    - Coracobrachialis
    - Brachialis
    - Pectoralis major and pectoralis minor
    - Deltoid
    - Triceps brachii (including anconeus)
    - Latissimus dorsi
    - Teres major.
- Muscular septa between:
    - Long and lateral heads of triceps brachii
    - Triceps brachii and teres major, and triceps brachii and teres minor
    - Triceps brachii and brachialis
    - Triceps brachii and biceps brachii

Visual Presentation of the Treatment Unit

Recommended treatment protocol

Rehydration Technique (ReT)

- Deltoid and triceps brachii
- Deltoid and pectoralis major
- Pectoralis major and pectoralis minor.

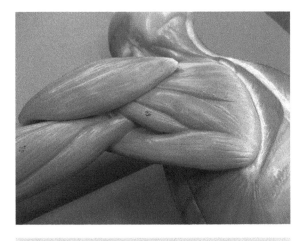

Figure 6.32 Brachial fascia: cranial part

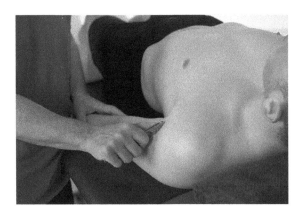

Figure 6.31 Brachial fascia

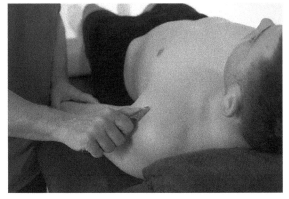

Figure 6.33 Long tendon of biceps brachii

Pain Relief Technique (PRT)

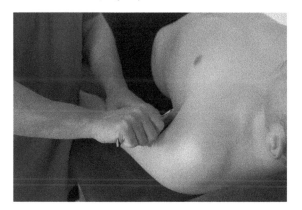

Figure 6.34 Myotendinous transition of biceps brachii and the long tendon

Regulation of Tone Technique (RoT)

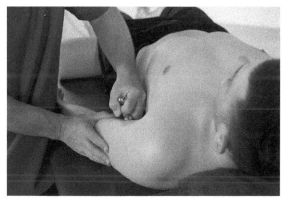

Figure 6.36 Biceps brachii (long head; the short head is not shown)

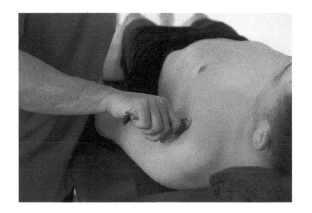

Figure 6.35 Long tendon of biceps brachii

Mobilization Technique (MoT)

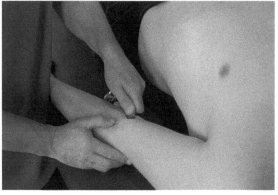

Figure 6.37 Biceps brachii (tenoperiosteal and myotendinous junctions)

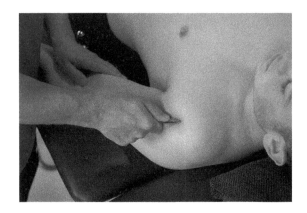

Figure 6.38 Long head of biceps brachii

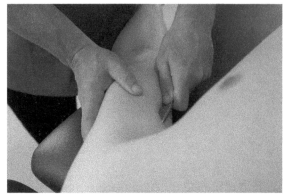

Figure 6.40 Biceps brachii (short head) and coracobrachialis

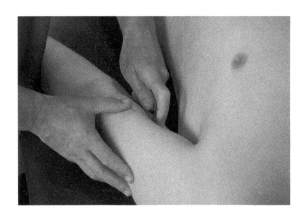

Figure 6.39 Both heads of biceps brachii

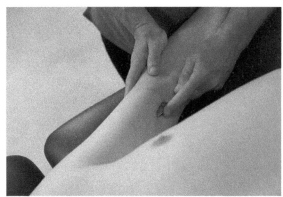

Figure 6.41 Biceps brachii and brachialis

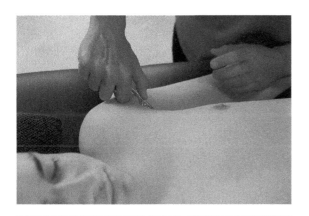

Figure 6.42 Biceps brachii and pectoralis major

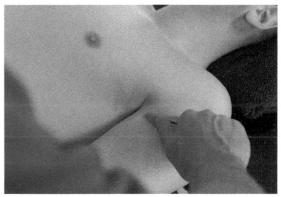

Figure 6.44 Long tendon of biceps brachii

Optional treatment protocol

Metabolization Technique (MeT)

Regulation of Tone Technique (RoT)

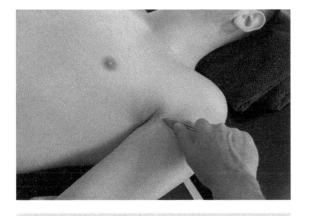

Figure 6.43 Myotendinous transition of biceps brachii and the long tendon

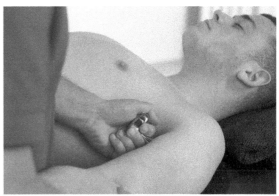

Figure 6.45 Coracobrachialis

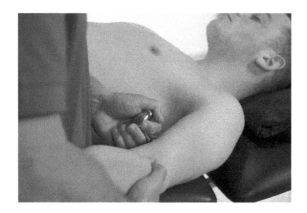

Figure 6.46 Brachialis

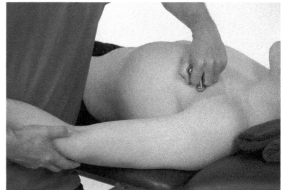

Figure 6.48 Pectoralis minor

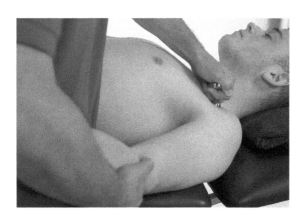

Figure 6.47 Pectoralis major

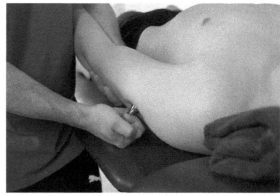

Figure 6.49 Triceps brachii

Mobilization Technique (MoT)

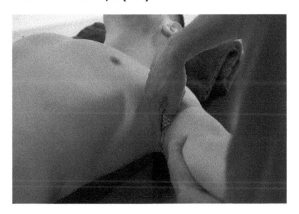

Figure 6.50 Coracobrachialis

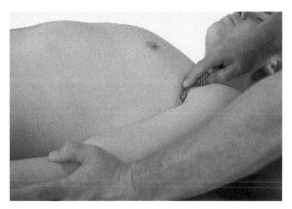

Figure 6.52 Pectoralis major

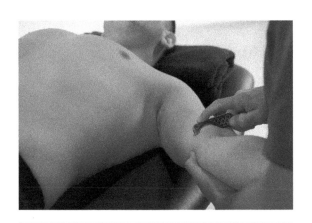

Figure 6.51 Brachialis

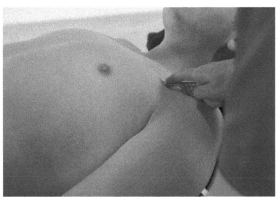

Figure 6.53 Pectoralis minor

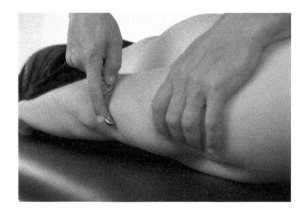

Figure 6.54 Triceps brachii (including anconeus)

Duration

Approximately 20 minutes.

Evaluation

- Numeric rating scale (NRS).
- Provocation tests (e.g. palm-up test, speed test, O'Brian test).
- ROM glenohumeral and elbow joint.
- End-feel shoulder and elbow extension.
- Analysis of standing position with scapula setting and position of the shoulder.
- Scapula dynamics.

Exercise progression

- Tissue stretch: stretch starting position: shoulder (and elbow) extension.

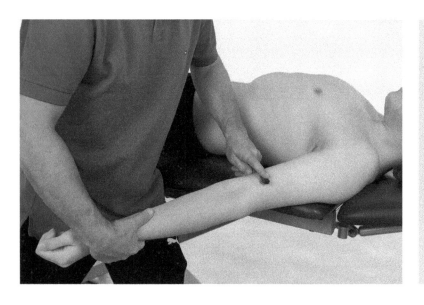

Figure 6.55 Treatment in stretch starting position: shoulder (and elbow) extension

- Tissue dynamics: active movements of the elbow: flexion–extension.

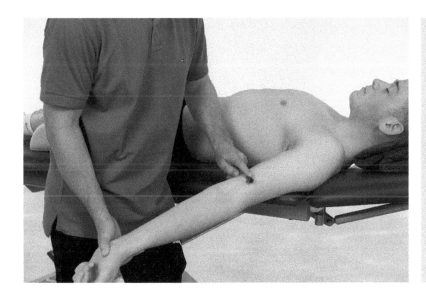

Figure 6.56 Tissue dynamics: extension

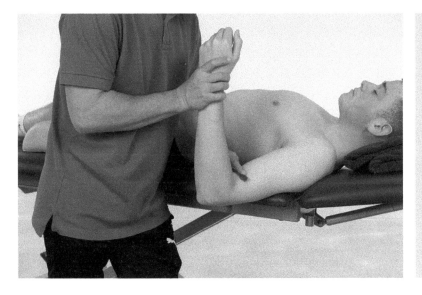

Figure 6.57 Tissue dynamics: flexion

- Tissue dynamics+: resistive movement against elastic resistance.

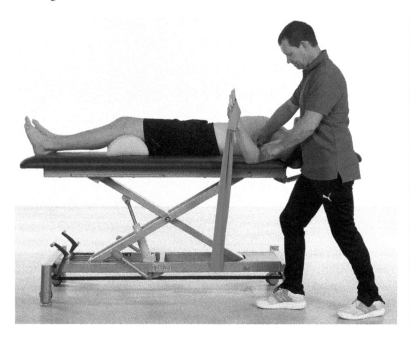

Figure 6.58 Resistive movement against elastic resistance

- Tissue loading: functionality of the starting position: (e.g. sitting or standing).
- Tissue loading+: use of tools, e.g. bands, oscillating bar (FlexBar® or Bioswing) and so on.

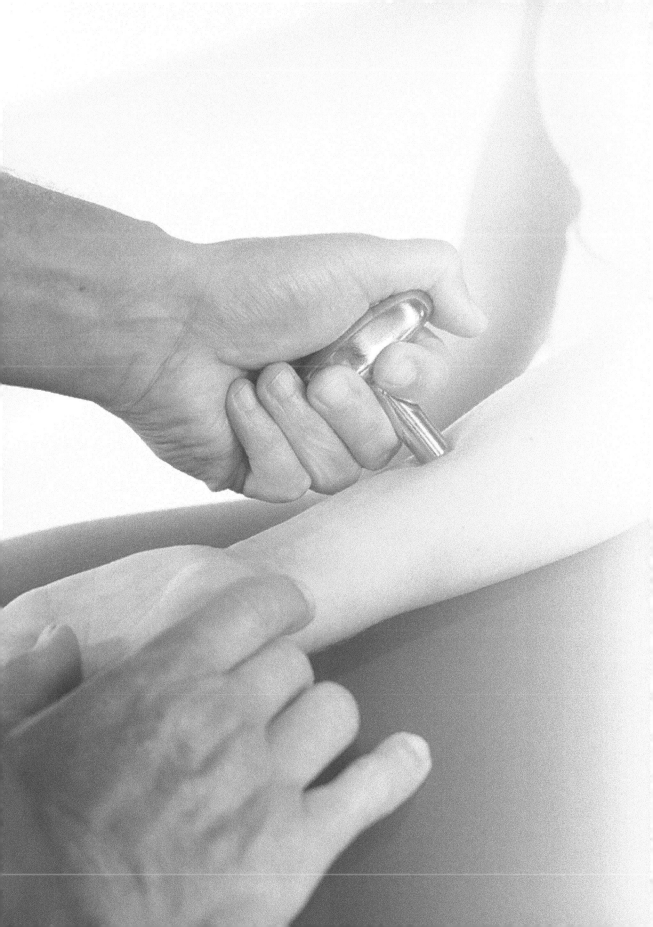

Two frequent and thus practice-relevant diagnoses have been selected for this chapter: epicondylopathy of the lateral humerus (also known as tennis elbow or lateral epicondylitis) and carpal tunnel syndrome (CTS). These diagnoses are representative of the range of musculoskeletal pathology in the elbow and the hand; treatment is adapted according to the symptoms and the potential causes. However, in this chapter, the authors also wanted to present the treatment of another fascial pathology that is representative of similar connective tissue diseases in the whole body: Dupuytren's contracture, also known as Morbus Dupuytren, Dupuytren's disease, Viking disease, or Celtic hand. This will allow description of the treatment of the intrinsic muscles of the hand. Analogous to the foot, this is a key region in the myofascial system and its potential for developing various chronic pain conditions in the upper extremity is correspondingly high.

Epicondylopathy of the Lateral Humerus (Tennis Elbow, Lateral Epicondylitis)

Detailed Description of the Treatment

Epicondylopathy of the lateral humerus involves the muscles that have their origin at the lateral epicondyle: extensor carpi radialis longus and brevis. The other extensors of the wrist (extensor carpi ulnaris, extensor digitorum, extensor digiti minimi, abductor pollicis longus, extensor pollicis longus, extensor pollicis brevis, and extensor indicis) are affected too, along with the adjacent structures of the antebrachial fascia, biceps brachii, supinator, brachioradialis, and the ligaments of the elbow joint (lateral collateral and anular ligaments).

The patient sits next to the therapy table; the entire forearm lies relaxed and pronated and is best supported distally with a cushion. The elbow is slightly bent. The supine or prone positions are alternatives but are rarely used.

The therapy starts with a Rehydration Technique, by performing large-area sliding of the area of the lateral forearm: from the wrist to the elbow joint (humeral lateral epicondyle to supracondylar ridge). This is best done with the convex side of a curved instrument. In rare cases, a longer curved instrument is used for very bulky forearms. The pressure is proportional to the actual thickness of the soft tissue layers. The more tissue under the instrument, the higher the pressure can be, although uniformity of the pressure is important. The technique is repeated several times, then the painful area at the lateral epicondyle is treated, from the myotendinous transition cranially to the origin of the wrist extensors. These origins are not only at the lateral epicondyle; they are broad and ascend following the humeral supracondylar ridge. It is best to use a relatively short part of an instrument for treatment: the edge of the hook is well designed for this task. Although the application pressure in this area should be low because the tenoperiosteal junction is located directly on the bone, it is advisable for the therapist to work with one hand and stabilize the patient's forearm with the other hand.

After the Rehydration Technique, the Pain Relief Technique is usually performed. It is also possible to start with this; however, beginning therapy with the gentle and rather pleasant Rehydration Technique has been used successfully by the authors. The technique is, naturally, limited to the painful area(s). Experience has shown that the most common areas are the tenoperiosteal transition and the myotendinous transition; the treatment can begin at either point. In order to achieve the greatest pain relief, the painful areas are provided with a high degree of mechanical stimulation through scraping. The technique is performed directly over the painful areas with a progressive pressure that should not increase the pain already present. This pressure is applied in both directions: away from the treated area and then on the return. If there are several pain points, they are treated one after the other.

The next technique applied is the Regulation of Tone. Application is again dependent on the physiotherapeutic findings. The hypertonic muscles are identified and immediately treated accordingly. In the area of the elbow, they are usually located in the extensor carpi radialis longus and brevis muscles, more rarely in extensor carpi ulnaris. Nevertheless, all the wrist and finger extensors (including abductor pollicis longus, supinator, brachioradialis and biceps brachii) should be examined for local hypertonicity. Once the therapist has located a hypertonic area, they place a short elongated instrument on the point, apply vertical pressure to the tissue, and maintain this pressure until the tone subsides. The therapist then has the impression that they can penetrate deeper into the tissue. At the new point of tension, the pressure is held again, and the therapist waits for a new release. The technique can be completed by small movements of the instrument. In this case, the therapist moves the instrument back and forth on the spot or performs small circular movements. Often, this "melting technique" brings an additional relaxing effect and thus increases the overall benefit.

The next technique applied is the Mobilization Technique. The experienced therapist will have no difficulty locating the hypomobile tissues of the lateral elbow. The superficial hypomobilities involve the antebrachial fascia and the bicipital aponeurosis. They are treated according to the standard protocol: first identified by the displacement test, then treated accordingly. The importance of these superficial hypomobilities is often underestimated in the opinion of the authors, as their treatment is integral to IAMT.

Special attention should be paid to the direction of the tissue mobility limitation. This is not necessarily identical over the entire course of the same structure; moreover, several or even all directions can be affected. The limitation can be determined by a simple test of displaceability using the therapist's hand or the instrument. In our experience, there is seldom a single point, but the loss of mobility usually extends to the entire structure. These characteristics vary between patients. Depending on the structure, the mobilization is carried out with the hook or the short, flat side of the instrument. It is important that the instrument always remains in contact with the same area. The instrument is not pushed over the skin, but the anatomical structure is moved in the restricted direction. The return movement is then done without pressure and is described as returning to the starting position.

The tenoperiosteal junction at the humerus is often chosen as an entry point for mobilization. Here the therapist mobilizes the tenoperiosteal junction with the edge of an instrument, while the tendon and the muscle are more easily mobilized with the edge of the same instrument; the advantage is that you can mobilize a little more selectively and therefore more precisely. The therapist then works along extensor carpi radialis longus and brevis from hypomobility to hypomobility further caudally. In addition to these muscles, the following muscular septa are also affected:

- between extensor carpi radialis longus and brevis
- between extensor carpi radialis brevis and extensor digitorum
- between extensor digitorum and extensor carpi ulnaris.

The last technique applied in this standard treatment session is the Metabolization Technique. The therapist scrapes with the instrument over the area to be treated. The pressure is relatively high but varies according to the volume of the tissue: the greater the volume (that is, the thicker the layer of tissue), the greater the pressure can be. The pressure is applied in one direction only and the speed of execution is also relatively high. The pain already present must not be increased.

An additional Pain Relief Technique may be performed directly over the painful areas or at a short distance from them. The most common areas treated are the tenoperiosteal transition and the myotendinous transition, which are worked on consecutively. The authors recommend ending the treatment with the most painful point.

In addition to the "standard treatment" described above, other procedures can be of benefit. Because of the holistic nature of the myofascial system, such treatment is recommended, particularly when the symptoms have been present for a long period of time. In chronic myofascial pain, the lesion becomes more involved and affects additional structures. In the case of tennis elbow, several structures often have localized hypertonicity that should be treated as described above. These structures are involved because of their anatomical proximity and their functional interaction within the execution of movement. The Regulation of Tone Technique may be effective on the following structures: brachioradialis, biceps brachii, extensor digitorum, extensor digiti minimi, abductor pollicis longus, extensor pollicis longus, extensor pollicis brevis, extensor indicis, and supinator. The tendons of all these muscles should be mobilized if necessary. Furthermore, the lateral collateral and anular ligaments should be rehydrated and mobilized.

Myofascial Connected System (MCS) (Figure 7.1)

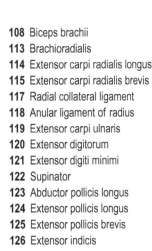

108 Biceps brachii
113 Brachioradialis
114 Extensor carpi radialis longus
115 Extensor carpi radialis brevis
117 Radial collateral ligament
118 Anular ligament of radius
119 Extensor carpi ulnaris
120 Extensor digitorum
121 Extensor digiti minimi
122 Supinator
123 Abductor pollicis longus
124 Extensor pollicis longus
125 Extensor pollicis brevis
126 Extensor indicis

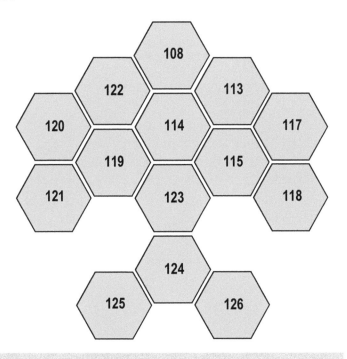

Figure 7.1 Epicondylopathy of the lateral humerus: representation of the MCS

Schematic Representation of the Treatment

Diagnosis

Epicondylopathy of the lateral humerus (tennis elbow, lateral epicondylitis).

Primary structure affected (Figure 7.2)

Extensor carpi radialis longus and brevis.

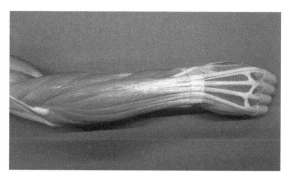

Figure 7.3 Epicondylopathy of the lateral humerus: secondary structures affected

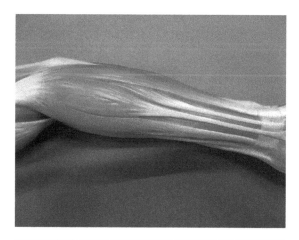

Figure 7.2 Epicondylopathy of the lateral humerus: primary structures affected

Secondary structures frequently affected (Figure 7.3)

- Antebrachial fascia.
- Extensor carpi ulnaris.
- Extensor digitorum.
- Extensor digiti minimi.
- Abductor pollicis longus.
- Extensor pollicis longus.
- Extensor pollicis brevis.
- Extensor indicis.
- Biceps brachii.
- Supinator.
- Brachioradialis.
- Lateral collateral ligament and anular ligament.

Initial position

The patient sits next to the therapy table; the forearm lies relaxed and pronated (supported distally with a cushion); the elbow is slightly bent.

Material

- Recommended: combination curved, straight short instrument.
- Optional: straight elongated instrument, curved instrument.

Technique

- Recommended: Rehydration, Pain Relief, Regulation of Tone, Mobilization, Metabolization.
- Optional: none.

Recommended treatment protocol (Table 7.1)

Rehydration Technique (ReT)

- Antebrachial fascia: lateral side of the forearm.
- Extensor carpi radialis longus and brevis: from the myotendinous transition cranially to the insertions.

Pain Relief Technique (PRT)

- Extensor carpi radialis longus and brevis: tenoperiosteal transition and myotendinous transition.

Table 7.1 Epicondylopathy of the lateral humerus: summary of recommended treatment protocol					
ReT	**PRT**	**RoT**	**MoT**		**MeT**
Antebrachial fascia	Painful area	Extensor carpi radialis longus	Antebrachial fascia		Painful area
Extensor carpi radialis longus and brevis		Extensor carpi radialis brevis	Extensor carpi radialis longus		
			Extensor carpi radialis brevis		
			Septa between: • extensor carpi radialis longus and brevis • extensor carpi radialis brevis and extensor digitorum • extensor digitorum and extensor carpi ulnaris		

Regulation of Tone Technique (RoT)

- Extensor carpi radialis longus.
- Extensor carpi radialis brevis.

Mobilization Technique (MoT)

- Antebrachial fascia and bicipital aponeurosis.
- Extensor carpi radialis longus.
- Extensor carpi radialis brevis.
- Muscular septa between:
  - extensor carpi radialis longus and brevis
  - extensor carpi radialis brevis and extensor digitorum
  - extensor digitorum and extensor carpi ulnaris.

Metabolization Technique (MeT)

- Extensor carpi radialis longus and brevis: myotendinous transition.

Optional treatment protocol (Table 7.2)

Regulation of Tone Technique (RoT)

- Extensor carpi ulnaris.
- Extensor digitorum.
- Extensor digiti minimi.
- Abductor pollicis longus.

Table 7.2 Epicondylopathy of the lateral humerus: summary of optional treatment protocol	
RoT	**MoT**
Extensor carpi ulnaris	Extensor carpi ulnaris
Extensor digitorum	Extensor digitorum
Extensor digiti minimi	Extensor digiti minimi
Abductor pollicis longus	Abductor pollicis longus
Extensor pollicis longus	Extensor pollicis longus
Extensor pollicis brevis	Extensor pollicis brevis
Extensor indicis	Extensor indicis
Biceps brachii	Biceps brachii
Supinator	Supinator
Brachioradialis	Brachioradialis
	Lateral collateral ligament
	Anular ligament

- Extensor pollicis longus.
- Extensor pollicis brevis.
- Extensor indicis.
- Biceps brachii.
- Supinator.
- Brachioradialis.

Mobilization Technique (MoT)

- Extensor carpi ulnaris.
- Extensor digitorum.
- Extensor digiti minimi.
- Abductor pollicis longus.
- Extensor pollicis longus.
- Extensor pollicis brevis.
- Extensor indicis.
- Biceps brachii.
- Supinator.
- Brachioradialis.
- Lateral collateral ligament.
- Annular ligament.

Visual Presentation of the Treatment Unit

Recommended treatment protocol

Rehydration Technique (ReT)

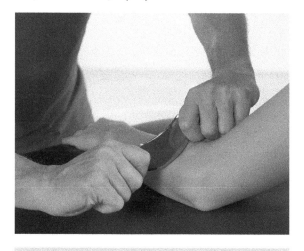

Figure 7.4 Antebrachial fascia: lateral side of the forearm

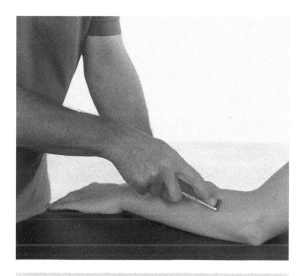

Figure 7.5 Extensor carpi radialis longus and brevis: from the myotendinous transition cranially to the insertions

Pain Relief Technique (PRT)

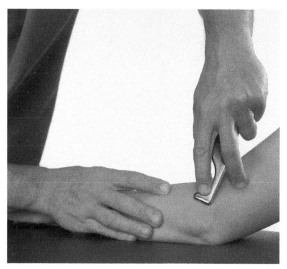

Figure 7.6 Extensor carpi radialis longus and brevis: tenoperiosteal transition

Regulation of Tone Technique (RoT)

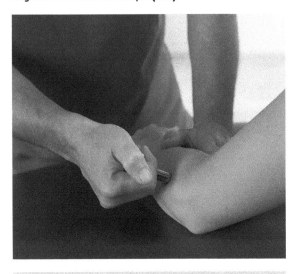

Figure 7.7 Extensor carpi radialis longus

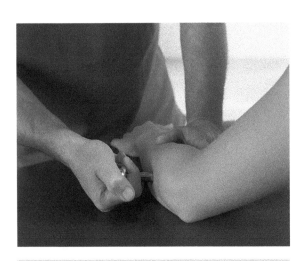

Figure 7.8 Extensor carpi radialis brevis

Mobilization Technique (MoT)

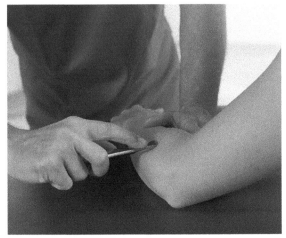

Figure 7.9 Antebrachial fascia

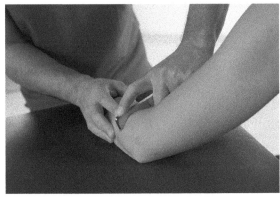

Figure 7.10 Extensor carpi radialis longus

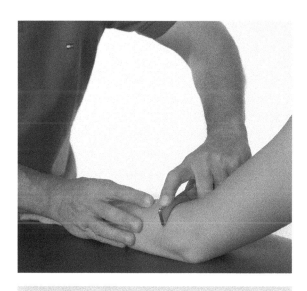

Figure 7.11 Extensor carpi radialis brevis

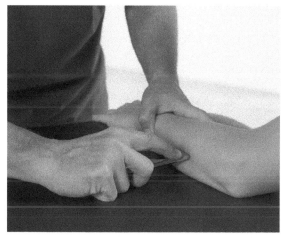

Figure 7.13 Septum between extensor carpi radialis brevis and extensor digitorum

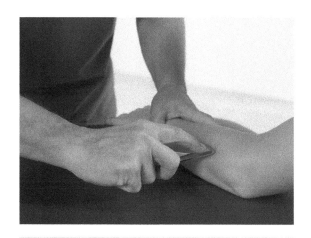

Figure 7.12 Septum between extensor carpi radialis longus and brevis

Metabolization Technique (MeT)

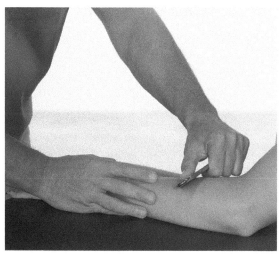

Figure 7.14 Extensor carpi radialis longus and brevis: myotendinous transition

Optional treatment protocol

Regulation of Tone Technique (RoT)

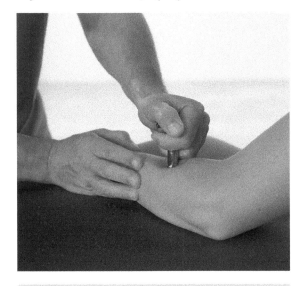

Figure 7.15 Extensor digitorum

Mobilization Technique (MoT)

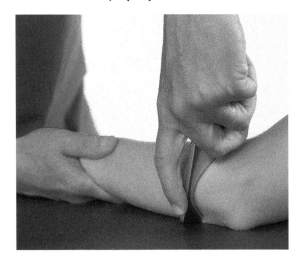

Figure 7.16 Extensor carpi ulnaris

Duration

Approximately 20 minutes.

Evaluation

- Numeric rating scale (NRS).
- Provocation tests (Cozen's test – also called Thompson test; reverse Cozen's test – also called Mill's test, chair-lift test).
- ROM wrist.
- End-feel wrist flexion.

Progression

- Tissue stretch: stretch starting position in wrist flexion.
- Tissue dynamics: active movements of the wrist (flexion–extension, radial–ulnar abduction).
- Tissue dynamics+: resistive movement against elastic resistance.
- Tissue loading+: use of tools, such as PC or smartphone.

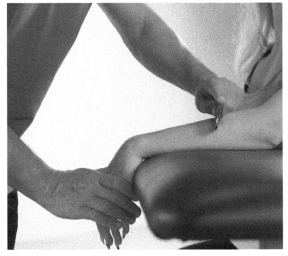

Figure 7.17 Treatment in stretched starting position (wrist flexion)

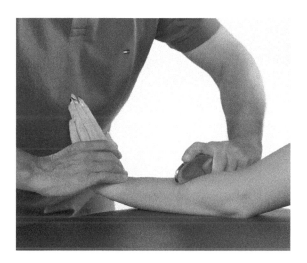

Figure 7.18 Tissue dynamics: active movements of the wrist (flexion–extension, radial–ulnar abduction)

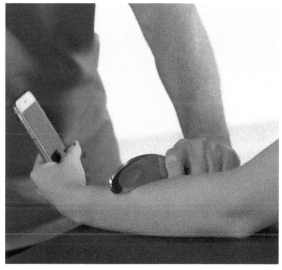

Figure 7.20 Tissue loading+: use of smartphone

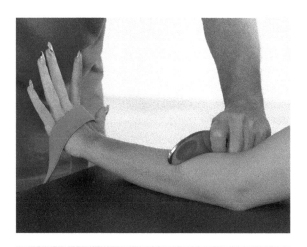

Figure 7.19 Tissue dynamics+: resistive movement against elastic resistance

Epicondylopathy of the medial humerus

For epicondylopathy of the medial humerus (also called "golfer's elbow"), the treatment is analogous to that of lateral epicondylopathy; the structures affected in this case are:

- Antebrachial fascia.
- Pronator teres.
- Flexor digitorum superficialis.
- Flexor carpi radialis.
- Palmaris longus.
- Flexor carpi ulnaris and the adjacent structures flexor digitorum profundus, flexor pollicis longus, and pronator quadratus.
- Ulnar collateral ligament.

Carpal Tunnel Syndrome

Detailed Description of the Treatment

Carpal tunnel syndrome (CTS) is a compression of the median nerve under the palmar flexor retinaculum. The primary symptoms are neurologic in nature: sensory and motor disturbances. Pain is rather rare. The treatment presented in this chapter assumes that CTS is caused by thickening of the flexor tendons due to overuse; the therapeutic goal is to reduce this pressure. We accordingly describe the goals of rehydration, tone regulation, and mobilization. Myofascial treatment alone is rarely sufficient. Other therapy options should be considered: nerve mobilizations and muscle stretching, among others.

The primary structure affected is the median nerve. The assumed cause is inflammation of the tendons of the flexor digitorum superficialis and profundus muscles, as well as the tendon of flexor pollicis longus in its passage under the flexor retinaculum. Adjacent structures that are often affected are the flexors of the wrist and the fingers (palmaris longus, flexor carpi radialis, and flexor carpi ulnaris, as well as the ulnar collateral ligament at its cranial insertions), the pronators (pronator teres and pronator quadratus), and the antebrachial fascia and palmar aponeurosis.

The patient sits next to the therapy table; the entire forearm lies relaxed and supinated, and is best supported distally with a cushion. The elbow is slightly bent.

The therapy starts with the Rehydration Technique using large-area sliding of the area of the lateral forearm (from the wrist to the elbow joint – medial epicondyle) and the hand. This is best done with the convex side of an instrument. The pressure is proportional to the thickness of the soft tissue layers. The more tissue under the instrument, the higher the pressure can be; however, uniformity of the pressure is important. The technique can be repeated several times. Next, the flexor retinaculum is treated in a transverse direction on the palmar surface. It is best to use a relatively short part of the instrument for treatment of the retinaculum: the edge of the hook is well designed for this. Although the pressure applied in the area is

low, the therapist should work with one hand and stabilize the patient's hand and forearm with the other hand.

The next technique applied is the Regulation of Tone. Application is again dependent on the physiotherapeutic findings. The hypertonic muscles are identified and immediately treated accordingly. In the area of the elbow, they are usually located in the flexor digitorum superficialis and profundus muscles, as well as in flexor pollicis longus. Nevertheless, all the wrist and finger flexors should be examined for local tightness. Once the therapist has located a hypertonic point, they place the rounded end of the short instrument on the point, apply vertical pressure to the tissue, and maintain this pressure until the tone subsides. The therapist may then feel they can penetrate deeper into the tissue. At the new point of tension, the pressure is held again and the therapist waits for a new release. The technique can be completed by small movements of the instrument. In this case, the therapist moves the instrument back and forth on the spot or performs small circular movements. Often, this "melting technique" brings an additional relaxing effect and thus increases the overall benefit.

The last technique applied is the Mobilization Technique. The experienced therapist will have no difficulty locating the hypomobile zones of the lateral elbow. The superficial hypomobilities involve the antebrachial fascia and the palmaris longus muscle. They are treated according to the standard protocol: first sensed by the displacement test, then treated accordingly. The importance of these superficial hypomobilities is often underestimated, in the authors' opinion, as their treatment is integral to IAMT.

Special attention should be paid to the direction of the limitation. This is not necessarily identical over the entire course of the same structure; moreover, several or even all directions can be affected. The limitation can be determined by a simple test of displaceability using the therapist's hand or the instrument. In the authors' experience, there is seldom a single point, but the loss of mobility usually extends to the entire structure. The characteristics can vary from one patient to another. Depending on the structure, mobilization is carried out with the hook or the short, flat side of the instrument. It is important that the instrument always remains in contact with the same area. The instrument is not pushed over the skin but the anatomical structure is moved in the restricted direction. The return movement is then done without pressure and is described as returning to the starting position. The flexor retinaculum is often chosen as an entry point for mobilization. Here, the therapist mobilizes the tendons with the edge of an instrument, the advantage being that one can mobilize a little more selectively and therefore more precisely.

The therapist then works along the flexors from hypomobility to hypomobility, further cranially in direction of the elbow. Then, the retinaculum is again chosen as the starting point for mobilization of the four tendons of the finger flexors.

In addition to the "standard treatment" described above, various procedures can be beneficial. Because of the holistic nature of the myofascial system, other structures should be assessed and treated because of their anatomical proximity and their functional interaction within the execution of movement. In the case of CTS, other localized hypertonic structures should be treated with Regulation of Tone, as described above. These structures include palmaris longus, flexor carpi radialis, and flexor carpi ulnaris, as well as pronator teres and pronator quadratus. The tendons of all these muscles (except the pronators) should be mobilized if necessary. Furthermore, the following

116 Ulnar collateral ligament
127 Palmaris longus
128 Flexor digitorum superficialis
129 Flexor digitorum profundus
130 Flexor carpi radialis
131 Flexor carpi ulnaris
132 Flexor pollicis longus
133 Pronator teres
134 Pronator quadratus
135 Palmar aponeurosis
136 Flexor retinaculum

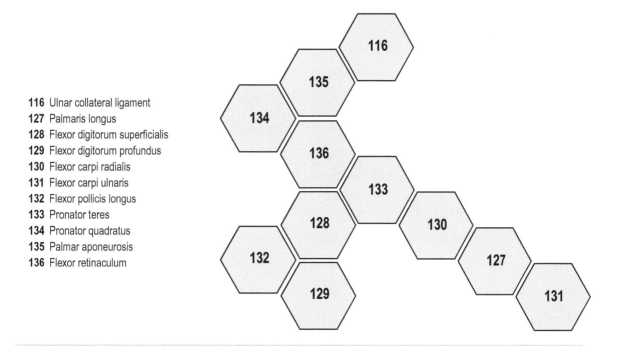

Figure 7.21 Carpal tunnel syndrome: representation of the MCS

fascial structures should be rehydrated and mobilized: the ulnar collateral ligament and palmar aponeurosis.

Myofascial Connected System (MCS) (Figure 7.21)

Schematic Representation of the Treatment

Diagnosis

Carpal tunnel syndrome (CTS).

Primary structures affected (Figure 7.22)

- Median nerve.
- Flexor digitorum superficialis and profundus.
- Flexor pollicis longus.

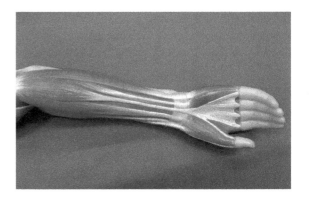

Figure 7.23 Carpal tunnel syndrome: secondary structures frequently affected – forearm and hand (anterior view)

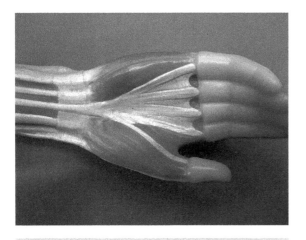

Figure 7.22 Carpal tunnel syndrome: primary structures affected

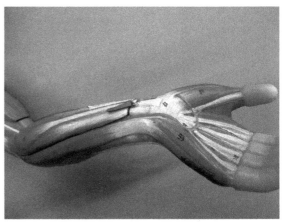

Figure 7.24 Carpal tunnel syndrome: secondary structures frequently affected – wrist and hand (palmar view)

Secondary structures frequently affected (Figures 7.23 and 7.24)

- Antebrachial fascia.
- Palmaris longus.
- Flexor carpi radialis.
- Flexor carpi ulnaris.
- Ulnar collateral ligament.
- Pronator teres.
- Pronator quadratus.
- Palmar aponeurosis.

Initial position

The patient sits next to the therapy table; the forearm lies relaxed and supinated (supported distally with a cushion); the elbow is slightly bent.

Material

- Recommended: combination curved, straight short instrument.
- Optional: straight elongated instrument, curved instrument.

Technique

- Recommended: Rehydration, Regulation of Tone, Mobilization.
- Optional: none.

Recommended treatment protocol (Table 7.3)

Rehydration Technique (ReT)

- Antebrachial fascia.

- Palmar aponeurosis.
- Flexor retinaculum.

Regulation of Tone Technique (RoT)

- Flexor digitorum superficialis.
- Flexor digitorum profundus.
- Flexor pollicis longus.

Mobilization Technique (MoT)

- Antebrachial fascia.
- Flexor digitorum superficialis.
- Flexor digitorum profundus.
- Flexor pollicis longus.
- Palmar aponeurosis.

Table 7.3 Carpal tunnel syndrome: summary of recommended treatment protocol				
ReT	**PRT**	**RoT**	**MoT**	**MeT**
Antebrachial fascia		Flexor digitorum superficialis	Antebrachial fascia	
Palmar aponeurosis		Flexor digitorum profundus	Flexor digitorum superficialis	
Flexor retinaculum		Flexor pollicis longus	Flexor digitorum profundus	
			Flexor pollicis longus	
			Palmar aponeurosis	

Table 7.4 Carpal tunnel syndrome: summary of optional treatment protocol	
RoT	**MoT**
Palmaris longus	Palmaris longus
Flexor carpi radialis	Flexor carpi radialis
Flexor carpi ulnaris	Flexor carpi ulnaris
Pronator teres	Ulnar collateral ligament
Pronator quadratus	Palmar aponeurosis

Optional treatment protocol (Table 7.4)

Regulation of Tone Technique (RoT)

- Palmaris longus.
- Flexor carpi radialis.
- Flexor carpi ulnaris.
- Pronator teres.
- Pronator quadratus.

Mobilization Technique (MoT)

- Palmaris longus.
- Flexor carpi radialis.

- Flexor carpi ulnaris.
- Ulnar collateral ligament.
- Palmar aponeurosis.

Visual Presentation of the Treatment Unit

Recommended treatment protocol

Rehydration Technique (ReT)

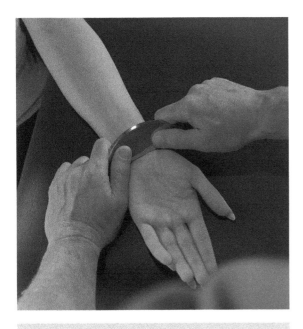

Figure 7.25 Flexor retinaculum

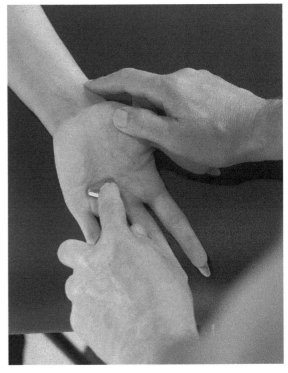

Figure 7.26 Palmar aponeurosis

Regulation of Tone Technique (RoT)

Mobilization Technique (MoT)

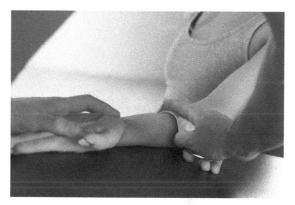

Figure 7.29 Flexor digitorum superficialis

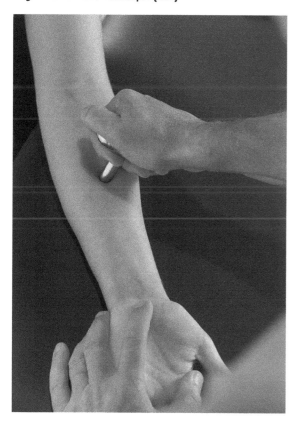

Figure 7.27 Flexor digitorum superficialis

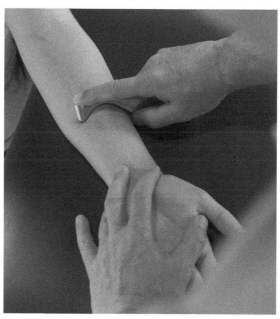

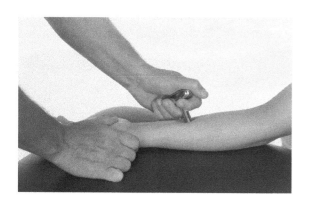

Figure 7.28 Flexor digitorum profundus

Figure 7.30 Flexor digitorum profundus

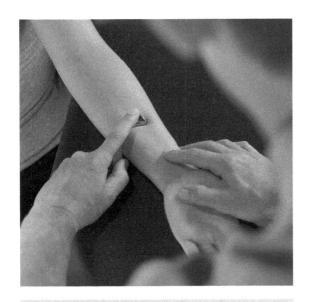

Figure 7.31 Flexor pollicis longus

Optional treatment protocol

Regulation of Tone Technique (RoT)

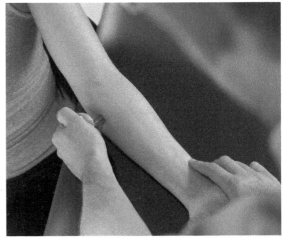

Figure 7.33 Flexor carpi ulnaris

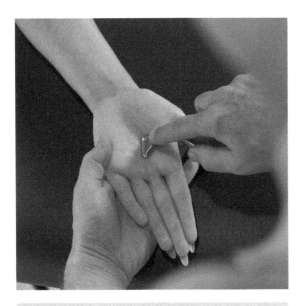

Figure 7.32 Palmar aponeurosis

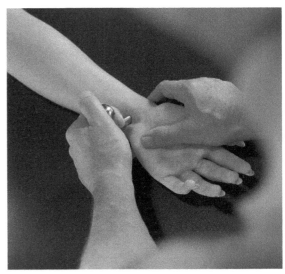

Figure 7.34 Pronator quadratus

Mobilization Technique (MoT)

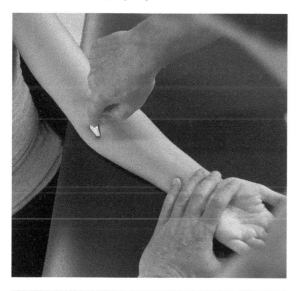

Figure 7.35 Palmaris longus

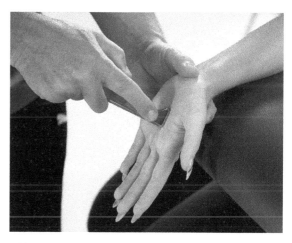

Figure 7.36 Treatment in stretched position (wrist extension)

Duration

Approximately 15 minutes.

Evaluation

- Numeric rating scale (NRS).
- Provocation tests (carpal compression test, Phalen's test, reverse Phalen's, Hoffmann–Tinel test).
- ROM wrist.
- End-feel wrist extension.

Exercise Progression

- Tissue stretch: stretch starting position in wrist extension.
- Tissue dynamics: active movements of the wrist (flexion–extension).
- Tissue dynamics+: resistive movement against elastic resistance.
- Tissue loading+: use of tools, such as PC, smartphone.

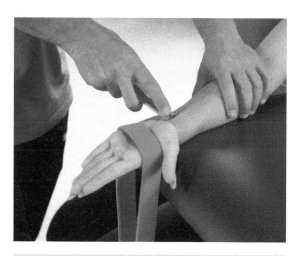

Figure 7.37 Resistive movement against elastic resistance

Dupuytren's Contracture

Detailed Description of the Treatment

Dupuytren's contracture (also known as Morbus Dupuytren, Dupuytren's disease, Viking disease, and Celtic hand) results from a formation of abnormal fascial tissue in the palmar aponeurosis. The authors believe that conservative treatment, including IAMT, is a worthwhile therapy, at least in the early stages of the condition. The leading symptoms are contractures and finger malposition with movement restrictions and loss of function. Pain is rather rare. The IAMT treatment is applied for the goals of rehydration, tone regulation, and mobilization.

The treatment presented here can also be applied pre-operatively or post-operatively, taking into account the wound-healing phases and the surgeon's instructions. The therapeutic goal is to stop or even improve the loss of function. The cosmetic aspect should also be improved with treatment. However, this myofascial treatment alone is rarely sufficient. Other therapy options should be considered, such as manual therapy and muscle stretching.

The primary structure affected is the palmar aponeurosis. The cause of loss of function and of the malposition in finger flexion (especially digits 4 and 5) is contracture of the aponeurosis and the closely related flexor tendons (flexor digitorum superficialis and profundus, but also palmaris longus and brevis). The IAMT therapy starts at both structures. The adjacent structures that are often affected can be divided into two groups: extrinsic hand muscles (flexor carpi radialis, flexor carpi ulnaris, pronator teres, pronator quadratus, including the antebrachial fascia) and intrinsic hand muscles. While the treatment of the extrinsic muscles has already been described, the treatment of the intrinsic muscles will be presented in detail here. These are the muscles of the thenar eminence (abductor pollicis brevis, flexor pollicis brevis, adductor pollicis brevis, and opponens

pollicis), the muscles of the hypothenar eminence (abductor digiti minimi, flexor digiti minimi, and opponens digiti minimi), and the muscles of the metacarpals (palmar interossei, dorsal interossei, and lumbricals).

The patient sits next to the therapy table; the entire forearm lies relaxed and supinated, and is best supported distally with a cushion. The elbow is slightly bent.

The therapy starts with a Rehydration Technique using small-area sliding of the palmar side of the hand (from the wrist to the fingers; with the edge of the hook of an instrument) and larger-area sliding of the anterior part of the forearm (from the wrist to the elbow; with the concave side of an instrument). The pressure is proportional to the thickness of the soft tissue layers. The more tissue under the instrument, the higher the pressure can be; however, uniformity of the pressure is important. The technique is repeated several times. Next, the triangular area between the flexor retinaculum and the metacarpophalangeal (MCP) joints is treated. This is also done with the edge of the pick (tip) of an instrument. The longitudinal fibers of the palmar aponeurosis at the level of these joints are treated particularly intensively, as are the interphalangeal ligaments and the tendons between these joints. Although the pressure in the area is low, the therapist should work with one hand and stabilize the patient's hand and forearm with the other hand.

The next technique applied is the Regulation of Tone. Application is again dependent on the physiotherapeutic findings. The hypertonic muscles are identified and treated accordingly. In the area of the hand, they are usually located in the thenar eminence (abductor pollicis brevis, flexor pollicis brevis, adductor pollicis brevis, and opponens pollicis) and the muscles of the hypothenar eminence (abductor digiti minimi, flexor digiti minimi, and opponens digiti minimi). Tightness can also be noted in the muscles of the metacarpals (palmar interossei, lumbrical muscles, and dorsal interossei), although this is rarer and less pronounced. Differentiation of the individual muscles in the palm is difficult; nevertheless, the extrinsic muscles of the hand (see above) should be examined for local hypertonicity. Once the therapist has located a hypertonic point, they place the instrument (straight short device) on the point, apply vertical pressure to the tissue, and maintain this pressure until the tone subsides. The therapist may then feel they can penetrate deeper into the tissue. At the new point of tension, the pressure is again held and the therapist waits for a new release. The technique can be completed by small movements of the instrument. In this case, the therapist moves the instrument back and forth on the spot or performs small circular movements. Often, this "melting technique" brings an additional relaxing effect and thus increases the overall benefit.

The last technique applied is the Mobilization Technique. The experienced therapist will have no difficulty locating the hypomobile zones of the hand. The superficial hypomobilities involve the palmar aponeurosis and the palmaris longus muscle. They are treated following the protocol previously described: first sensed by the displacement test, then treated accordingly. The importance of these superficial hypomobilities is often underestimated, in the authors' opinion, as their treatment is integral to IAMT.

Special attention should be paid to the direction of the limitation. This is not necessarily identical over the entire course of the same structure; moreover, several or even all directions can be affected. The limitation can be determined by a simple test of displaceability using the therapist's hand or the instrument. In the authors' experience, there is seldom a single point, but the loss of mobility usually extends to the entire structure. The characteristics vary, of course, from one patient to another. Depending on the structure, mobilization is carried out with the hook or the short, flat side of the instrument. It is important that the instrument always remains in contact with the same area. The instrument is not pushed over the skin, but the anatomical structure is moved in the restricted direction. The return movement is then done without pressure and is described as returning to the starting position.

The flexor retinaculum is often chosen as an entry point for mobilization. From here, the therapist mobilizes the tendons with the edge of an instrument, the advantage being that mobilization is more selective and therefore more precise. The therapist then works along the flexors from hypomobility to hypomobility, distally in direction of the fingertips.

In addition to the "standard treatment" described above, various procedures can be beneficial for the entire myofascial system. In Dupuytren's contracture, several other structures near the hand or involved in hand function often exhibit local hypertonicity that should be treated as described above. The Regulation of Tone Technique may be applied to the extrinsic muscles (including the antebrachial fascia): palmaris longus, flexor carpi radialis, flexor carpi ulnaris, pronator teres, and pronator quadratus.

The Mobilization Technique may then be applied to palmaris longus, flexor carpi radialis, and flexor carpi ulnaris.

Myofascial Connected System (MCS) (Figure 7.38)

Schematic Representation of the Treatment

Diagnosis

Dupuytren's contracture (Morbus Dupuytren, Dupuytren's disease, Viking disease, Celtic hand).

Primary structure affected

- Palmar aponeurosis.
- Flexor digitorum superficialis and profundus, palmaris longus and brevis.
- Anterior part of antebrachial fascia.

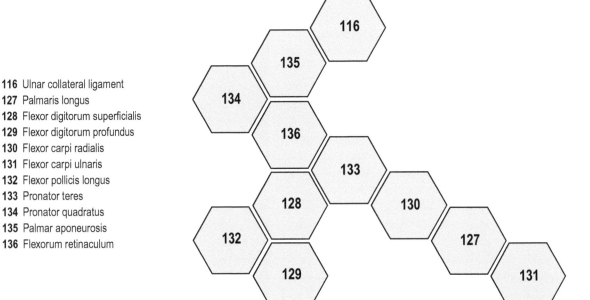

116 Ulnar collateral ligament
127 Palmaris longus
128 Flexor digitorum superficialis
129 Flexor digitorum profundus
130 Flexor carpi radialis
131 Flexor carpi ulnaris
132 Flexor pollicis longus
133 Pronator teres
134 Pronator quadratus
135 Palmar aponeurosis
136 Flexorum retinaculum

Figure 7.38 Dupuytren's contracture: representation of the MCS

Secondary structures frequently affected
- Extrinsic muscles (including the antebra-chial fascia):
  - ○ Flexor carpi radialis
  - ○ Flexor carpi ulnaris
  - ○ Pronator teres
  - ○ Pronator quadratus.
- Intrinsic muscles:
  - ○ Thenar muscles: abductor pollicis brevis, flexor pollicis brevis, adductor pollicis brevis, opponens pollicis
  - ○ Hypothenar muscles: abductor digiti minimi, flexor digiti minimi, opponens digiti minimi
  - ○ Metacarpal muscles: palmar interossei, lumbricals, dorsal interossei.

Initial position
The patient sits next to the therapy table; the fore-arm lies relaxed and supinated (supported distally with a cushion); the elbow is slightly bent.

Material
- Recommended: combination curved, straight short instrument.
- Optional: straight elongated instrument, curved instrument.

Technique
- Recommended: Rehydration, Regulation of Tone, Mobilization.
- Optional: none.

Recommended treatment protocol (Table 7.5)

Rehydration Technique (ReT)
- Palmar aponeurosis.
- Anterior part of antebrachial fascia.

Regulation of Tone Technique (RoT)
- Flexor digitorum superficialis.
- Flexor digitorum profundus.
- Thenar muscles:

Table 7.5 Dupuytren's contracture: summary of recommended treatment protocol

ReT	PRT	RoT	MoT	MeT
Palmar aponeurosis		Flexor digitorum superficialis	Palmar aponeurosis	
Anterior part of antebrachial fascia		Flexor digitorum profundus	Flexor digitorum superficialis	
		Abductor pollicis brevis	Flexor digitorum profundus	
		Flexor pollicis brevis		
		Adductor pollicis brevis		
		Opponens pollicis		
		Abductor digiti minimi		
		Flexor digiti minimi		
		Opponens digiti minimi		
		Palmar interossei		
		Lumbricals		
		Dorsal interossei		

- ° Abductor pollicis brevis
- ° Flexor pollicis brevis
- ° Adductor pollicis brevis
- ° Opponens pollicis.
- Hypothenar muscles:
  - ° Abductor digiti minimi
  - ° Flexor digiti minimi
  - ° Opponens digiti minimi.
- Metacarpal muscles:
  - ° Palmar interossei
  - ° Lumbrical muscles
  - ° Dorsal interossei.

Mobilization Technique (MoT)

- Palmar aponeurosis.
- Flexor digitorum superficialis.
- Flexor digitorum profundus.

Optional treatment protocol (Table 7.6)

Regulation of Tone Technique (RoT)

- Palmaris longus.

- Flexor carpi radialis.
- Flexor carpi ulnaris.
- Pronator teres.
- Pronator quadratus.

Mobilization Technique (MoT)

- Palmaris longus.
- Flexor carpi radialis.
- Flexor carpi ulnaris.

Table 7.6 Dupuytren's contracture: summary of optional treatment protocol

RoT	MoT
Palmaris longus	Palmaris longus
Flexor carpi radialis	Flexor carpi radialis
Flexor carpi ulnaris	Flexor carpi ulnaris
Pronator teres	
Pronator quadratus	

Visual Presentation of the Treatment Unit

Recommended treatment protocol

Rehydration Technique (ReT)

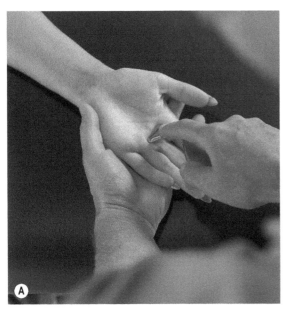

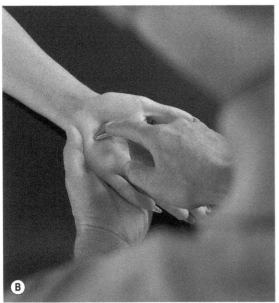

Figure 7.39 (A and B) Palmar aponeurosis

Regulation of Tone Technique (RoT)

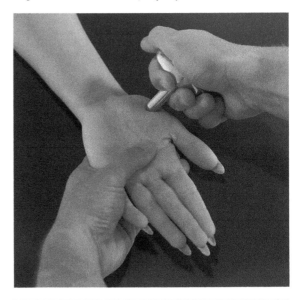

Figure 7.40 Abductor pollicis brevis

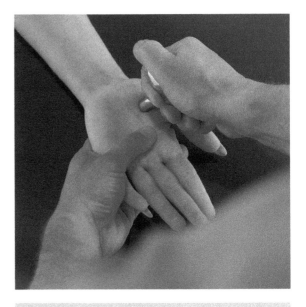

Figure 7.41 Opponens pollicis

Mobilization Technique (MoT)

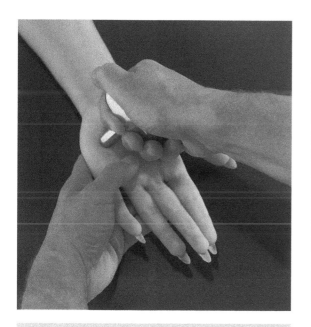

Figure 7.42 Opponens digiti minimi

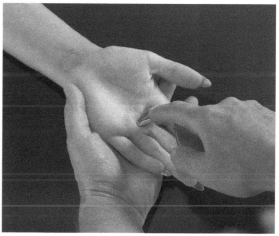

Figure 7.44 Palmar aponeurosis

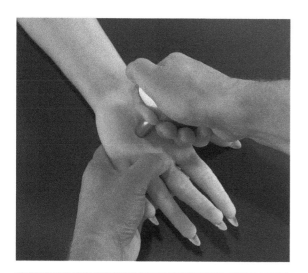

Figure 7.43 Palmar interossei, lumbricals

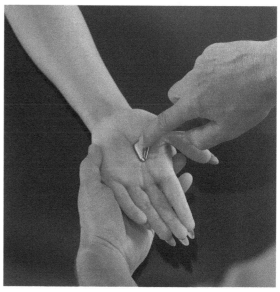

Figure 7.45 Flexor digitorum profundus

Duration

Approximately 10 minutes.

Evaluation

- Finger position.
- ROM fingers/wrist in extension.
- End-feel fingers/wrist extension.

Exercise Progression

- Tissue stretch: stretch starting position in finger/wrist extension.

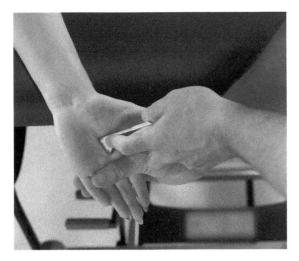

Figure 7.46 Treatment in stretched position (finger and wrist extension)

- Tissue dynamics: active movements of the finger/wrist (flexion–extension).
- Tissue dynamics+: resistive movement against elastic resistance.

Stenosing tenosynovitis

For so-called "trigger finger" (stenosing tenosynovitis), usually of the ring finger or the thumb, the treatment is analogous to that of Dupuytren's contracture. The structure affected in this case is the tendon of the corresponding finger (flexor digitorum profundus).

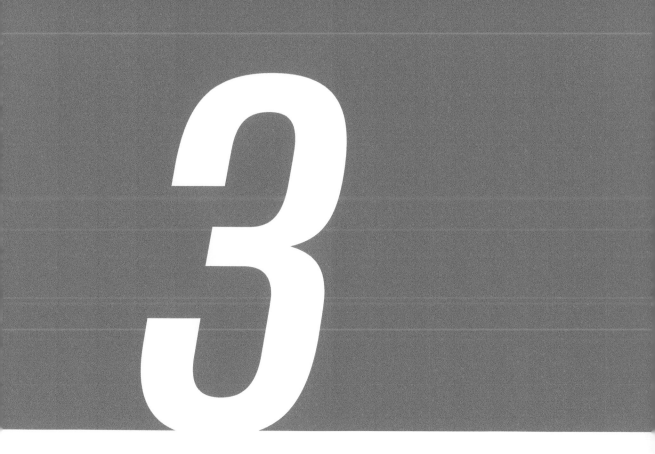

3

Clinical Applications of IAMT: Lower Quarter

As in the previous section, the chapters in Part 3 deal with the clinical application of the instruments on the patient: IAMT in daily practice. The lower quarter is described here. We continue to strive for good readability and high relevance to everyday practice, and follow the same structure, which allows the reader to tackle each chapter separately and still be able to apply the corresponding therapy directly.

At least two important – and common – diseases have been selected for each area. A detailed description of the treatment is given first, followed by a schematic representation of the treatment with numerous illustrations, for immediate and optimal implementation of the therapy in the reader's practice. A treatment protocol is provided, which has proven itself in practice. Of course, it can and should always be adapted to the patient or the condition. Sometimes not all steps are necessary; sometimes a certain part of the treatment must be carried out more intensively. However, especially when the therapist is still gaining experience with IAMT, it is advisable to follow the protocols; they lend a certain structure and often give the therapist a corresponding sense of security. They also increase comparability between patients.

A visual representation of the treatment is also provided, for quick reference. Finally, the authors give information on the possible duration of the therapy, suggest evaluation tests, and present possibilities for progression as well as pre- and post-treatment techniques. In the latter case, reference should always be made to Chapter 4 since these techniques are almost always identical.

Clinical Applications of IAMT: Lower Quarter

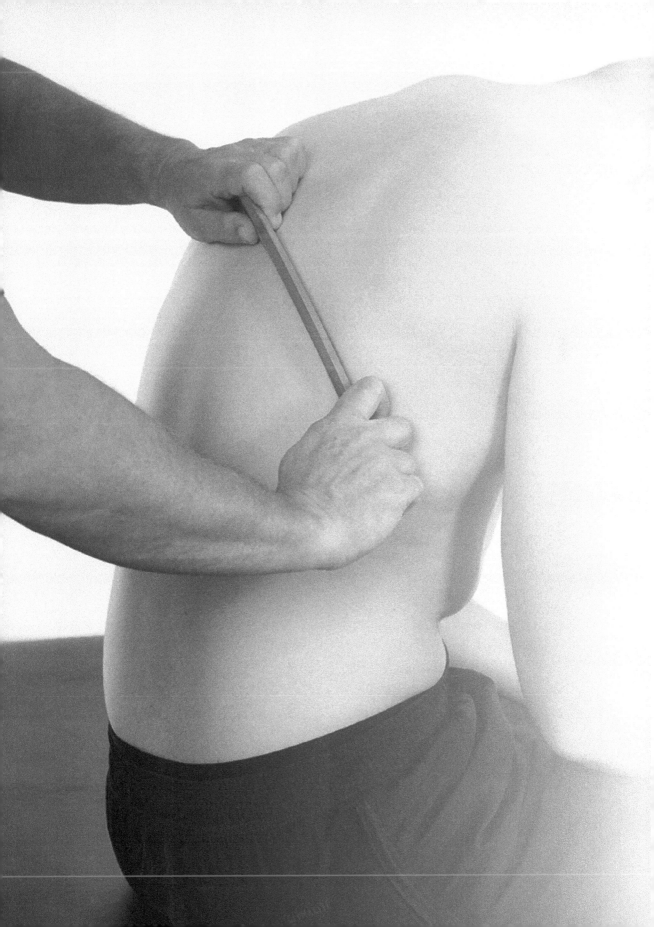

Pain and disease in the thoracic spine and thoracic region are encountered less frequently than in the lumbar and cervical spine in the authors' experience; therefore, only one clinical protocol is presented here. The treatment selected for this area is "dorsalgia," non-specific back pain in the thoracic spine, which is representative of the range of musculoskeletal pathologies in the thoracic spine and the chest. Dorsalgia treatment is adapted according to the symptoms and the suspected causes. In this chapter, both the dorsal and ventral surfaces of the thoracic region will be discussed in the management of dorsalgia. For purely didactic reasons, the authors have chosen to present them separately in two treatment units but it is not always necessary to treat both dorsal and ventral surfaces. Usually, the therapist starts with the treatment of the dorsal structures and then addresses the ventral structures in a second session. Of course, it is also possible to treat both areas within one treatment, although experience has shown that this is quite stressful for the patient. Dosage is often the key to success; thus, individual techniques from both regions can be combined.

The reader will find a detailed description of the treatment of adjacent structures in the corresponding chapters; in addition to the table of contents, Figure I.1 in the Introduction is suitable for quickly finding the corresponding structures in the book. Through the Myofascial Connected System, the therapist is also guided in a clear way through the entire body-wide network of fascial structures. In this way, a holistic treatment of the human body is provided, even for seemingly local problems.

Treatment of the Dorsal Structures of the Thoracic Spine

Detailed Description of the Treatment

Dorsalgia is characterized by non-specific back pain in the thoracic spine. The structures affected are the erector spinae, trapezius (descending/upper part), rhomboid major and rhomboid minor, serratus posterior superior, and the intercostal muscles, as well as the ligaments of the spine (interspinous and supraspinous ligaments) and costovertebral joints (superior and lateral costotransverse ligaments). The adjacent structures of the thoracolumbar fascia and latissimus dorsi and serratus anterior muscles may also be involved.

The patient lies prone, with ankle joints supported (relaxation of the treated structure) or feet in overhang. The arms should be relaxed next to the body. The patient's head is rotated. Equilateral rotation is advantageous for relaxation of most of the structures to be treated. However, it may also be useful to change the position of the head during treatment. If it is necessary and the head or cervical spine does not allow sufficient rotation or is painful, the patient's face should lie in the designated nasal slit. The seated position on a massage chair may be an alternative.

The therapy starts with a Rehydration Technique using large-area sliding of the entire area of the thoracic spine. Starting from the last ribs, the technique is performed in a cranial direction, up toward the shoulder and the cervicothoracic junction. This area is usually not large; therefore, it is useful to treat it all at the same time, although it may sometimes be necessary to treat the lateral side of the thorax separately. It is best treated with the convex side of a curved instrument.

Due to the thoracic anatomy (presence of the scapula), the area is treated in several phases: from the lower ribs to the scapula, between the scapula and the spine, the posterior side of the scapula, and possibly the supraspinatus fossa. Initially, the instrument is applied caudally and parallel to the ribs at a slightly oblique angle. It is then pushed cranially; the edge of the instrument is slightly higher laterally than medially so that the instrument is horizontal at the inferior angle of the scapula. At this point, the medial end is immobilized, while the lateral end is pushed in a circular motion further upward to the axilla. Next, the area between the scapula and the spine is treated. Due to the area available for treatment, the convex side of a curved instrument is used. Alternatively, it is also possible to use a combination curve instrument. The muscle-covered posterior side of the scapula between the inferior angle and the spine should also be treated. Typically, both the affected side of the thoracic spine and the unaffected or non-painful side are treated. The anatomical connections – for example, the insertions and locations of the trapezius muscle and the thoracolumbar fascia – as well as the localization of the spine itself in the center of the body justify this procedure, as does the functional unity of the spine as an organ of protection, support, and movement. Furthermore, experience shows that dorsalgia is often bilateral and vague, and not usually limited to one point with one side more affected than the other.

When treating elderly patients (particularly females), therapists may encounter a rather unique situation near C7. In some older adults, a circumscribed thickening forms at the cervicothoracic junction. This is often a connective tissue thickening in response to chronic postural stress, thus stimulating a remodeling process. While it is rarely the trigger or the cause of dorsalgia, it is part of the clinical picture, in the experience of the authors. This tissue fulfills a postural holding function but is otherwise obstructive to the reduction of pain and correction of posture, as it tends to hold the thoracic spine in a flexed malposition. Since it is fascial tissue, treatment with the Rehydration Technique is particularly recommended. At this point, the entire area is intensively rehydrated over a large area.

After the Rehydration Technique, the Pain Relief Technique is usually performed. Of course, it is possible to start with this; however, beginning therapy with the gentle and rather pleasant Rehydration Technique has proven to be effective in the authors' experience. The technique is, naturally, limited to the painful area(s). Pain localization, as discussed above, is usually vague and bilateral; thus, the areas that the patient defines as painful are treated. To achieve the greatest relief, the painful areas are treated with a high degree of mechanical stimulation through scraping. The technique is performed directly over the painful areas with a progressive pressure (which should not, however, increase the pain already present). The pressure is applied in both treatment directions: away from the treated area and then on the return. If there are several pain points, they are treated consecutively. The tissue layer in the thoracic spine is generally thinner than elsewhere on the body, and the therapist and patient may have the feeling of rubbing over the ribs. This can be perceived as unpleasant and so the pressure must be reduced accordingly. An alternative is to limit this technique to the area between the ribs (intercostal spaces). Straight, short instruments are suitable for this purpose.

The next technique applied is Regulation of Tone. Application is again dependent on the physiotherapeutic findings. The hypertonic muscles are identified and treated accordingly. In the area of the thoracic spine, hypertonic muscles include erector spinae, rhomboids major and minor, and the intercostals. Nevertheless, all the muscles of the thoracic spine should be examined for local hypertonicity. Once the therapist has located a hypertonic muscle, they place the (straight, short) instrument on the point, apply vertical pressure to the tissue, and maintain this pressure until the tone subsides. The therapist may then have the impression that they can penetrate deeper into the tissue. At the new point of tension, the pressure is held again, and the therapist waits for a new release. The technique can be completed by small movements of the instrument. In this case, the therapist moves the instrument back and forth on the spot or performs small circular movements. Often, this "melting technique" brings an additional relaxing effect and thus increases the overall benefit.

The next technique applied is the Mobilization Technique. The experienced therapist will have no difficulty locating the hypomobile areas of the thoracic spine. The superficial hypomobilities typically involve the thoracolumbar fascia. They are treated according to the protocol already described: first sensed by the displacement test, then treated accordingly. The importance of these superficial hypomobilities is often underestimated in the authors' view, as their treatment is integral to IAMT.

The deeper hypomobilities are somewhat more difficult to locate; they are mostly in the erector spinae muscle and at the insertions (tenoperiosteal junction) of the descending (upper) part of trapezius, rhomboids major and minor, and serratus posterior superior, as well as in the interspinal and supraspinal ligaments, and the superior and lateral costotransverse ligaments. In addition, the following muscular septa should be mobilized:

- between erector spinae and rhomboids
- between erector spinae and serratus posterior superior
- between trapezius (descending part) and rhomboids
- between trapezius (descending part) and latissimus dorsi.

Special attention should be paid to the direction of the tissue mobility limitation. This is not necessarily identical over the entire course of the same structure; moreover, several or even all directions can be affected. The limitation can be determined by a simple test of displacement using the therapist's hand or the instrument. In our experience, there is seldom a single point, but the loss of mobility usually extends to the entire structure. These characteristics can vary from one patient to another. Depending on the structure, the mobilization is carried out with the hook or the short, flat side of the instrument. It is important that the instrument always remains in contact with the same area. The instrument is not pushed over the skin, but the anatomical structure is moved in the restricted direction. The return movement is then done without pressure and is described as returning to the starting position.

The tenoperiosteal junctions of the erector spinae muscle should always be mobilized and they are often chosen as an entry point for mobilization. This is done either more locally with the end of a straight instrument, or more regionally with the convex side of a curved instrument or a combination curve instrument. The therapist then works along the spine from hypomobility to hypomobility further cranially.

In the typical back pain patient, flexion is severely limited and it is often very difficult for the therapist to treat these structures initially. Therefore, the ligaments of the spine (interspinous and supraspinous) and those of the ribs (superior and lateral costotransverse) also require treatment. Treatment of the spinal ligaments is best done in the lateral position due to the limited opening of the intervertebral spaces. The patient's spine is flexed (with hips and knees flexed) and the chin placed on the chest, if possible, to open the dorsal area as much as possible. The treatment is best done with the hook of an instrument for the ligaments of the spine or with a straight, short instrument for the ligaments of the ribs.

The last technique applied in this standard treatment session is the Metabolization Technique. The therapist scrapes the instrument over the area to be treated. The pressure is relatively high and varies according to the volume of the tissue: the greater the volume (that is, the thicker the layer of tissue), the greater the pressure can be.

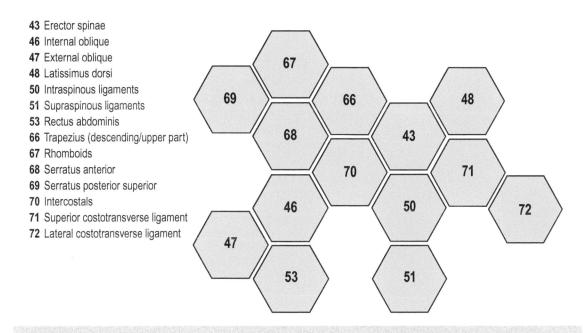

43 Erector spinae
46 Internal oblique
47 External oblique
48 Latissimus dorsi
50 Intraspinous ligaments
51 Supraspinous ligaments
53 Rectus abdominis
66 Trapezius (descending/upper part)
67 Rhomboids
68 Serratus anterior
69 Serratus posterior superior
70 Intercostals
71 Superior costotransverse ligament
72 Lateral costotransverse ligament

Figure 8.1 Treatment of the dorsal structures of the thoracic spine: representation of the MCS

The pressure is applied in one direction only and the speed of execution is also relatively high. The pain already present must, under no circumstances, be increased.

The Pain Relief Technique may be repeated at the end, as described previously. The authors recommend finishing the session with the most painful treatment. The therapist can limit this technique to the intercostal spaces when the classical approach does not seem ideal.

Myofascial Connected System (MCS) (Figure 8.1)

Schematic Representation of the Treatment

Diagnosis

Dorsalgia (non-specific back pain in the thoracic spine).

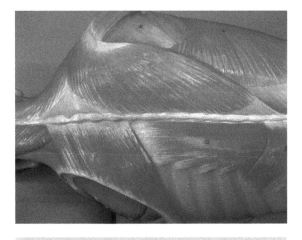

Figure 8.2 Dorsal structures of the thoracic spine: primary structures affected

Primary structures affected (Figure 8.2)

- Thoracolumbar fascia.
- Erector spinae.
- Trapezius (upper portion).
- Rhomboid major and minor.
- Serratus posterior superior.
- Intercostal muscles.
- Interspinous ligament.
- Supraspinous ligament.
- Superior costotransverse ligament.
- Lateral costotransverse ligament.

Secondary structures frequently affected

- Latissimus dorsi.
- Serratus anterior.

Initial position

- Lying prone:
  - ankle joints supported (relaxation of the treated structure) or feet in overhang
  - arms relaxed next to the body
  - head rotated or in nasal slit.
- Seated on a massage chair as an alternative.

Material

- Recommended: straight elongated instrument, curved instrument, combination curved, straight short instrument.
- Optional: none.

Technique

- Recommended: Rehydration, Pain Relief, Regulation of Tone, Mobilization, Metabolization.
- Optional: none.

Recommended treatment protocol (Table 8.1)

Rehydration Technique (ReT)

- Entire area of the thoracic spine, including scapulae.
- Eventually, cervicothoracic junction.

Table 8.1 Treatment of the dorsal structures of the thoracic spine: summary of recommended treatment protocol

ReT	PRT	RoT	MoT	MeT
Entire area of the thoracic spine, including scapulae	Painful area	Erector spinae	Thoracolumbar fascia	Painful area
Eventually, cervicothoracic junction		Rhomboids	Erector spinae	
		Intercostals	Trapezius (descending/upper part)	
			Rhomboids	
			Serratus posterior superior	
			Interspinous ligament Supraspinous ligament	
			Superior costotransverse ligament Lateral costotransverse ligament	
			Muscular septa between: • erector spinae and rhomboids • erector spinae and serratus posterior superior • trapezius (descending part) and rhomboids • trapezius (descending part) and latissimus dorsi	

Pain Relief Technique (PRT)

- Regional: entire area of the thoracic spine.
- Alternatively, limited to the intercostal spaces.

Regulation of Tone Technique (RoT)

- Erector spinae.
- Rhomboids.
- Intercostals.

Mobilization Technique (MoT)

- Thoracolumbar fascia.
- Erector spinae.
- Trapezius (descending/upper part).
- Rhomboids.
- Serratus posterior superior.
- Interspinous ligament.
- Supraspinous ligament.
- Superior costotransverse ligament.
- Lateral costotransverse ligament.
- Muscular septa between:
  - erector spinae and rhomboids
  - erector spinae and serratus posterior superior
  - trapezius (descending part) and rhomboids
  - trapezius (descending part) and latissimus dorsi.

Metabolization Technique (MeT)

- Regional: entire area of the thoracic spine.
- Alternatively, limited to the intercostal spaces.

Visual Presentation of the Treatment Unit

Recommended treatment protocol

Rehydration Technique (ReT)

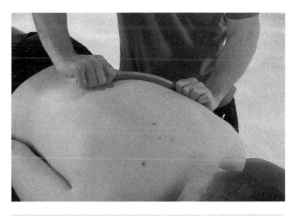

Figure 8.3 Thoracolumbar fascia, under scapula: starting position

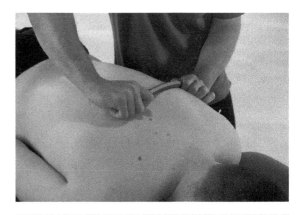

Figure 8.4 Thoracolumbar fascia, under scapula: end position

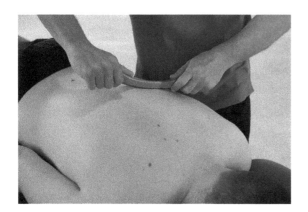

Figure 8.5 Between scapula and spine: starting position

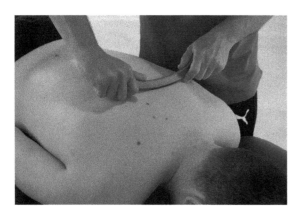

Figure 8.6 Between scapula and spine: end position

Pain Relief Technique (PRT)

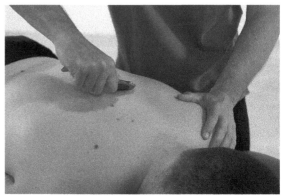

Figure 8.7 Thoracic spine

Regulation of Tone Technique (RoT)

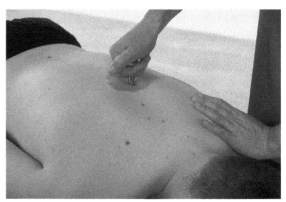

Figure 8.8 Erector spinae

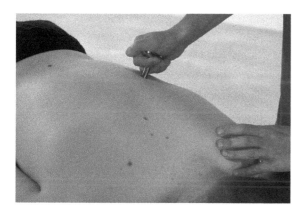

Figure 8.9 Intercostal muscles

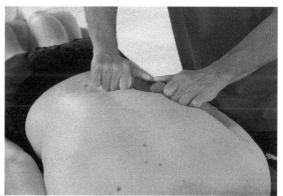

Figure 8.11 Trapezius (ascending part)

Mobilization Technique (MoT)

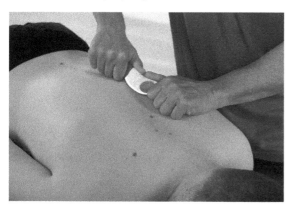

Figure 8.10 Erector spinae

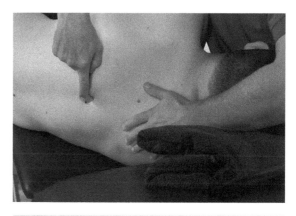

Figure 8.12 Interspinous and supraspinous ligaments

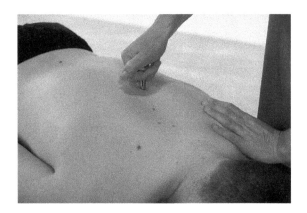

Figure 8.13 Superior costotransverse ligament and lateral costotransverse ligament

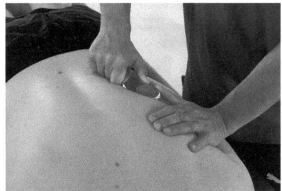

Figure 8.15 Muscular septum between trapezius and latissimus dorsi

Metabolization Technique (MeT)

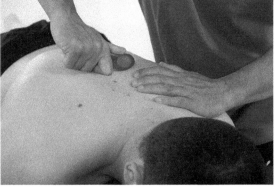

Figure 8.14 Muscular septum between erector spinae and rhomboids

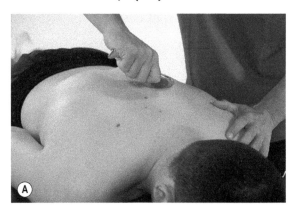

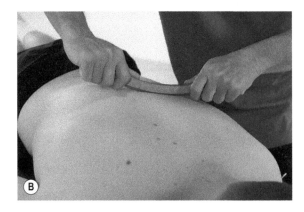

Figure 8.16 (A and B) Thoracic spine: different instruments

Duration
Approximately 10 minutes.

Evaluation
- Numeric rating scale (NRS).
- Distance sternum–wall.
- Schober–Ott test.
- Segmental mobility tests of the thoracic spine.

Exercise progression
- Tissue stretch: stretch starting position in flexion (or in rotation):
  - Lying on the side in flexion
  - Sitting on the stool
  - Prone position on the large exercise ball
  - Standing position (flabby posture)
  - Side lying in rotation.

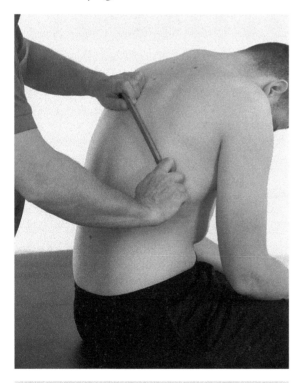

Figure 8.17 Treatment in stretched starting position (flexion), seated

- Tissue dynamics: active movements of the lumbar spine:
  - Lying on the side (flexion–extension)
  - Sitting on the stool (flexion–extension, rotation).

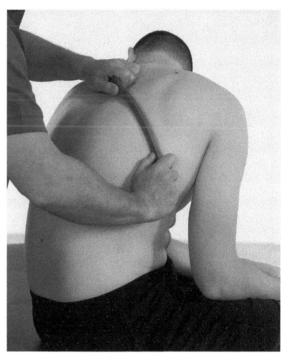

Figure 8.18 Treatment with active movements (flexion and rotation), seated

- Tissue loading: functionality of the starting position:
  - Sitting on the stool
  - In standing position.
- Tissue loading+: use of tools:
  - Elastic bands
  - Weights.

Treatment of the Ventral Structures of the Thoracic Spine and the Chest

Detailed Description of the Treatment

Treatment of the ventral structures of the thoracic spine and the chest is usually performed unilaterally for technical reasons. If both sides are affected, they are treated one after the other. Different issues sometimes complicate the treatment for female patients. The anatomical localization of the cranial insertions of the abdominal muscles and of the pectoralis major muscle, as well as the existence of the breast, can lead to potentially difficult situations. The authors recommend discussing this with the patient beforehand. In case of doubt, we recommend not performing the treatment. Furthermore, the breast can be an obstacle to effective therapy with certain techniques (such as Rehydration, Pain Relief, and Metabolization). In this case, the authors suggest refraining from using these. It goes without saying that the female breast is not treated with the instruments in any way.

The structures affected are the pectoral fascia and the superficial abdominal fascia, the intercostals, pectoralis major, pectoralis minor, obliquus internus abdominis, obliquus externus abdominis, rectus abdominis, and serratus anterior, as well as the ligaments of the costosternal joints.

The patient lies supine, with knee joints and head supported (relaxation of the treated structure). The arms should be relaxed next to the body or folded on the abdomen.

The therapy starts with large-area sliding of the entire area of the chest. However, the parts below and above the breast and the inferior border of the pectoralis major muscle are treated separately from each other. Starting from the last ribs, the technique is performed in a cranial direction, up towards the shoulder and the clavicle. While this area is not usually large, it may be necessary to treat the lateral side of the thorax separately to reach the insertions of obliquus externus abdominis and serratus anterior. The area is best treated with the convex side of a curved instrument. Initially, the instrument is applied caudally and parallel to the ribs (slightly oblique). It is then pushed cranially at a slightly higher speed laterally than medially, so that the instrument is horizontal at the inferior border of the pectoralis major muscle. The treatment is continued above the breast with a curved or a combination curve instrument. The upper limit of the treatment area is the clavicle or the jugular fossa; note that the jugular fossa is never treated with the instruments. In addition, the insertions of pectoralis major and rectus abdominis on the sternum should be treated separately. These are frequently strained in patients with dorsalgia. In addition, the sternalis muscle is located in this region. The therapist best rehydrates this area by treating it with the edge of the back of a curved or a combination curve instrument from the xyphoid process to the manubrium of the sternum.

After the Rehydration Technique, the Pain Relief Technique is performed. However, musculoskeletal pain in the region of the chest is very rare in relation to back problems. Patients occasionally express pain in the area of the rib cartilage; if so, the Pain Relief Technique can be employed.

The next technique applied is the Regulation of Tone. Application is again dependent on the physiotherapeutic findings. The hypertonic muscles are identified and treated accordingly. In the area of the chest, they are usually located in the intercostal muscles, pectoralis major, and pectoralis minor. However, all muscles of the chest should be examined for local hypertension. Once the therapist has located a hypertonic point, they place the instrument (short instrument) on the point, apply vertical pressure to the tissue, and maintain this pressure until the tone subsides. The therapist then has the impression that they can penetrate deeper into the tissue. At the new point of tension, the pressure is held again, and the therapist waits for a new release.

The technique can be completed with small movements of the instrument. In this case, the therapist moves the instrument back and forth on the spot or performs small circular movements. Often, this "melting technique" brings an additional relaxing effect and thus increases the overall benefit.

The next technique applied is the Mobilization Technique. The experienced therapist will have no difficulty locating the hypomobile areas of the thoracic spine. The superficial hypomobilities involve the pectoral fascia and are somewhat less pronounced in the superficial abdominal fascia. They are treated according to the protocol already described: first sensed by the displacement test, then treated accordingly.

The deeper hypomobilities are somewhat more difficult to locate; they are mostly in the intercostal muscles, pectoralis major (particularly at the sternum), pectoralis minor (especially at the ribs), obliquus internus abdominis, obliquus externus abdominis, rectus abdominis, and serratus ante-

rior, as well as the sternocostal ligaments. Furthermore, the muscular septum between pectoralis major and minor should be mobilized.

Special attention should be paid to the direction of the tissue mobility limitation. The limitation is not necessarily identical over the entire course of the same structure; moreover, several or even all directions can be affected. The limitation can be determined by a simple test of displacement using the therapist's hand or the instrument. In the authors' experience, there is seldom a single point, but the loss of mobility usually extends to the entire structure. Depending on the structure, mobilization is carried out with the hook or the short, flat side of the instrument. It is important that the instrument always remains in contact with the same area. The instrument is not pushed over the skin, but the anatomical structure is moved in the restricted direction. The return movement is then done without pressure and is described as returning to the starting position. The tenoperiosteal junctions of the

46 Internal oblique
47 External oblique
53 Rectus abdominis
68 Serratus anterior
70 Intercostals
73 Pectoralis major
74 Pectoralis minor
75 Radiate sternocostal ligaments

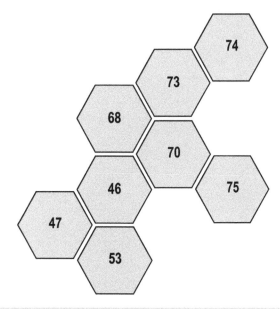

Figure 8.19 Treatment of the ventral structures of the thoracic spine: representation of the MCS

pectoralis muscle should always be mobilized and they are often chosen as an entry point for mobilization. The technique is done either more locally with the end of a straight elongated instrument, or more regionally with the convex side of a curved or a combination curve instrument.

Usually, the last technique applied in this standard treatment session is Metabolization; however, this is generally not applied in this region.

Myofascial Connected System (MCS) (Figure 8.19)

Schematic Representation of the Treatment

Diagnosis

Dorsalgia (non-specific back pain in the thoracic spine).

Primary structures affected (Figures 8.20–8.22)
- Pectoral and superficial abdominal fascia.
- Intercostal muscles.
- Pectoralis major and pectoralis minor.
- Obliquus internus abdominis, obliquus externus abdominis, and rectus abdominis.
- Serratus anterior.
- Sternocostal ligament.

Initial position
- Lying supine, with knee joints and head supported (relaxation of the treated structure).
- Arms relaxed next to the body or folded on the abdomen.

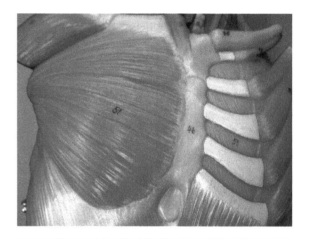

Figure 8.21 Affected structures at the breast

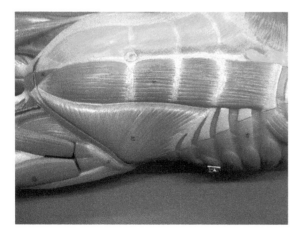

Figure 8.20 Affected structures in the abdomen

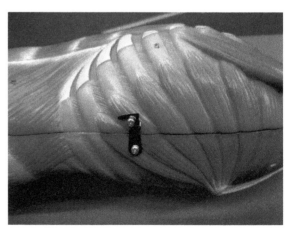

Figure 8.22 Affected structures on the lateral side of the thorax

Material

- Recommended: straight elongated instrument, curved instrument, combination curved, straight short instrument.
- Optional: none.

Technique

- Recommended: Rehydration, Regulation of Tone, Mobilization.
- Optional: Pain Relief, Metabolization.

Recommended treatment protocol (Table 8.2)

Rehydration Technique (ReT)

- Entire area of the chest (except for the breast and nipple area).

Regulation of Tone Technique (RoT)

- Intercostal muscles.
- Pectoralis major.
- Pectoralis minor.

Mobilization Technique (MoT)

- Pectoral and superficial abdominal fascia.
- Intercostal muscles.
- Pectoralis major (especially at the sternum).
- Pectoralis minor (especially at the ribs).
- Obliquus internus abdominis.
- Obliquus externus abdominis.
- Rectus abdominis.
- Serratus anterior.
- Sternocostal ligaments.
- Muscular septum between pectoralis major and minor.

Table 8.2 Treatment of the ventral structures of the thoracic spine: summary of recommended treatment protocol

ReT	PRT	RoT	MoT	MeT
Entire area of the chest (except for the breast and nipple area)	Painful area	Intercostal muscles	Pectoral and superficial abdominal fascia	
		Pectoralis major	Intercostal muscles	
		Pectoralis minor	Pectoralis major (especially at the sternum)	
			Pectoralis minor (especially at the ribs)	
			Obliquus internus abdominis	
			Obliquus externus abdominis	
			Rectus abdominis	
			Serratus anterior	
			Sternocostal ligaments	
			Muscular septum between pectoralis major and minor	

Visual Presentation of the Treatment Unit

Recommended treatment protocol

Rehydration Technique (ReT)

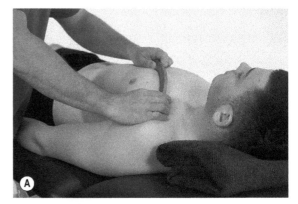

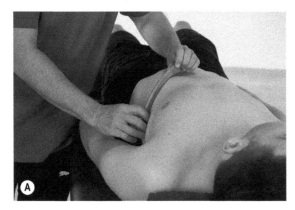

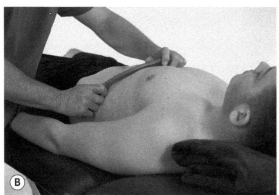

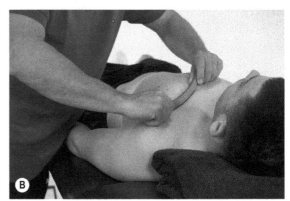

Figure 8.23 (A and B) Pectoral fascia: below breast

Figure 8.24 (A and B) Pectoral fascia: above breast

Regulation of Tone Technique (RoT)

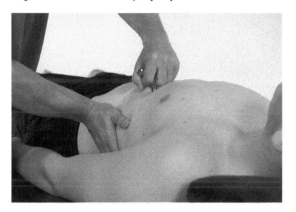

Figure 8.25 Intercostal muscles

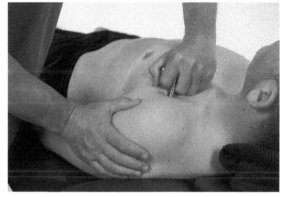

Figure 8.27 Pectoralis minor

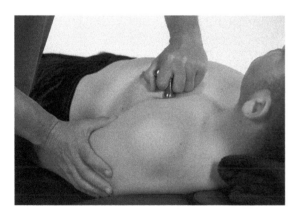

Figure 8.26 Pectoralis major

Mobilization Technique (MoT)

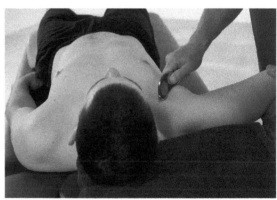

Figure 8.28 Pectoral fascia

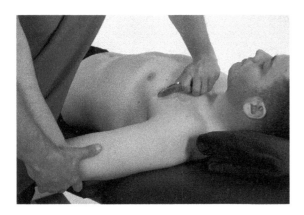

Figure 8.29 Pectoralis major

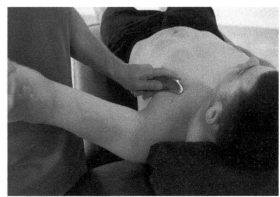

Figure 8.30 Treatment in stretched starting position (arm in elevation), lying supine

Duration

Approximately 10 minutes.

Evaluation

- Numeric rating scale (NRS).
- Distance sternum–wall.
- Schober–Ott test.
- Segmental mobility tests of the thoracic spine.
- Position of the ribs.
- Respiratory motion and movement amplitude.

Exercise progression

- Tissue stretch: stretch starting position in extension (or in rotation):
  - Lying supine with arms in elevation
  - Lying supine with a pillow under the thoracic spine
  - Supine position on the large exercise ball
  - Lying on the side in rotation
  - Rotation–stretching position
  - C-position
  - In maximum inspiration (or expiration) position of the ribs (end-respiratory break).

- Tissue dynamics: active movements of the thoracic spine:
  - Lying supine: rotation or lateral flexion
  - Sitting on the stool: flexion–extension, rotation or lateral flexion
  - Standing: flexion–extension, rotation or lateral flexion.

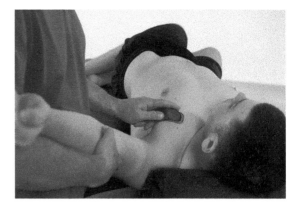

Figure 8.31 Treatment with active movements of the thoracic spine (rotation), lying supine

- Tissue loading: functionality of the starting position:
  - Sitting on the stool
  - In standing position
  - Starting positions in a specific context, e.g. serving position (tennis).

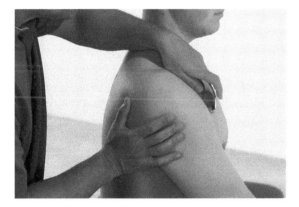

Figure 8.32 Treatment in a functional starting position (sitting)

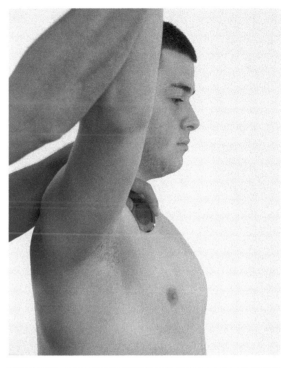

Figure 8.33 Treatment in a specific starting position (sitting with elevation of the arm)

- Tissue loading+: use of tools:
  - Elastic bands
  - Weights.

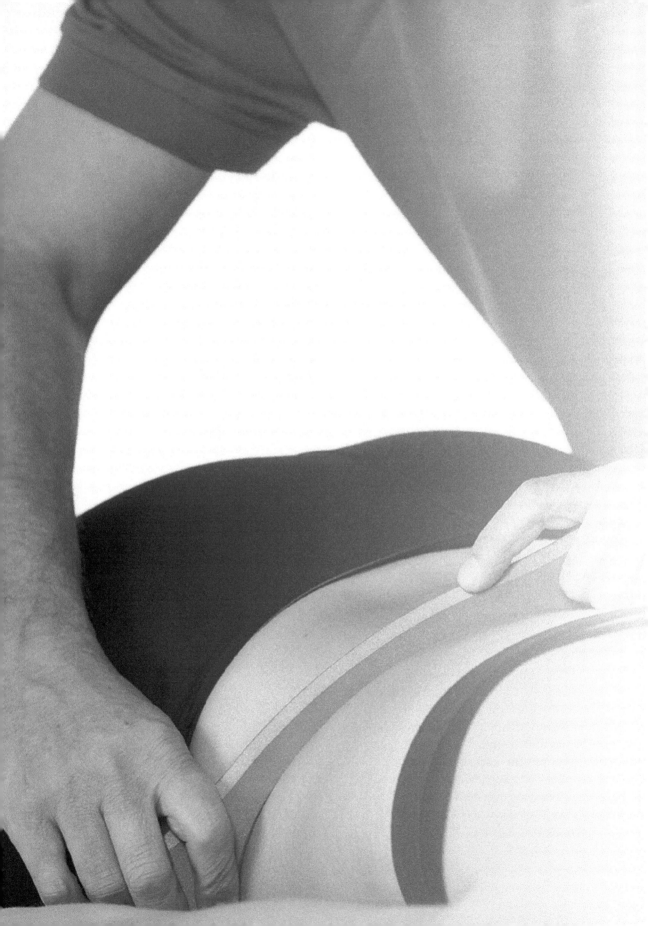

Low back pain (non-specific) and sacroiliac joint dysfunction (that is, sacroiliac blockage or sacroiliac syndrome) are representative of the range of pathology in the lumbar spine and sacroiliac joint. Treatment is adapted according to the symptoms of individual patients and the suspected causes.

Low Back Pain (Non-specific)

Detailed Description of the Treatment

The diagnosis of low back pain without a specific origin affects the lumbar spine and its myofascial structures: the thoracolumbar fascia and the erector spinae, latissimus dorsi, and serratus posterior inferior muscles, as well as the interspinous, supraspinous, and intertransverse ligaments. The adjacent structures are the gluteal and superficial abdominal fascia, gluteus maximus, transversus abdominis, quadratus lumborum, internal oblique, external oblique, rectus abdominis, psoas major, iliacus, and the diaphragm.

The term erector spinae is used here to refer to the group of superficial spinal muscles (iliocostalis, longissimus, and spinalis). A differentiated treatment for these individual muscles is neither necessary nor practical in low back pain.

In most chapters, a standard treatment (for the primary structures affected) and an additional treatment (for the secondary structures affected) are presented at this point. For low back pain, two parts of the treatment are described due to the complexity of the lumbar area and the clinical diagnosis. It is not always necessary to perform both parts of the treatment consecutively. Usually, the therapist starts with the treatment of the dorsal structures and then addresses the ventral structures during the second treatment. Of course, it is also possible to treat both areas within one treatment; however, experience has shown that this is

quite stressful for the patient and so individual techniques from both parts of the treatment can be combined.

Treatment of the dorsal structures of the lumbar spine

The patient lies prone, with ankle joints supported or feet in overhang to relax the treatment area. The therapy starts with large-area sliding of the entire area of the lumbar spine. Starting from the iliac crest at the level of the sacrum, the technique is performed in a cranial direction up to the ribs and the thoracolumbar junction. Of course, this area is rather large; therefore, it is best treated with the convex side of a curved or a combination curve instrument. It is also advisable to treat the area in two parts. One approach has proven effective in practice: the therapist applies the instrument parallel to the iliac crest; the lateral end remains relatively immobile, while the medial end is moved cranially so that the device makes a "windshield wiper"-type movement. Thus, the entire area (of one side of the trunk) is treated at once. The pressure is proportional to the thickness of the soft tissue layers: the more tissue under the instrument, the higher the pressure can be. However, uniformity of the pressure is important. Each of these parts is treated several times.

Next the painful areas of the lumbar spine are treated; there are usually several pain points here. It is best to use a relatively short part of the instrument for this local treatment. The pressure applied in this area can be relatively high because of the thickness of the structures and the strength of the thoracolumbar fascia in the lumbar region. A relatively large amount of pressure is required to reach the deep aspects of the thoracolumbar fascia.

While rehydration is a technique that can be used on large areas of the lumbar spine, different areas may be difficult to reach. This is where the value of the equipment and its special properties become apparent. The lumbar spine is often affected in both easily accessible areas, but also in areas that are small in size and embedded between bony structures, such as between the ilium, the sacrum, and the L4 or L5 vertebrae. Therefore, the therapist may attempt to rehydrate this area with a narrow instrument. The muscular attachments (tenoperiosteal junctions) on the iliac crest should also be treated. The authors' experience suggests that non-specific back pain is often deep, broad-based, and bilateral; usually, one side is more affected than the other. Therefore, both the affected side of the lumbar spine and the unaffected or non-painful side are treated. The lumbar spine's function as an organ of protection and support for movement, as well as its anatomy (the location and insertion of the abdominal muscles and thoracolumbar fascia, along with the localization of the spine itself in the center of the body), support the rationale for bilateral treatment.

After the Rehydration Technique, the Pain Relief Technique is usually performed. Of course, it is also possible to start with this technique; however, beginning therapy with the Rehydration Technique has proven to be effective, in the experience of the authors. The technique is, naturally, limited to the painful area(s). Pain localization, discussed above, is often deep lumbar (over L4 and L5), broad-based, and bilateral. These painful areas, which the patient can often identify precisely, are then treated accordingly. The area may extend along the thoracolumbar fascia and even beyond into the gluteal fascia.

In order to achieve the greatest pain relief, the painful areas are provided with a high degree of mechanical stimulation through scraping. The technique is performed directly over the painful areas with a progressive pressure that should not increase the pain already present. This pressure is applied in both treatment directions: away from the treated area and then on the return. If there are several pain points, they are treated consecutively, often along the thoracolumbar fascia and into the gluteal fascia. In these cases, the patient does not always specify a main pain point; thus, the entire area is treated. However, the individual movements of the instrument on the patient's skin should not be longer than 10–15 cm (4–5 inches). The authors recommend performing the technique with both hands and slightly reducing the speed.

The next technique applied is Regulation of Tone. Application is again dependent on the physiotherapeutic findings. The hypertonic muscles are identified and treated accordingly. In this area, they are usually located in the entire section of the lumbar spine (erector spinae, latissimus dorsi, serratus posterior) and in the insertions of the gluteus maximus and abdominal muscles (transversus abdominis, quadratus lumborum, internal oblique, external oblique), at the iliac crest. Once the therapist has located a hypertonic point, they place the straight, short instrument on it, apply vertical pressure to the tissue, and maintain this pressure until the tone subsides. The therapist may then sense that they can penetrate deeper into the tissue. At the new point of tension, the pressure is held again, and the therapist waits for a new release. The technique can be completed by small movements of the instrument. In this case, the therapist moves the instrument back and forth on the spot or performs small, circular movements. Often this "melting technique" brings an additional relaxing effect and thus increases the overall benefit. Although for most areas the length of the straight short instrument is sufficient to reach the structures, for the deep abdominal muscles (quadratus lumborum) the use of a straight short instrument that is a bit longer (like Artzt Vitality Fazer 5, for example) is recommended, particularly when the tissue layers are thicker: for example, in obese patients or athletes.

The next technique applied is the Mobilization Technique. The experienced therapist will have no difficulty locating the hypomobile areas of the lumbar spine, particularly the superficial hypomobilities of the thoracolumbar fascia. The hypomobilities are treated according to the protocol already described: first sensed by the displacement test, then treated accordingly. The authors feel that the treatment of superficial hypomobility disorders is integral to IAMT.

The deeper hypomobilities are sometimes more difficult to locate; they are mostly in the erector spinae muscle and at the insertions (tenoperiosteal junction) of quadratus lumborum, transversus abdominis, internal oblique, and gluteus maximus. Furthermore, the following intermuscular septa are to be mobilized:

- between latissimus dorsi and the internal oblique

- between latissimus dorsi and erector spinae
- between erector spinae and serratus posterior inferior.

Special attention should be paid to the direction of the tissue mobility limitation, which may not be consistent throughout the structure; moreover, several or all directions can be affected. The limitation can be determined by a simple test of displaceability using the therapist's hand or the instrument. In the authors' experience, there is seldom a single point; the loss of mobility usually extends to the entire structure. Depending on the structure, the mobilization is carried out with the hook or the short, flat side of the instrument. It is important that the instrument always remains in contact with the same area. The instrument is not

17 Gluteus maximus
43 Erector spinae
44 Transversus abdominis
45 Quadratus lumborum
46 Internal oblique
47 External oblique
48 Latissimus dorsi
49 Serratus posterior inferior
50 Interspinous ligaments
51 Supraspinous ligaments
52 Intertransverse ligaments
53 Rectus abdominis
54 Psoas major
55 Iliacus
56 Diaphragm

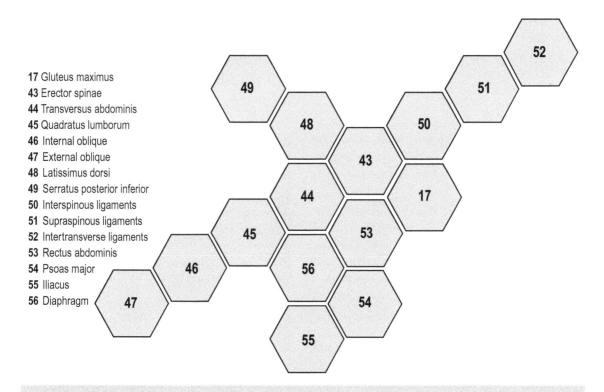

Figure 9.1 Low back pain: representation of the MCS

pushed over the skin, but the anatomical structure is mobilized in the restricted direction. The return movement is then done without pressure and is described as returning to the starting position.

The tenoperiosteal junction at the iliac crest is often chosen as an entry point for mobilization. At this point, the therapist can work with the short side of a curved or a combination curve instrument, the advantage being that mobilization can be a little more selective and therefore more precise. The therapist then works laterally along the iliac crest from hypomobility to hypomobility. In addition to the insertions, the muscle bellies are also treated; in order to address these structures precisely and with the necessary pressure, use of a curved instrument is recommended. Due to the longer lever arm, optimum pressure can be applied more effectively. The tenoperiosteal junctions of the erector spinae muscle should also be mobilized. This is done either more locally with the end of a curved or a combination curve instrument, or more regionally with the convex side of the same instrument.

The ligaments of the lumbar spine also may require treatment (interspinous, supraspinous, and intertransverse ligaments). Treatment of these structures is best done in the side-lying position. The patient's hips and knees are flexed to open the dorsal lumbar spine as much as possible. In the typical back pain patient, flexion is severely limited, and it is often very difficult for the therapist to treat these structures initially; however, mobility improves as the pain is reduced. The treatment is best done with the hook of a curved or a combination curve instrument (interspinous and supraspinous ligaments) or with the straight, short instrument (intertransverse ligaments).

The last technique applied in this standard treatment session is the Metabolization Technique. The therapist scrapes the instrument over the area to be treated. The pressure is relatively high and varies according to the volume of the tissue: the greater the volume (that is, the thicker the layer of tissue), the greater the pressure can be. The pressure is applied in one direction only and the speed of execution is also relatively high. The pain already present must, under no circumstances, be increased.

Myofascial Connected System (MCS) (Figure 9.1)

Schematic Representation of the Treatment

Diagnosis
Low back pain (non-specific).

Primary structures affected (Figure 9.2)
- Thoracolumbar fascia.
- Erector spinae.
- Latissimus dorsi.
- Serratus posterior inferior.
- Interspinous ligament.
- Supraspinous ligament.
- Intertransverse ligament.

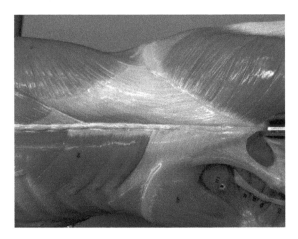

Figure 9.2 Low back pain: primary structures affected (dorsal)

Secondary structures frequently affected (Figure 9.3)

- Gluteal fascia.
- Superficial abdominal fascia.
- Gluteus maximus.
- Transversus abdominis.
- Quadratus lumborum.
- Internal oblique.
- External oblique.
- Rectus abdominis.
- Psoas major.
- Iliacus.
- Diaphragm.

Initial position

Lying prone, with ankle joints supported or feet in overhang.

Material

- Recommended: straight elongated instrument, straight short instrument, curved instrument.
- Optional: combination curve instrument.

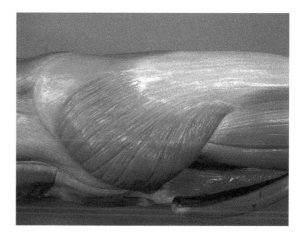

Figure 9.3 Low back pain: secondary structures affected (dorsal)

Technique

- Recommended: Rehydration, Pain Relief, Regulation of Tone, Mobilization, Metabolization.
- Optional: none.

Table 9.1 Low back pain: summary of recommended treatment protocol (dorsal structures)

ReT	PRT	RoT	MoT	MeT
Thoracolumbar fascia	Painful area	Erector spinae	Thoracolumbar fascia	Painful area
Gluteal fascia		Latissimus dorsi	Erector spinae	
		Serratus posterior	Latissimus dorsi	
		Gluteus maximus	Serratus posterior	
		Quadratus lumborum	Gluteus maximus	
		Transversus abdominis	Quadratus lumborum	
		External oblique	Transversus abdominis	
		Internal oblique	Internal oblique	
			Septa: • between latissimus dorsi and the internal oblique • between latissimus dorsi and erector spinae • between erector spinae and serratus posterior inferior	

Recommended treatment protocol (Table 9.1)

Rehydration Technique (ReT)

- Entire area of the lumbar spine (thoracolumbar fascia and gluteal fascia).

Pain Relief Technique (PRT)

- Local: deep lumbar over L4 and L5 (broad-based and bilateral).
- Regional: entire area of the lumbar spine.

Regulation of Tone Technique (RoT)

- Erector spinae.
- Latissimus dorsi.
- Serratus posterior.
- Gluteus maximus.
- Quadratus lumborum.
- Transversus abdominis.
- External oblique.
- Internal oblique.

Mobilization Technique (MoT)

- Thoracolumbar fascia.
- Erector spinae.
- Latissimus dorsi.
- Serratus posterior.
- Gluteus maximus.
- Quadratus lumborum.
- Transversus abdominis.
- Internal oblique.
- Muscular septa between:
  - latissimus dorsi and the internal oblique
  - latissimus dorsi and erector spinae
  - erector spinae and serratus posterior inferior.

Metabolization Technique (MeT)

- Entire area of the lumbar spine (thoracolumbar fascia and gluteal fascia).

Visual Presentation of the Treatment Unit

Recommended treatment protocol

Rehydration Technique (ReT)

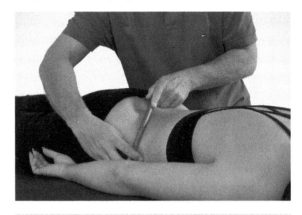

Figure 9.4 Lumbar spine: starting position

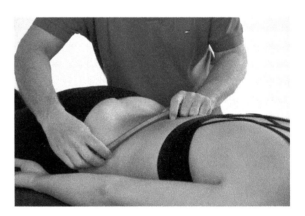

Figure 9.5 Lumbar spine: middle position

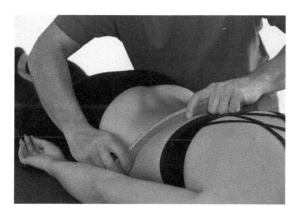

Figure 9.6 Lumbar spine: end position

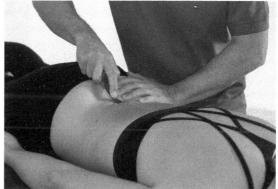

Figure 9.8 Lumbar spine: small area

Pain Relief Technique (PRT)

Regulation of Tone Technique (RoT)

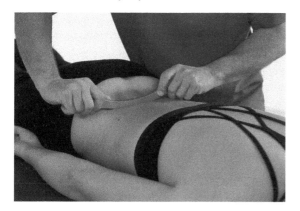

Figure 9.7 Lumbar spine: large area

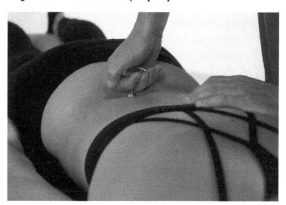

Figure 9.9 Erector spinae

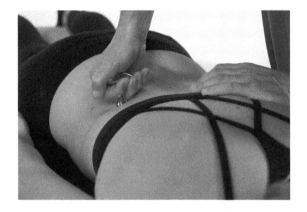

Figure 9.10 Latissimus dorsi

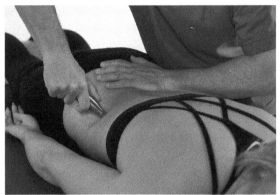

Figure 9.12 Quadratus lumborum

Mobilization Technique (MoT)

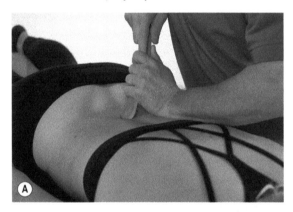

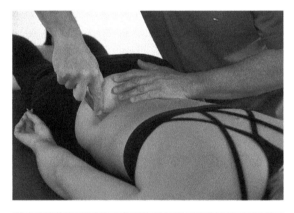

Figure 9.13 Transversus abdominis (iliac crest)

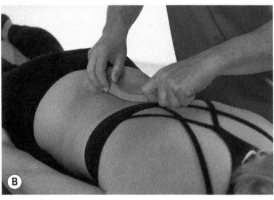

Figure 9.11 (A and B) Erector spinae

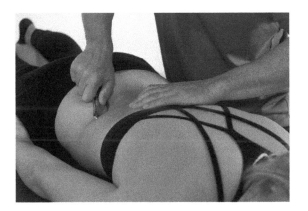

Figure 9.14 Muscular septum between latissimus dorsi and the internal oblique

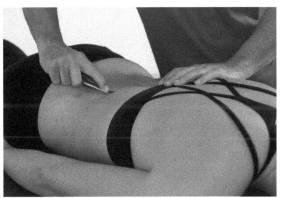

Figure 9.16 Muscular septum between erector spinae and serratus posterior inferior

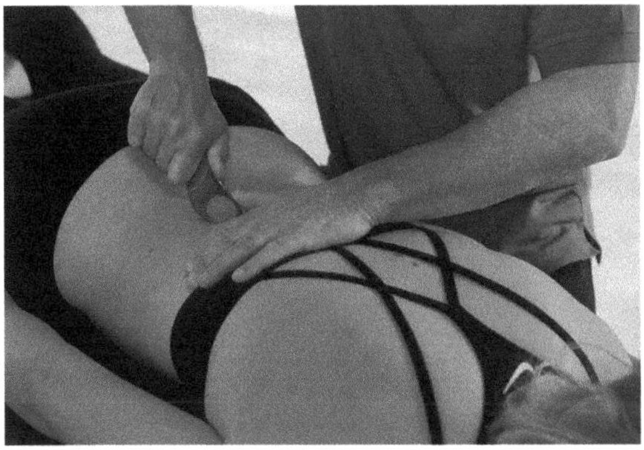

Metabolization Technique (MeT)

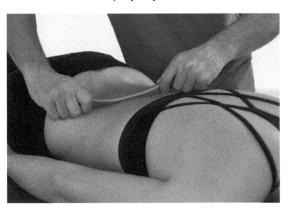

Figure 9.15 Muscular septum between latissimus dorsi and erector spinae

Figure 9.17 Lumbar spine

Duration

Approximately 20 minutes.

Evaluation

- Numeric rating scale (NRS).
- Finger-to-floor distance.
- Schober's test.
- Segmental mobility tests of the lumbar spine.

Exercise progression

- Tissue stretch: stretch starting position in flexion or in rotation:
  - ○ Lying on the side in flexion
  - ○ Sitting on the stool
  - ○ Prone position on the large exercise ball
  - ○ Standing position (bent forward)
  - ○ Side lying in rotation.

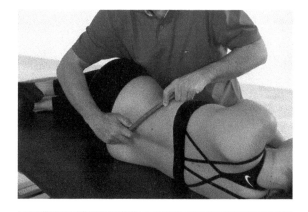

Figure 9.19 Treatment with active movements: in flexion of the lumbar spine

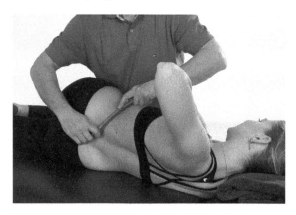

Figure 9.18 Treatment in stretch starting position: side lying in rotation

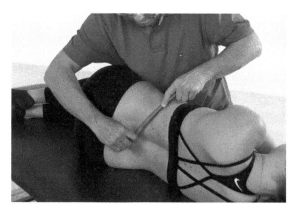

Figure 9.20 Treatment with active movements: in extension of the lumbar spine

- Tissue dynamics: active movements of the lumbar spine:
  - ○ Lying supine (lateral flexion)
  - ○ Side lying (flexion–extension)
  - ○ Sitting on the large exercise ball (flexion–extension)
  - ○ Prone position on the large exercise ball (flexion–extension).

- Tissue loading: functionality of the starting position:
  - ○ Sitting on the stool
  - ○ Standing position.
- Tissue loading+: use of tools:
  - ○ Elastic bands
  - ○ Weights.

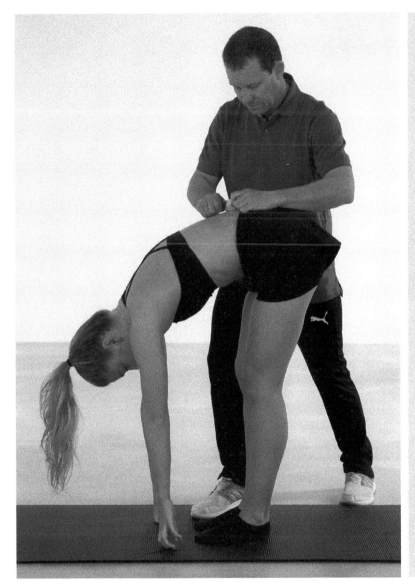

Figure 9.21 Treatment in a functional position (standing in flexion)

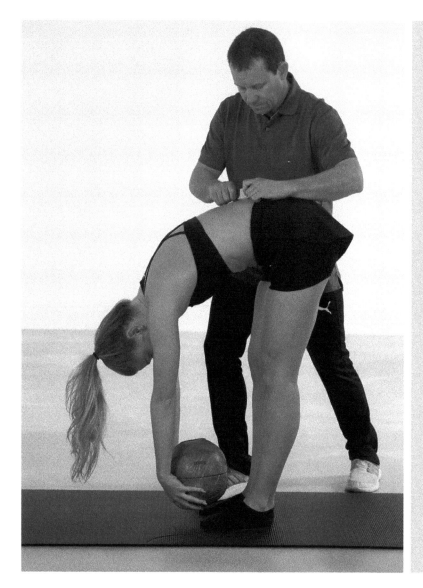

Figure 9.22 Treatment in loaded position (with weight)

Treatment of the ventral structures of the lumbar spine

The treatment of the ventral structures of the lumbar spine is usually performed unilaterally for technical reasons. If both sides are affected, they are treated one after the other. Different issues sometimes complicate the treatment. The anatomical localization of the caudal insertions, mainly of the rectus abdominis muscle at the pubis, can lead to potentially difficult situations. The authors recommend discussing this clearly with the patient at the beginning of the treatment. The thickness of the abdominal wall can also be an obstacle to effective therapy with certain techniques (such as Rehydration, Pain Relief, and Metabolization). In this case, the authors recommend refraining from using these.

The therapy starts with large-area sliding of the entire area of the abdomen (superficial abdominal fascia) between the inguinal ligament and the ribs. The technique is performed starting from the groin and working in a cranial direction up to the ribs and the sternum. Because this area is rather large, it is best treated with the convex side of a curved or a combination curve instrument. It is also advisable to treat the area in two parts, similarly to the dorsal lumbar spine. The therapist applies the instrument parallel to the groin; the lateral end remains relatively immobile, while the medial end is moved cranially, making a "windshield-wiper" movement. Thus, the entire area (of one side of the abdomen) is treated at once. The pressure is proportional to the thickness of the soft tissue layers; the more tissue under the instrument, the higher the pressure can be. Each of these areas is treated several times. The Rehydration Technique performed in the abdominal area is usually not very effective; nevertheless, the authors recommend the short and superficial sequence described.

After Rehydration, the Pain Relief Technique is performed. However, musculoskeletal pain in the abdominal region is very rare – at least in relation to lower back problems. Lumbar patients occasionally complain of pain in the pubic symphysis area. The Pain Relief Technique can be performed there in the standardized manner; however, this is the exception rather than the rule.

The next technique applied is the Regulation of Tone. Application is again dependent on the physiotherapeutic findings. The hypertonic muscles are identified and treated. In the area of the abdominal wall, they are usually located in all abdominal muscles (rectus abdominis, transversus abdominis, internal oblique, external oblique), as well as psoas major, iliacus, and the diaphragm. The hypertonicity is usually in the muscle belly; however, it is not uncommon to find several points in one muscle. The localization of these points is both superficial and deep. Pressure on the hypertonic points on relaxed structures is unpleasant for the patient in the abdominal area because the pressure is transferred to the internal organs due to the tissue's lack of resistance. For the therapist, the technique can also be unpleasant, as it is usually ineffective. Therefore, positioning and treating the structures directly while in relative tension is recommended. This is achieved for the rectus abdominis and transversus abdominis muscles by supporting the lumbar spine with a cushion; for the abdominal oblique muscles, a rotational position seems most effective.

In contrast, to reach psoas major, iliacus, and the diaphragm, the abdominal wall must necessarily be maximally relaxed. For psoas major and iliacus, this is achieved by elevating the trunk and by flexing the hip joints. To reach psoas major, it is best to use a slightly longer straight, short instrument (like the Artzt Vitality Fazer 5, for example).

For the diaphragm, relaxation of the abdominal wall is achieved by elevating the trunk and head or by treating the patient in a sitting position. In the latter position, the therapist stands behind the patient for treatment. The therapist places one arm over the patient's ipsilateral shoulder, bringing the patient not only into flexion but also into ipsilateral lateral flexion and slight rotation. This position allows maximum relaxation of the structures through which the therapist must penetrate to reach the diaphragm.

The instrument of choice depends on the depth of the structure to be reached, the thickness of the tissue layers, and therapist preference; the straight, short instrument is better for more superficial lesions or thin patients, while a slightly longer straight, short instrument (like the Artzt Vitality Fazer 5, for example) is better for deeper lesions or larger patients.

Once the therapist has located a hypertonic point, they place the instrument on the point, apply vertical pressure to the tissue, and maintain this pressure until the tone subsides. The therapist may then have the impression that they can penetrate deeper into the tissue. At the new point of tension, the pressure is held again, and the therapist waits for a new release. The technique can be completed by small movements of the instrument. In this case, the therapist moves the instrument back and forth on the spot or performs small, circular movements. Often, this "melting technique" brings an additional relaxing effect and thus increases the overall benefit.

The next technique applied is the Mobilization Technique. The experienced therapist will have no difficulty locating the hypomobile areas of the abdominal wall. The superficial hypomobilities are sometimes difficult to identify due to the thickness of the subcutaneous fat; from experience, they are rarely relevant because of this thick layer. In the case of scars (see Chapters 13 and 14), however, the situation is different; regardless of the tissue layer and its extent, scars are a leading factor for hypomobility. They should be treated accordingly in most cases.

The deeper hypomobilities are sometimes difficult to detect and treatment may be unpleasant for the patient. They are usually located at the insertions (tenoperiosteal junction) of psoas major, iliacus, rectus abdominis, transversus abdominis, the internal oblique, the external oblique, and the diaphragm. In addition, experience has shown that it is worth mobilizing the inguinal ligament and the linea alba.

Special attention should be paid to the direction of the tissue mobility limitation. This is not necessarily identical over the entire course of the same structure; moreover, several or even all directions can be affected. The limitation can be determined by a simple test of displacement using the therapist's hand or the instrument. In the authors' experience, there is seldom a single point, but the loss of mobility usually extends to the entire structure. Depending on the structure, the mobilization is carried out with the hook or the short, flat side of the instrument using a combination curve instrument or a curved instrument (for deeper structures). It is important that the instrument always remains in contact with the same area. The instrument is not pushed over the skin, but the anatomical structure is moved in the restricted direction. The return movement is then done without pressure and is described as returning to the starting position.

The tenoperiosteal junction at the anterior part of the iliac crest is often chosen as an entry point for mobilization. Here the therapist can work with the short side of a curved or a combination curve instrument, the advantage being that mobilization can be a little more selective and therefore more precise. The therapist then works posteriorly along the iliac crest from hypomobility to hypomobility. Finally, the tenoperiosteal transitions at the ribs, sternum, and the anterior structures of the lumbar spine are mobilized.

Usually, the last technique applied in a standard treatment session is the Metabolization Technique; however, it is rarely performed on the ventral surface of lumbar patients.

Schematic Representation of the Treatment

Diagnosis
Low back pain (non-specific).

Primary structures affected (Figure 9.23)
- Gluteal fascia.
- Superficial abdominal fascia.
- Gluteus maximus.
- Transversus abdominis.
- Quadratus lumborum.
- Internal oblique.
- External oblique.
- Rectus abdominis.
- Psoas major.
- Iliacus.
- Diaphragm.

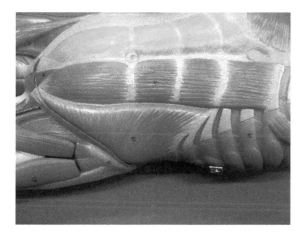

Figure 9.23 Low back pain: primary structures affected (ventral)

Initial position

Lying supine, knee joints and head supported (relaxation of the treated structure).

Material

- Recommended: straight elongated instrument, straight short instrument, curved instrument.
- Optional: combination curve instrument.

Technique

- Recommended: Rehydration, Regulation of Tone, Mobilization.
- Optional: Pain Relief Technique, Metabolization.

Recommended treatment protocol (Table 9.2)

Rehydration Technique (ReT)

- Entire area of the abdomen (superficial abdominal fascia).

Regulation of Tone Technique (RoT)

- Rectus abdominis.
- Transversus abdominis.
- Internal oblique.
- External oblique.
- Psoas major.
- Iliacus.
- Diaphragm.

Mobilization Technique (MoT)

- Superficial abdominal fascia.
- Rectus abdominis.
- Transversus abdominis.
- Internal oblique.
- External oblique.
- Psoas major.
- Iliacus.
- Diaphragm.

Table 9.2 Low back pain: summary of recommended treatment protocol (ventral structures)

ReT	PRT	RoT	MoT	MeT
Superficial abdominal fascia		Rectus abdominis	Rectus abdominis	
		Transversus abdominis	Transversus abdominis	
		Internal oblique	Internal oblique	
		External oblique	External oblique	
		Psoas major	Psoas major	
		Iliacus	Iliacus	
		Diaphragm	Diaphragm	

Visual Presentation of the Treatment Unit

Recommended treatment protocol

Rehydration Technique (ReT)

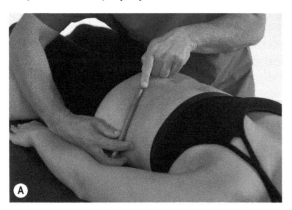

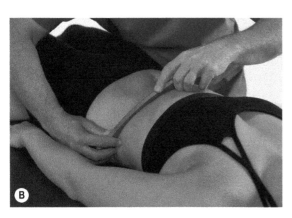

Figure 9.24 Abdominal wall (superficial abdominal fascia). (A) Start position. (B) End position.

Regulation of Tone Technique (RoT)

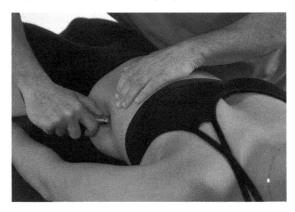

Figure 9.25 Transversus abdominis

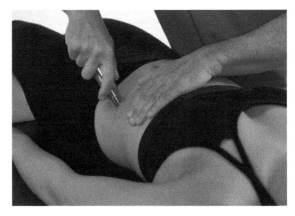

Figure 9.26 Internal oblique

Mobilization Technique (MoT)

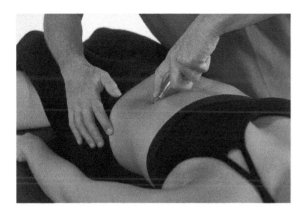

Figure 9.27 External oblique

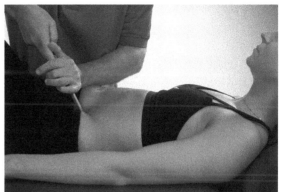

Figure 9.29 Internal oblique

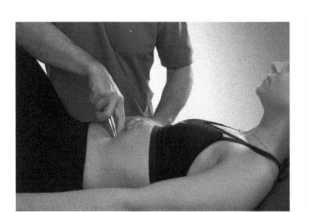

Figure 9.28 Psoas major

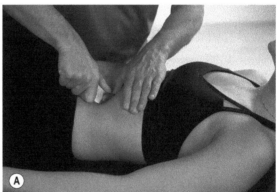

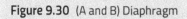

Figure 9.30 (A and B) Diaphragm

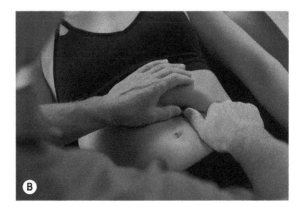

Duration

Approximately 10 minutes.

Evaluation

- Numeric rating scale (NRS).
- Finger-to-floor distance.
- Sternum wall test.
- Schober's test.
- Segmental mobility tests of the lumbar spine.

Exercise progression

A general abdominal exercise progression is recommended.

Sacroiliac Joint Dysfunction

Detailed Description of the Treatment

Sacroiliac joint dysfunction (SIJD) often involves the thoracolumbar and gluteal fascia, sacral ligaments (posterior sacroiliac, sacrospinous, sacrotuberous, and iliolumbar), and the gluteus maximus, gluteus medius, gluteus minimus, piriformis, gemellus superior, gemellus inferior, and obturator internus muscles.

The patient lies prone, with ankle joints supported (relaxation of the treated structure) or feet in overhang.

The therapy starts with the Rehydration Technique. For the sacroiliac joint, the area to be treated is divided into two: one part below the iliac crest and one part above the iliac crest. This is recommended because the technique is applied in opposite directions. The part above the iliac crest is rehydrated using the "windshield-wiper" technique, as described above. Starting from the iliac crest in line with the sacrum, the technique is performed in a cranial direction, up to the ribs and the thoracolumbar junction, with the convex side of a curved or a combination curve instrument. The therapist applies the instrument parallel to the iliac crest; the lateral end remains relatively immo-

bile, while the medial end is moved cranially with a "windshield wiper" movement. Thus, the entire area (of one side of the trunk) is completely treated at one time. The part below the iliac crest is rehydrated in the opposite direction: that is, the device is moved from cranio-lateral to caudo-medial to facilitate treating the thickness of the tissue layer. The pressure is proportional to the thickness of the soft tissue layers: the more tissue under the instrument, the higher the pressure can be. Each of these parts is treated several times. Next, the painful area of the sacroiliac joint is treated; this is usually located at the sacroiliac joint line. It is best to use a relatively short part of a curved or a combination curve instrument for this local treatment. The muscular attachments (tenoperiosteal junctions) at the sacrum and at the greater trochanter of the femur should be treated as well.

After Rehydration, the Pain Relief Technique (PRT) is usually performed. Of course, it is also possible to start with this technique; however, the patient may benefit from beginning with the gentle and rather pleasant Rehydration Technique. The Pain Relief Technique is naturally limited to the painful area(s). The authors' experience suggests that there is usually only one painful point: just over the sacroiliac joint line. In order to achieve the greatest pain relief, the painful area is provided with a high degree of mechanical stimulation through scraping. The technique is performed directly over the painful area with a progressive pressure (which should not increase the pain already present). This pressure is applied in both treatment directions: away from the treated area and then on the return. If there are several pain points, these are treated one after the other.

The next technique applied is Regulation of Tone. Application is again dependent on the physiotherapeutic findings. The hypertonic muscles are identified and treated accordingly. In the area of the sacroiliac joint, they are usually located in the gluteal muscles (gluteus maximus, gluteus medius, gluteus minimus) and in piriformis, as well as in gemellus superior, gemellus inferior, and obturator internus. All muscles surrounding the sacroiliac joint should be examined for local hypertension. Once the therapist has located a hypertonic point, they place the instrument (usually a straight short instrument) on it, apply vertical pressure to the tissue, and maintain this pressure until the tone subsides. The therapist then has the impression that they can penetrate deeper into the tissue. At the new point of tension, the pressure is held again, and the therapist waits for a new release. The technique can be completed by small movements of the instrument. In this case, the therapist moves the instrument back and forth on the spot or performs small, circular movements. Often, this "melting technique" brings an additional relaxing effect and thus increases the overall benefit.

The next technique applied is the Mobilization Technique. The superficial hypomobilities involve the thoracolumbar and gluteal fasciae. They are treated according to the protocol already described: first sensed by the displacement test, then treated accordingly.

The experienced therapist will have no difficulty locating the deeper hypomobile zones of the sacroiliac joint and the surrounding fascial ligaments (posterior sacroiliac, sacrospinous, sacrotuberous, and iliolumbar). Special attention should be paid to the direction of the tissue mobility limitation. This is not necessarily identical over the entire course of the same structure; often, several or even all directions can be affected. The limitation can be determined by a simple test of displacement using the therapist's hand or the instrument. In the authors' experience, there is seldom a single point, but the loss of mobility usually extends to the entire structure. Depending on the structure, the mobilization is carried out with the hook or the short, flat side of the instrument using a curved or a combination curve instrument. It is important that the instrument always remains in contact with the same area. The instrument is not pushed over the skin, but the anatomical structure is moved in the restricted direction. The return movement is then done without pressure and is described as returning to the starting position.

The iliolumbar ligament is often chosen as an entry point for mobilization. From here, the therapist can work with the short side of a curved or a combination curve instrument or with a straight, short instrument, the advantage being that mobilization can be more selective and therefore more precise. The therapist then treats the sacroiliac ligament along the posterior side of the sacrum from hypomobility to hypomobility further caudally. Finally, two longer ligaments are mobilized: the sacrotuberous ligament and the sacrospinous ligament, two ligaments which are very commonly involved in SIJD. While their treatment is not easy due to their deep anatomical position underneath the thick muscle layer, the therapist and patient may find it worthwhile to treat them.

The last technique applied in this standard treatment session is the Metabolization Technique. The therapist scrapes with the instrument over the area to be treated. The pressure is relatively high and varies according to the volume of the tissue: the greater the volume (that is, the thicker the layer of tissue), the greater the pressure can be. The pressure is applied in one direction only and the speed of execution is also relatively high. The pain already present must not be increased.

In the case of SIJD, no additional treatment is presented. If further therapy is required, this will involve treatment of either the dorsal hip structures or the lumbar spine.

Myofascial Connected System (MCS) (Figure 9.31)

Schematic Representation of the Treatment

Diagnosis

Sacroiliac joint dysfunction (blockage, syndrome).

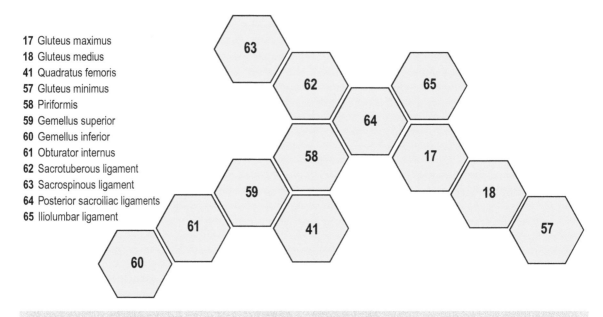

17 Gluteus maximus
18 Gluteus medius
41 Quadratus femoris
57 Gluteus minimus
58 Piriformis
59 Gemellus superior
60 Gemellus inferior
61 Obturator internus
62 Sacrotuberous ligament
63 Sacrospinous ligament
64 Posterior sacroiliac ligaments
65 Iliolumbar ligament

Figure 9.31 Sacroiliac joint dysfunction: representation of the MCS

Primary structures affected (Figures 9.32–9.34)

- Thoracolumbar and gluteal fascia.
- Posterior sacroiliac ligament.
- Sacrospinous ligament.
- Sacrotuberous ligament.
- Iliolumbar ligament.
- Gluteus maximus, gluteus medius, and gluteus minimus.
- Piriformis.
- Gemellus superior, gemellus inferior, and obturator internus.

Initial position

Lying prone, with ankle joints supported (relaxation of the treated structure) or feet in overhang.

Material

- Recommended: straight elongated instrument, combination curve instrument, straight short instrument.
- Optional: curved instrument.

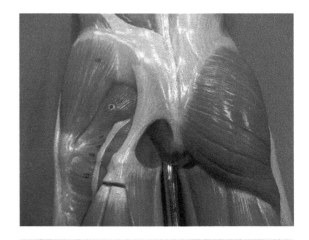

Figure 9.32 Sacroiliac joint dysfunction: primary structures affected in the iliosacral region (superficial layer)

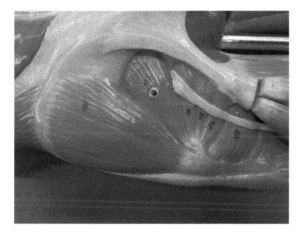

Figure 9.33 Primary affected structures (muscles) in the iliosacral region (deeper layer)

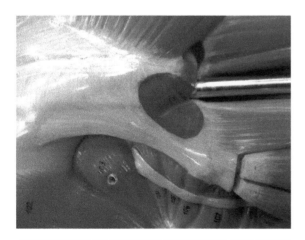

Figure 9.34 Primary affected structures (ligaments) in the iliosacral region (superficial layer, sacroiliac ligament)

Technique

- Recommended: Rehydration, Pain Relief, Regulation of Tone, Mobilization, Metabolization.
- Optional: none.

Recommended treatment protocol (Table 9.3)

Rehydration Technique (ReT)

- Area below and area above the iliac crest.
- Tenoperiosteal junction at the sacrum and at the greater trochanter.

Pain Relief Technique (PRT)

- Sacroiliac joint (joint gap).

Regulation of Tone Technique (RoT)

- Gluteus maximus.
- Gluteus medius.
- Gluteus minimus.
- Piriformis.
- Gemellus superior, gemellus inferior, and obturator internus.

Mobilization Technique (MoT)

- Thoracolumbar and gluteal fascia.
- Posterior sacroiliac ligament.
- Sacrospinous ligament.
- Sacrotuberous ligament.
- Iliolumbar ligament.

Metabolization Technique (MeT)

- Area below and area above the iliac crest.

Table 9.3 Sacroiliac joint dysfunction: summary of recommended treatment protocol				
ReT	**PRT**	**RoT**	**MoT**	**MeT**
Area below and area above the iliac crest	Painful area	Gluteus maximus	Thoracolumbar and gluteal fascia	Painful area
Tenoperiosteal junction at the sacrum and at the greater trochanter		Gluteus medius	Posterior sacroiliac ligament	
		Gluteus minimus	Sacrospinous ligament	
		Gemellus superior, gemellus inferior, and obturator internus	Sacrotuberous ligament	
			Iliolumbar ligament	

Visual Presentation of the Treatment Unit

Recommended treatment protocol

Rehydration Technique (ReT)

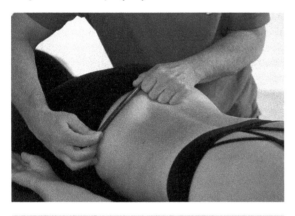

Figure 9.35 Starting position

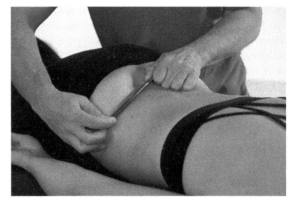

Figure 9.36 End position

Pain Relief Technique (PRT)

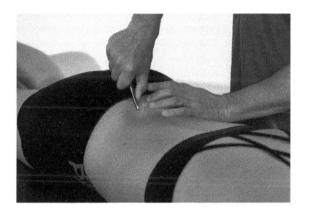

Figure 9.37 Treatment at the tenoperiosteal junction at the sacrum

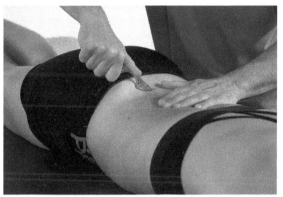

Figure 9.39 Sacroiliac junction

Regulation of Tone Technique (RoT)

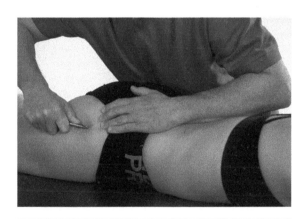

Figure 9.38 Treatment at the greater trochanter

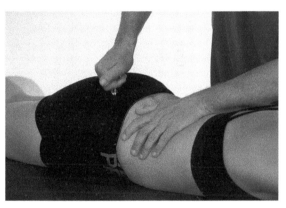

Figure 9.40 Gluteus medius

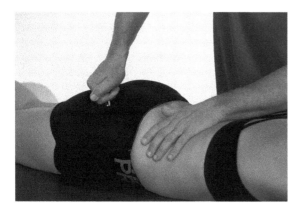

Figure 9.41 Piriformis

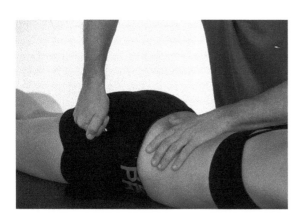

Figure 9.42 Gemellus superior, gemellus inferior, and obturator internus

Mobilization Technique (MoT)

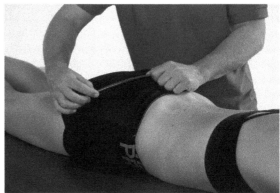

Figure 9.43 Gluteal fascia

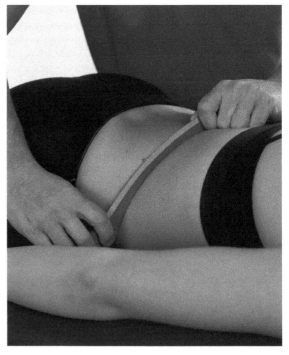

Figure 9.44 Thoracolumbar fascia

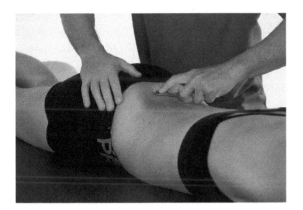

Figure 9.45 Posterior sacroiliac ligament

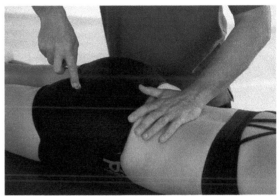

Figure 9.47 Sacrotuberous ligament

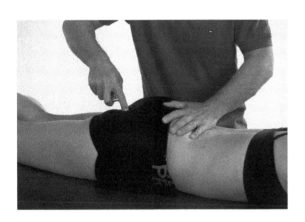

Figure 9.46 Sacrospinous ligament

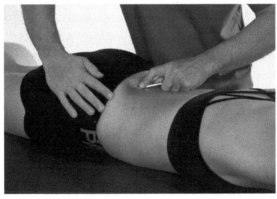

Figure 9.48 Iliolumbar ligament

Metabolization Technique (MeT)

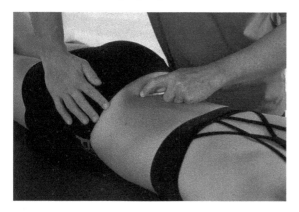

Figure 9.49 Sacroiliac joint

Duration

Approximately 20 minutes.

Evaluation

- Numeric rating scale (NRS).
- Finger-to-floor distance.
- Mobility tests of the sacroiliac joint.
- Provocation tests (compression, distraction, thigh thrust, sacral thrust, Gaenslen's test).
- Analysis of standing position.
- Analysis of gait.

Exercise progression

- Tissue stretch: stretch starting position in flexion or in rotation:
  - Lying on the side in flexion
  - Sitting on the stool
  - Prone position on the large exercise ball
  - Standing position (bent forward)
  - Side lying in rotation.
- Tissue dynamics: active movements of the lumbar spine:
  - Prone position: pushing the leg down (depression–elevation of coccyx).
- Tissue loading: functionality of the starting position:
  - Sitting on the stool
  - In standing position.
- Tissue loading+: use of tools:
  - Elastic bands around a foot (gait simulation).

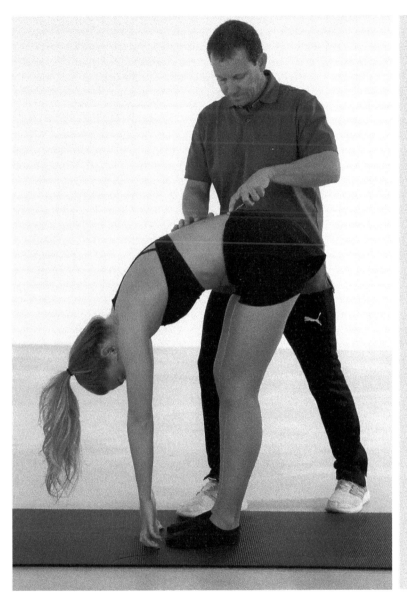

Figure 9.50 Tissue stretch: treatment in stretch starting position (flexion)

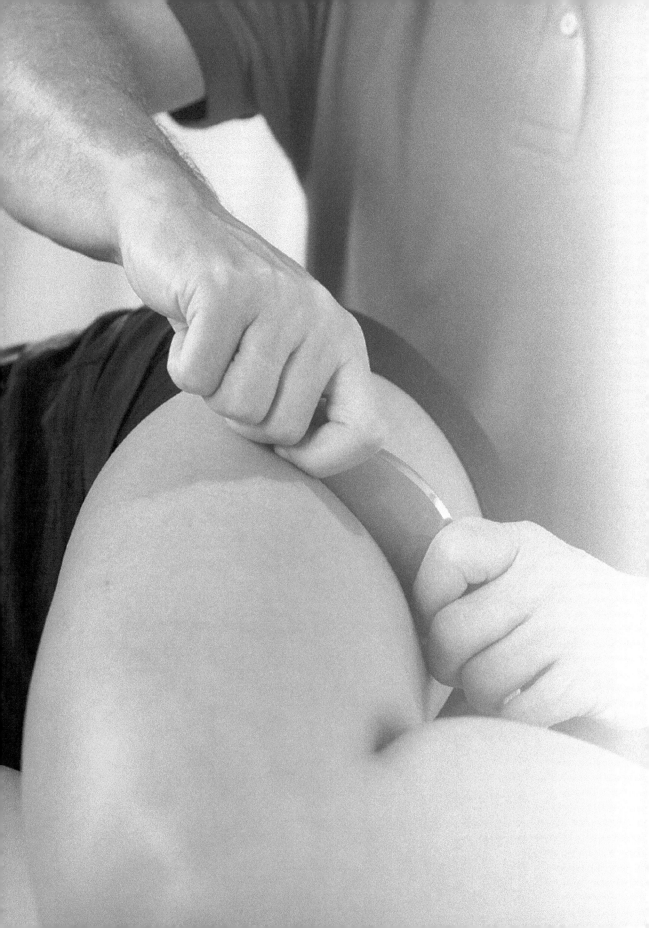

Tendinopathy of the adductors (pubalgia or groin pain) and tendinopathy of the hamstrings are representative of the musculoskeletal pathologies in the hip, thigh, and pelvis region.

Tendinopathy of the Adductors (Pubalgia, Groin Pain)

Detailed Description of the Treatment

Pubalgia (groin pain) involves the tendons of the hip adductors (pectineus, adductor longus, gracilis, adductor brevis, and adductor magnus muscles) and also the adjacent structures: the fascia lata, inguinal ligament, semitendinosus, semimembranosus, and sartorius, as well as the abdominal muscles (rectus abdominis, including the linea alba and pyramidalis, internal oblique, and external oblique).

The patient is supine, with knee joints and head supported (relaxation of the treated structure). The leg to be treated is slightly flexed, abducted, and externally rotated to make the areas treated more accessible.

The therapy starts with the Rehydration Technique using large-area sliding of the entire inner thigh, from the inner side of the knee joint (adductor tubercle) to the groin. The attachments of the adductors at the pubis rarely coincide with the lower edge of the patient's underwear but lie further cranially. However, experience has shown that treatment of the muscular attachments at the pubis is essential for success. Because of the sensitive location, the patient must be informed before treatment and consent obtained. The insertions of the gracilis muscle and the semitendinosus muscle on the medial side of the tibia are not treated initially; because they are located directly above the periosteum, they are addressed separately with less pressure applied. Treatment of the inner side of the thigh, on the other hand, requires significantly greater pressure with a longer instrument. The same applies to the more sensitive area of the adductor attachments to the pubis. The pressure is proportional to the thickness of the soft tissue layers: the more tissue under the instrument, the higher the pressure can be. Treating the inner thigh in two parts (ventro-medial and dorso-medial) is recommended, depending on the instrument and the circumference of the thigh. Each of these two parts is treated several times. Then, the affected areas – the insertions of the adductors on the inferior ramus of the pubis – are worked on. The same technique is used here; however, only the upper third of the thigh is treated. A long, curved instrument is ideal for this; while it is long and wide enough to treat the insertions of the entire adductors in one movement, its size allows treatment of these sensitive areas.

Then, after the Rehydration Technique, the Pain Relief Technique is usually performed. Of course, it is also possible to start with the Pain Relief Technique; however, beginning therapy with the Rehydration Technique has been proven to be clinically beneficial. The Pain Relief Technique is, naturally, limited to the painful area(s). Experience has shown that the insertions of the adductors on the pubis are the most painful areas (tenoperiosteal transition). Normally, treatment would begin at these points; however, in the authors' experience and with special consideration of the sensitivity of the areas to be treated, indirect treatment is recommended. If the therapist still chooses a direct technique, the pressure should be less than usual, due to the localization of the insertions directly over the bone and its well innervated periosteum. A combination curved or a straight, elongated instrument is ideally suited to this small-area treatment. It is best to use the short, convex end of the instrument. This allows one hand to control movement of the instrument and the other hand to hold the tension of the structures to avoid moving the soft tissues back and forth. In order to achieve the greatest pain relief, the painful areas are provided with a high degree of mechanical stimulation through scraping. The technique is performed directly over the painful areas with a progressive pressure (which should not increase the pain already present). This pressure is applied in both treatment directions: away from the treated area and then on the return. If there are several pain points, they are treated consecutively.

If the therapist should choose an indirect technique, it can be performed with correspondingly increased or "normal" pressure on the surrounding structures. In this case, a straight, elongated or a combination curve instrument is ideally suited. It is best to use the long, convex side of the instrument. This allows one hand to move the instrument and the other hand to hold the tension of the structures to avoid moving the soft tissues back and forth. The results of this indirect application may not be as effective as a direct application, but it should be considered as an alternative in acute conditions or very painful cases.

The next technique applied is Regulation of Tone. Application is dependent on the physiotherapeutic findings. The hypertonic muscles are identified and immediately treated. The hypertonic zones are usually found at the attachments in the proximal area of the thigh, close to the inguinal ligament. Hypertonic zones are also frequently distributed over the entire muscle bellies of the adductors down to the knee joint (adductor magnus and gracilis). Nevertheless, all the adductors should be examined for local hypertonicity. Once the therapist has located a hypertonic point, they place the instrument (straight, short instrument) on it, apply vertical pressure to the tissue, and maintain this pressure until the tone subsides. The therapist may then feel they can penetrate deeper into the tissue. At the new point of tension, the pressure is held again and the therapist waits for a new release. The technique can be completed by

small movements of the instrument. In this case, the therapist moves the instrument back and forth on the spot or performs small, circular movements. Often, this "melting technique" brings an additional relaxing effect and thus increases the overall benefit. Usually, a straight, short instrument is chosen. However, in larger patients, the length of this instrument is sometimes not sufficient to reach the deeper layers; in this case, use of a slightly longer straight, short instrument (like the Artzt Vitality Fazer 5, for example) is recommended.

The next technique applied is the Mobilization Technique. The superficial hypomobilities involve the fascia lata. They are treated according to the protocol already described: first sensed by the displacement test, then treated accordingly. The experienced therapist will have no difficulty locating the deeper hypomobile zones in the adductor muscles.

Special attention should be paid to the direction of the tissue mobility limitation, which is not necessarily identical over the entire course of the same structure; moreover, several or even all directions can be affected. The limitation can be determined by a simple test of displacement using the therapist's hand or the instrument. In the authors' experience, there is seldom a single point, but the loss of mobility usually extends to the entire structure. Depending on the structure, the mobilization is carried out with the hook or the short, flat side of the instrument. It is important that the instrument always remains in contact with the same area. The instrument is not pushed over the skin, but the anatomical structure is moved in the restricted direction. The return movement is then done without pressure and is described as returning to the starting position.

Mobilization is best started at the tenoperiosteal transitions at the pubis. While the superficial muscles (pectineus and adductor longus) are relatively easy to differentiate, the deeper muscles are more difficult. However, differentiation is not really necessary; the adductor attachments are mobilized in their entirety as deeply as possible. For this purpose, it is best to use the hook of the instrument for the proximal areas close to the bone. The adductor muscles should be examined and treated for hypomobilities throughout their entire course. This should be done up to their insertion at the adductor tubercle on the femur (adductor magnus) or up to the pes anserinus (gracilis). Furthermore, the following muscular septa should be checked for hypomobility and treated if necessary:

- between pectineus and sartorius, and between adductor longus and sartorius
- between adductor magnus and semitendinosus
- between adductor magnus and gracilis
- between gracilis and sartorius
- between gracilis and semimembranosus.

For large-scale mobilization of the muscle mass of the adductors as a whole, the convex part of an instrument (straight, elongated or curved or combination curve) can be used. However, in order to treat these structures precisely and with the necessary pressure, it is advisable to use a long, curved instrument. Due to the longer lever arm, optimum pressure can be efficiently applied.

The last technique applied in this standard treatment session is the Metabolization Technique. The therapist scrapes with the instrument over the area to be treated. The pressure is relatively high and varies according to the volume of the tissue: the greater the tissue volume (that is, the thicker the layer of tissue), the greater the pressure can be. The pressure is applied in one direction only and the speed of execution is relatively high. The pain already present must not be increased.

In addition to the "standard treatment" described above, various procedures can be added due to the holistic nature of the myofascial system, particu-

larly with longstanding symptoms affecting multiple structures. These structures are affected because of both their spatial (anatomical) proximity and their functional interaction within the execution of movement. Tone reduction may be beneficial on the following structures: fascia lata, inguinal ligament, semitendinosus, semimembranosus, and sartorius, as well as the abdominal muscles (rectus abdominis, including the linea alba and pyramidalis, internal oblique, and external oblique). The tendons of all these muscles should be mobilized if necessary. See the respective chapters for specific treatment of these areas.

Myofascial Connected System (MCS) (Figure 10.1)

Schematic Representation of the Treatment

Diagnosis

Tendinopathy of the adductors (pubalgia, groin pain).

Primary structures affected (Figure 10.2)
- Tendons of the hip adductors (pectineus, adductor longus, gracilis, adductor brevis, and adductor magnus).

Secondary structures frequently affected (Figure 10.3)
- Fascia lata.
- Inguinal ligament.
- Semitendinosus.
- Semimembranosus.
- Sartorius.
- Abdominal muscles (rectus abdominis, including the linea alba and pyramidalis, internal oblique, external oblique).

Initial position

Lying supine, with knee joints and head supported (relaxation of the treated structure); the leg to be treated is slightly flexed, abducted, and externally rotated to make the areas to be treated more accessible.

28 Inguinal ligament
29 Rectus abdominis
30 Linea alba, pyramidalis
31 Internal oblique
32 External oblique
33 Sartorius
34 Pectineus
35 Adductor longus
36 Gracilis
38 Adductor brevis
39 Adductor magnus

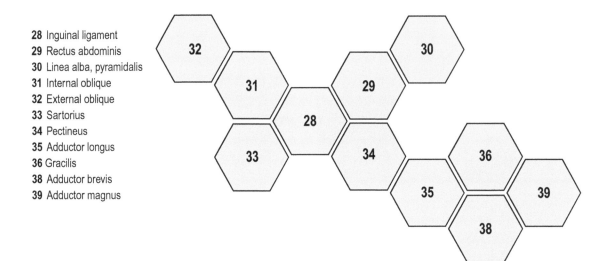

Figure 10.1 Tendinopathy of the adductors (pubalgia, groin pain): representation of the MCS

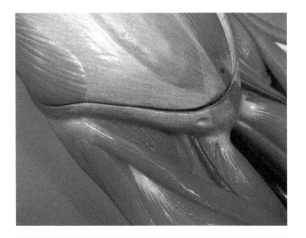

Figure 10.2 Tendinopathy of the adductors: primary structures affected

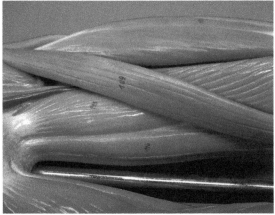

Figure 10.3 Tendinopathy of the adductors: secondary structures affected

Material
- Recommended: straight elongated instrument, curved instrument, combination instrument.
- Optional: longer straight short instrument.

Technique
- Recommended: Rehydration, Pain Relief, Regulation of Tone, Mobilization, Metabolization.
- Optional: none.

Recommended treatment protocol (Table 10.1)

Rehydration Technique (ReT)

- Hip adductors:
  - Pectineus
  - Adductor longus
  - Gracilis
  - Adductor brevis
  - Adductor magnus.

Pain Relief Technique (PRT)

- Insertions of the adductors on the pubis are the most painful areas (tenoperiosteal transition).
- Use an indirect technique if necessary.

Regulation of Tone Technique (RoT)

- Hip adductors:
  - Pectineus
  - Adductor longus
  - Gracilis
  - Adductor brevis
  - Adductor magnus.

Mobilization Technique (MoT)

- Fascia lata.
- Proximal insertions of the adductors on the pubis are the most painful areas (tenoperiosteal transition).
- Distal insertions of the adductors at the adductor tubercle (adductor magnus) and the pes anserinus (gracilis).
- Muscular septa between:
  - pectineus and sartorius, and between adductor longus and sartorius
  - adductor magnus and semitendinosus
  - adductor magnus and gracilis
  - gracilis and sartorius
  - gracilis and semimembranosus.

Metabolization Technique (MeT)

- Insertions of the adductors on the pubis are the most painful areas (tenoperiosteal transition).

Table 10.1 Tendinopathy of the adductors (pubalgia, groin pain): summary of recommended treatment protocol

ReT	PRT	RoT	MoT	MeT
Pectineus	Painful area	Pectineus	Fascia lata	Painful area
Adductor longus		Adductor longus	Proximal insertions of the adductors on the pubis are the most painful areas (tenoperiosteal transition)	
Gracilis		Gracilis	Distal insertions of the adductors at the adductor tubercle (adductor magnus) and the pes anserinus (gracilis)	
Adductor brevis		Adductor brevis	Muscular septa between: • pectineus and sartorius, and between adductor longus and sartorius • adductor magnus and semitendinosus • adductor magnus and gracilis • gracilis and sartorius • gracilis and semimembranosus	
Adductor magnus		Adductor magnus		

Table 10.2 Tendinopathy of the adductors (pubalgia, groin pain): summary of optional treatment protocol

RoT	MoT
Semitendinosus	Semitendinosus
Semimembranosus	Semimembranosus
Sartorius	Sartorius
Rectus abdominis	Inguinal ligament
Internal oblique	Linea alba
External oblique	

Optional treatment protocol (Table 10.2)

Regulation of Tone (RoT)

- Semitendinosus.
- Semimembranosus.
- Sartorius.
- Rectus abdominis.
- Internal oblique.
- External oblique.

Mobilization Technique (MoT)

- Semitendinosus.
- Semimembranosus.
- Sartorius.
- Inguinal ligament.
- Linea alba.

Visual Presentation of the Treatment Unit

Recommended treatment protocol

Rehydration Technique (ReT)

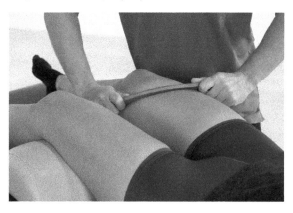

Figure 10.4 Medial thigh (hip adductors): start position

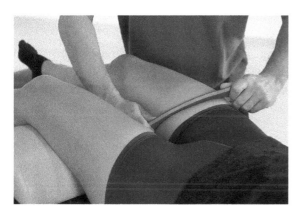

Figure 10.5 Medial thigh (hip adductors): end position

Regulation of Tone Technique (RoT)

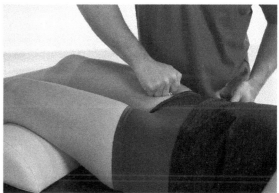

Figure 10.7 Pectineus

Pain Relief Technique (PRT)

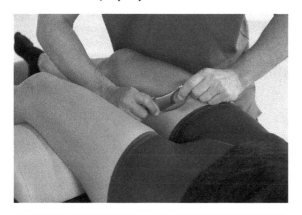

Figure 10.6 Insertions of the adductors on the pubis. These are the most painful areas (tenoperiosteal transition): use an indirect technique if necessary

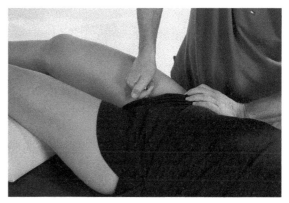

Figure 10.8 Adductor longus

Mobilization Technique (MoT)

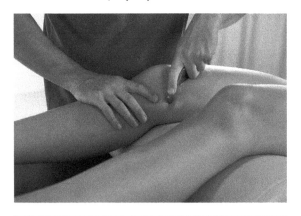

Figure 10.9 Distal insertions of the adductors at the adductor tubercle (hook)

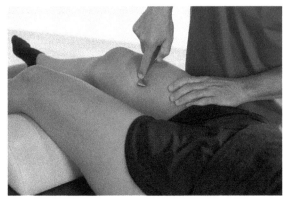

Figure 10.11 Gracilis and sartorius

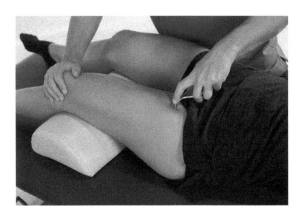

Figure 10.10 Muscular septa between pectineus and sartorius (edge)

Metabolization Technique (MeT)

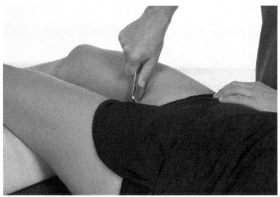

Figure 10.12 Insertions of the adductors on the pubis: these are the most painful areas (tenoperiosteal transition)

Optional treatment protocol

Regulation of Tone Technique (RoT)

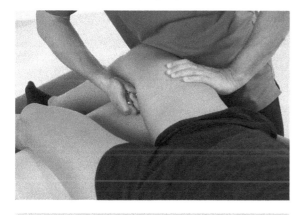

Figure 10.13 Semitendinosus

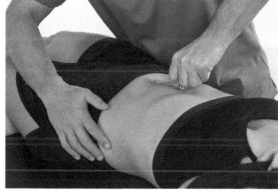

Figure 10.15 Rectus abdominis

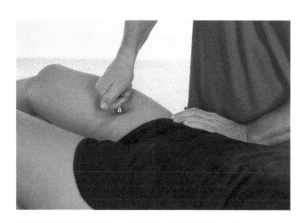

Figure 10.14 Sartorius

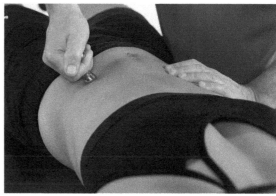

Figure 10.16 External oblique

Mobilization Technique (MoT)

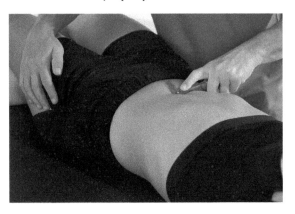

Figure 10.17 Linea alba

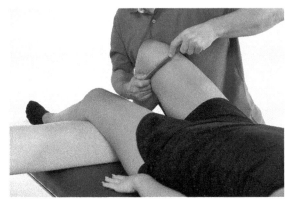

Figure 10.18 Treatment in middle abduction

Duration

Approximately 20 minutes.

Evaluation

- Numeric rating scale (NRS).
- ROM hip joint (adduction, extension).
- End-feel (adduction, extension).
- Pain provocation test in lying (hip adduction against resistance).
- Pain provocation test in standing: lateral lunge.
- Analysis of gait.
- Analysis of running.

Exercise progression

- Tissue stretch: stretch starting position: lying supine; hip in middle abduction, then in full abduction.
- Tissue dynamics: active movements of the hip (abduction–adduction).
- Tissue dynamics+: active movements of the hip (abduction–adduction) against elastic resistance.
- Tissue loading: functionality of the starting position: e.g. lateral lunge.

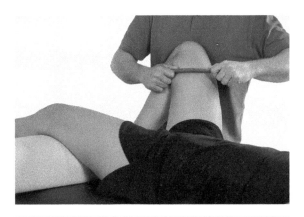

Figure 10.19 Treatment in full abduction

- Tissue loading+: use of tools: e.g. bands, stability trainer.

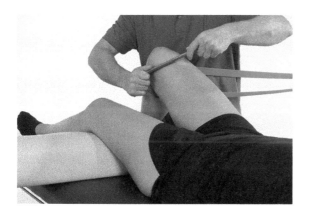

Figure 10.20 Tissue dynamics+: treatment with active movements against elastic resistance (starting position)

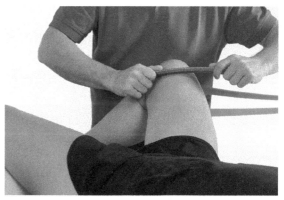

Figure 10.21 Tissue dynamics+: treatment with active movements against elastic resistance (end position)

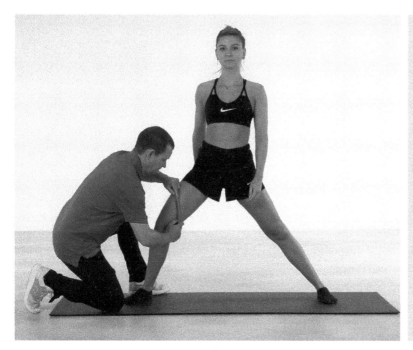

Figure 10.22 Tissue loading: treatment in functional position – lateral lunge

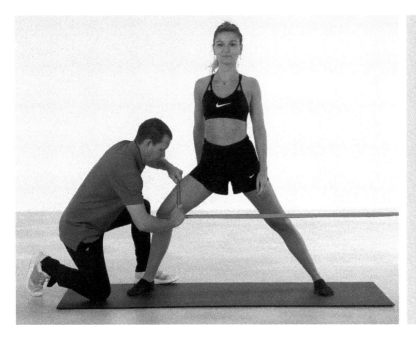

Figure 10.23 Tissue loading+: treatment in functional position – lateral lunge against elastic resistance

Tendinopathy of the Hamstrings
Detailed Description of the Treatment

Tendinopathy of the hamstrings affects the semitendinosus, semimembranosus, and biceps femoris muscles, as well as the adjacent structures: fascia lata, iliotibial tract (or iliotibial band, ITB), peroneus longus (fibularis longus), gastrocnemius, vastus lateralis, sartorius, gracilis, adductor magnus, gluteus maximus, vastus medialis, and the short quadratus femoris and popliteus.

The patient is prone, with ankle joints supported (relaxation of the treated structure). Slight adduction (relaxation of the "semis") or external rotation (relaxation of biceps femoris) may be appropriate for maximum relaxation of certain structures.

The therapy starts with the Rehydration Technique using large-area sliding of the entire dorsal thigh, from the knee joint (above the popliteal fossa) to the ischial tuberosity. The attachments of the hamstrings at the ischial tuberosity rarely coincide with the inferior border of the gluteus maximus muscle but lie much further proximally. As with the attachments of the adductors, it is best for the therapist to explain this to the patient before starting the treatment. The short head of biceps femoris (inserting on the middle third of the lateral lip of the linea aspera) is also treated, even if this area is rarely affected by tendinopathy. If the area is painful, the rounded side of a straight, elongated or curved instrument is suitable for rehydration. Due to its very deep location, the pressure applied must be correspondingly high. The insertions of the following muscles at the tibia or the fibula are initially left out and treated separately: proximal insertions at the ischial tuberosity and distal insertions at the tibia at the pes anserinus (semitendinosus, semimembranosus) and biceps femoris at the fibula. Since they are located directly above the periosteum, the pressure must be adjusted. Treatment of the posterior thigh with the long curved instrument, on the other hand, requires significantly greater pressure.

Treating the dorsal side of the thigh in at least three parts (dorso-medial, dorsal, and dorso-lateral) is recommended, depending on the instrument and the circumference of the thigh. Each of these three parts is treated several times. Then, the affected areas – the insertions of the hamstrings at the ischial tuberosity – are treated. The same technique is used here; however, only the upper third of the thigh is treated. A curved instrument is ideal for this treatment; while it is long and wide enough to treat the insertions of the entire hamstrings in one movement, its size allows effective treatment of these sensitive areas.

Then, after rehydration, the Pain Relief Technique is usually performed. Of course, it is possible to start with this; however, beginning therapy with the gentle and rather pleasant Rehydration Technique has been used successfully. The technique is, naturally, limited to the painful area(s). Experience has shown that the insertions of the hamstrings at the ischial tuberosity are the most painful areas (tenoperiosteal transition). Sometimes, the transition between the tendon and the muscle (myotendinous transition) is also painful. The short head of the biceps (insertion in the middle third of the lateral lip of the linea aspera) is rarely affected by tendinopathy, but if it is painful, the rounded side of a straight, elongated or curved instrument is suitable for pain relief. Due to its very deep location, the pressure applied must be correspondingly high. In order to achieve the greatest pain relief, the painful areas are provided with a high degree of mechanical stimulation through scraping. The technique is performed directly over the painful areas with a progressive pressure (which should not increase the pain already present). This pressure is applied in both treatment directions: away from the treated area and then on the return. If there are several pain points, they are treated consecutively.

The next technique applied is the Regulation of Tone. Application is dependent on the physio-therapeutic findings. The hypertonic muscles are identified and immediately treated accordingly. In the case of the hamstrings, they are usually located in the distal half of the muscle bellies (in the lower third of the thigh), in both the "semis" and the long head of the biceps, but rarely in the deeper-lying short head. Nevertheless, all three (or four) parts of the hamstring muscles should be examined for local hypertonicity. Once the therapist has located a hypertonic point, they place the instrument (straight, short instrument) on it, apply vertical pressure to the tissue, and maintain this pressure until the tone subsides. The therapist then has the impression that they can penetrate deeper into the tissue. At the new point of tension, the pressure is held again and the therapist waits for a new release. The technique can be completed by small movements of the instrument. In this case, the therapist moves the instrument back and forth on the spot or performs small, circular movements. Often, this "melting technique" brings an additional relaxing effect and thus increases the overall benefit.

The next technique applied is the Mobilization Technique. The superficial hypomobilities usually involve the fascia lata. They are treated according to the protocol already described: first identified by the displacement test, then treated accordingly. The experienced therapist will have no difficulty locating the deeper hypomobile zones of the hamstrings.

Special attention should be paid to the direction of the tissue mobility limitation. Limitations are not necessarily identical over the entire course of the same structure; moreover, several or even all directions can be affected. The limitation can be determined by a simple test of displacement using the therapist's hand or the instrument. In our experience, there is seldom a single point, but the loss of mobility usually extends to the entire structure.

Depending on the structure, focal mobilization is carried out with the hook or the short, flat side of an instrument. Smaller areas are treated with the convexity of an instrument; larger areas can be treated with the convexity of a long, curved instrument. Sometimes, the loss of mobility is greater with depth (between the two heads of the biceps femoris muscle and/or between semitendinosus and semimembranosus); thus the hypomobility is so pronounced that a long, curved instrument is used with its short side since the lever arm is longer and allows better mobilization.

The relatively long tendons of the long head of biceps femoris and semitendinosus can easily be mobilized with the flat edge of an instrument or its hook. It is important that the instrument always remains in contact with the same area. The instrument is not pushed over the skin, but the anatomical structure is moved in the restricted direction. The return movement is then done without pressure and is described as returning to the starting position.

Other hypomobilities are often located in the following muscular septa:

- between hamstrings and gluteus maximus
- between biceps femoris and the iliotibial tract
- between biceps femoris and semitendinosus
- between biceps femoris and vastus lateralis
- between semitendinosus and adductor magnus
- between semimembranosus and adductor magnus
- between semimembranosus and gracilis
- between semimembranosus and vastus medialis.

To treat these structures precisely and with the necessary pressure, it is advisable to use a long curved instrument. Due to the longer lever arm, optimum pressure can be applied efficiently.

The last technique applied in this standard treatment session is the Metabolization Technique. The therapist scrapes with the instrument over the area to be treated. The pressure is relatively high but varies according to the volume of the tissue: the greater the volume (that is, the thicker the layer of tissue), the greater the pressure can be. The pressure is applied in one direction only and the speed of execution is also relatively high. The pain already present must not be increased.

In addition to the "standard treatment" described above, various procedures can be added due to the holistic nature of the myofascial system, particularly with longstanding symptoms affecting multiple structures. In the case of tendinopathy of the hamstrings, the following structures often also have local hypertonicity, which should be treated as described above. These structures are affected because of both their spatial (anatomical) proximity and their functional interaction within the execution of movement. Regulation of Tone may be applied to the following structures: fascia lata, iliotibial tract, peroneus longus, gastrocnemius, vastus lateralis, sartorius, gracilis, adductor magnus, gluteus maximus, vastus medialis, quadratus femoris, and popliteus. See the respective chapters for specific treatment of these areas.

Myofascial Connected System (MCS) (Figure 10.24)

Schematic Representation of the Treatment

Diagnosis
Tendinopathy of the hamstrings.

Primary structures affected (Figures 10.25 and 10.26)
- Semitendinosus.
- Semimembranosus.
- Biceps femoris.

Secondary structures frequently affected (Figure 10.27)
- Fascia lata.
- Iliotibial tract (or iliotibial band, ITB).
- Peroneus longus.

3 Peroneus longus
4 Gastrocnemius
7 Iliotibial tract
8 Biceps femoris
17 Gluteus maximus
19 Vastus lateralis
24 Vastus medialis
33 Sartorius
36 Gracilis
37 Semitendinosus
39 Adductor magnus
40 Semimembranosus
41 Quadratus femoris
42 Popliteus

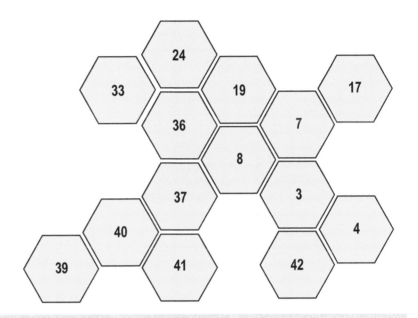

Figure 10.24 Tendinopathy of the hamstrings: representation of the MCS

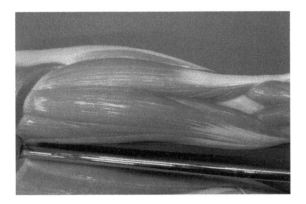

Figure 10.25 Tendinopathy of the hamstrings: primary structures affected – superficial layer

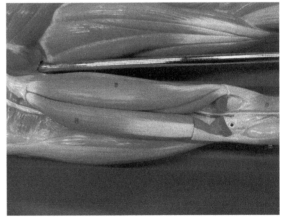

Figure 10.26 Tendinopathy of the hamstrings: primary structures affected – deep layer

- Gastrocnemius.
- Vastus lateralis.
- Sartorius.
- Gracilis.
- Adductor magnus.

- Gluteus maximus.
- Vastus medialis.
- Quadratus femoris.
- Popliteus.

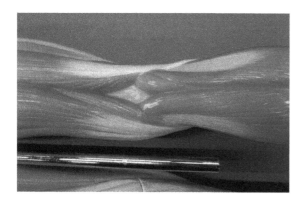

Figure 10.27 Tendinopathy of the hamstrings: secondary structures affected

Initial position

Lying prone, with a cushion underlying ankle joints (relaxation of the treated structure). Slight adduction (relaxation of the "semis") or exter-nal rotation (relaxation of the biceps) may be appropriate for maximum relaxation of certain structures.

Material
- Recommended: straight elongated instrument, curved instrument, straight short instrument.
- Optional: none.

Technique
- Recommended: Rehydration, Pain Relief, Regulation of Tone, Mobilization, Metabolization.
- Optional: none.

Recommended treatment protocol (Table 10.3)

Rehydration Technique (ReT)
- Thigh: dorsal side (in three parts: dorso-medial, dorsal, dorso-lateral).

Table 10.3 Tendinopathy of the hamstrings: summary of recommended treatment protocol				
ReT	**PRT**	**RoT**	**MoT**	**MeT**
Thigh: dorsal side (in three parts: dorso-medial, dorsal, dorso-lateral)	Painful area	Semitendinosus	Fascia lata	Painful area
Proximal insertions at ischial tuberosity and linea aspera (lower third)		Semimembranosus	Hamstrings: semitendinosus, semimembranosus, biceps femoris (muscle bellies and tendons)	
Distal insertions at the tibia (pes anserinus), semitendinosus, semimembranosus and the fibula (biceps femoris)		Biceps femoris	Between semitendinosus and semimembranosus	
			Between semitendinosus and semimembranosus	
			Muscular septa between: • hamstrings and gluteus maximus • biceps femoris and iliotibial tract • biceps femoris and semitendinosus • biceps femoris and vastus lateralis • semitendinosus and adductor magnus • semimembranosus and adductor magnus • semimembranosus and gracilis • semimembranosus and vastus medialis	

- Proximal insertions at the ischial tuberosity and linea aspera (lower third).
- Distal insertions at the tibia (pes anserinus), semitendinosus, semimembranosus and the fibula (biceps femoris).

Pain Relief Technique (PRT)

- Proximal insertions at the ischial tuberosity.

Regulation of Tone Technique (RoT)

- Hamstrings: semitendinosus, semimembranosus, biceps femoris – distal half of the muscle bellies (in the lower third of the thigh).

Mobilization Technique (MoT)

- Fascia lata.
- Hamstrings: semitendinosus, semimembranosus, biceps femoris (muscle bellies and tendons).
- Between the two heads of biceps femoris.
- Between semitendinosus and semimembranosus.
- Muscular septa between:
  - hamstrings and gluteus maximus
  - biceps femoris and the iliotibial tract
  - biceps femoris and semitendinosus
  - biceps femoris and vastus lateralis
  - semitendinosus and adductor magnus
  - semimembranosus and adductor magnus
  - semimembranosus and gracilis
  - semimembranosus and vastus medialis.

Metabolization Technique (MeT)

- Proximal insertions at the ischial tuberosity.

Optional treatment protocol (Table 10.4)

Regulation of Tone Technique (RoT)

- Iliotibial tract.
- Peroneus longus.
- Gastrocnemius.
- Vastus lateralis.

- Sartorius.
- Gracilis.
- Adductor magnus.
- Gluteus maximus.
- Vastus medialis.
- Quadratus femoris.
- Popliteus.

Mobilization Technique (MoT)

- Iliotibial tract.
- Vastus lateralis.
- Sartorius.
- Gracilis.
- Adductor magnus.
- Vastus medialis.

Table 10.4 Tendinopathy of the hamstrings: summary of optional treatment protocol

RoT	MoT
Iliotibial tract	Iliotibial tract
Peroneus longus	Vastus lateralis
Gastrocnemius	Sartorius
Vastus lateralis	Gracilis
Sartorius	Adductor magnus
Gracilis	Vastus medialis
Adductor magnus	
Gluteus maximus	
Vastus medialis	
Quadratus femoris	
Popliteus	

Visual Presentation of the Treatment Unit

Recommended treatment protocol

Rehydration Technique (ReT)

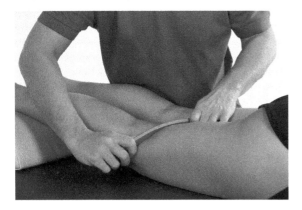

Figure 10.28 Thigh: dorsal side

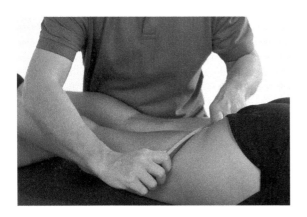

Figure 10.29 Proximal insertions at ischial tuberosity and linea aspera (lower third)

Pain Relief Technique (PRT)

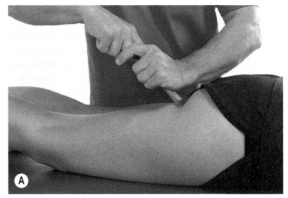

A

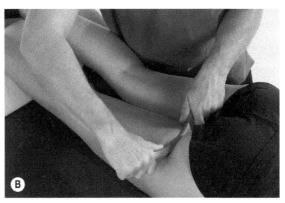

B

Figure 10.30 (A and B) Proximal insertions at the ischial tuberosity

Regulation of Tone Technique (RoT)

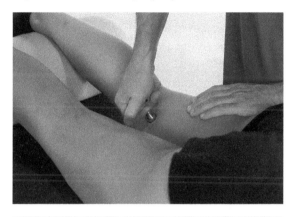

Figure 10.31 Semitendinosus

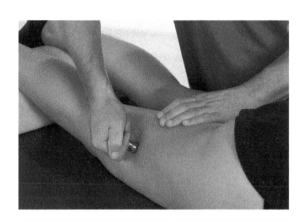

Figure 10.32 Biceps femoris

Mobilization Technique (MoT)

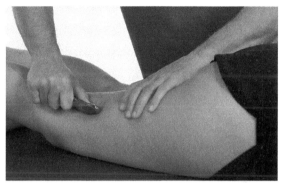

Figure 10.33 Between the two heads of biceps femoris

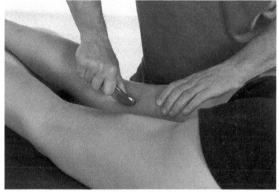

Figure 10.34 Between semitendinosus and semimembranosus

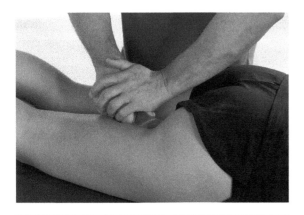

Figure 10.35 Between the hamstrings and gluteus maximus

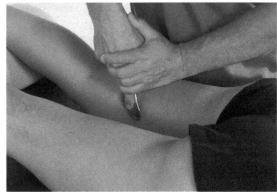

Figure 10.37 Semitendinosus and adductor magnus

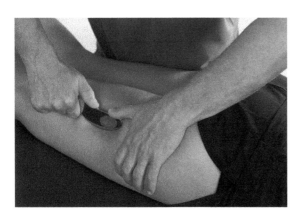

Figure 10.36 Biceps femoris and iliotibial tract

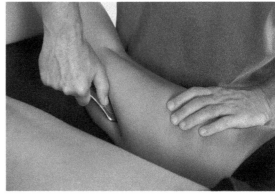

Figure 10.38 Semimembranosus and vastus medialis

Metabolization Technique (MeT)

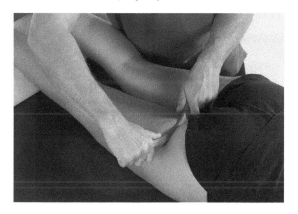

Figure 10.39 Proximal insertions at ischial tuberosity

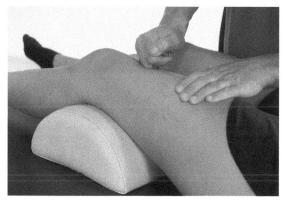

Figure 10.41 Vastus medialis

Optional treatment protocol

Regulation of Tone Technique (RoT)

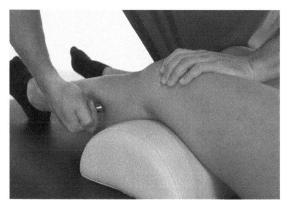

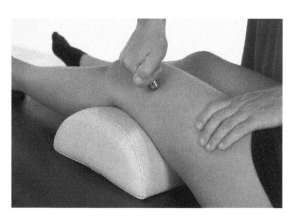

Figure 10.42 Vastus lateralis

Figure 10.40 Peroneus longus

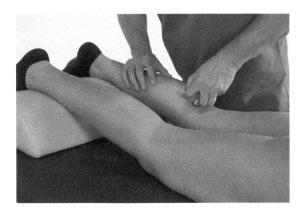

Figure 10.43 Popliteus

Mobilization Technique (MoT)

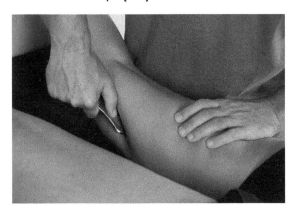

Figure 10.44 Gracilis

Duration

Approximately 20 minutes.

Evaluation

- Numeric rating scale (NRS).
- Straight leg raise or extension of the knee with hip flexed.
- End-feel (hip flexion, knee extension).
- Pain provocation test in lying (knee flexion against resistance).
- Pain provocation test in standing: ventral lunge.
- Analysis of gait.
- Analysis of running.

Exercise progression

- Tissue stretch: stretch starting position:
  ○ lying supine; hip in maximal flexion; knee bent (relaxed); the patient holds the leg with the hands or a sling in this position (tissue stress)
  ○ lying on the side: lateral position, leg supported on a pillow, hip flexed, knee extended.

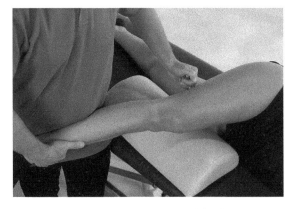

Figure 10.45 Tissue stretch: treatment in stretched position

- Tissue dynamics: active movements of the knee (flexion–extension).
- Tissue dynamics+: active movements of the knee (flexion–extension) against elastic resistance.

- Tissue loading: functionality of the starting position: e.g. ventral lunge.
- Tissue loading +: use of tools: e.g. bands, stability trainer.

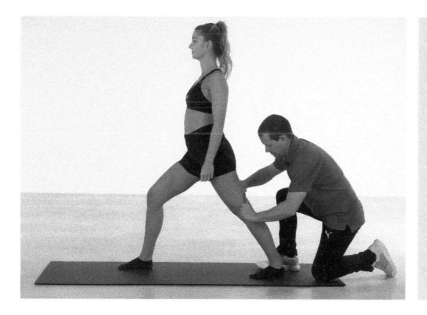

Figure 10.46 Tissue loading: treatment in a functional position (ventral lunge)

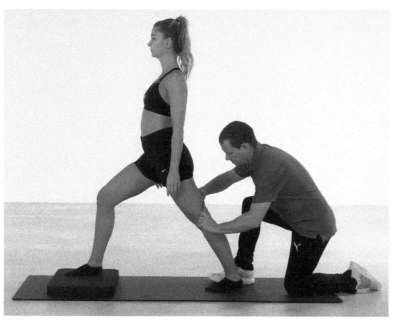

Figure 10.47 Tissue loading+: treatment standing on unstable surface

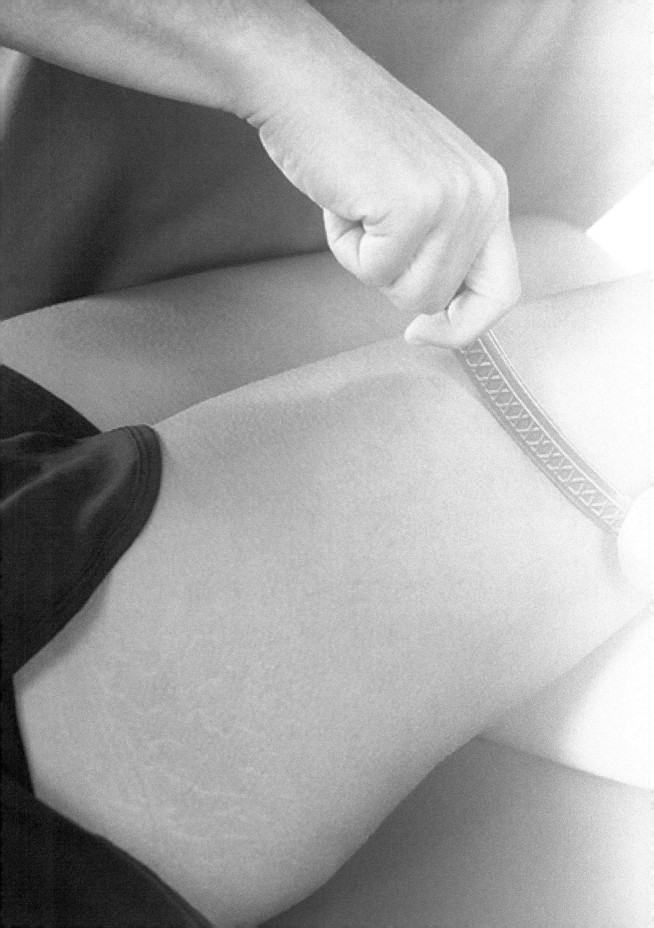

Two common knee diagnoses are presented here: iliotibial tract friction syndrome (IT band syndrome, runner's knee) and tendinopathy of the patellar ligament (patellar tendinopathy, jumper's knee). These diagnoses are representative of the range of musculoskeletal pathologies in the knee; treatment is adapted according to the symptoms and the suspected causes.

Iliotibial Tract Friction Syndrome
Detailed Description of the Treatment

Iliotibial tract friction syndrome (IT band syndrome, runner's knee) affects the iliotibial tract and the tensor fasciae latae, and also the adjacent structures: fascia lata and deep fascia of the leg (fascia cruris), tibialis anterior, gluteus maximus and gluteus medius, quadriceps femoris (vastus lateralis, rectus femoris), and biceps femoris (short head), as well as the lateral patellar retinaculum and the lateral collateral ligament.

The patient is supine with the knee joints supported, or lies prone with the ankle joint supported.

The therapy starts with the Rehydration Technique using large-area sliding of the entire iliotibial tract (IT band) from Gerdy's tubercle to the anterior superior iliac spine, as well as the connecting fibers of gluteus maximus. Starting from Gerdy's tubercule, the technique is performed in a cranial direction up to the vastus lateralis muscle. At this point, the iliotibial tract is rather narrow and runs closely over the bone; the technique is accordingly performed with little pressure and with the narrow edge of the hook of an instrument. As the therapist moves from this area, the technique can be performed with considerably more pressure and with a wider part of the instrument, as the iliotibial tract widens somewhat and no longer lies directly over a bony struc-

ture; here, the concave side of the instrument is preferred. Just below the greater trochanter, the iliotibial tract becomes even wider and radiates into the gluteus maximus muscle. Gluteal fibers with different orientations cross in this area. In the authors' experience, this is a site of great tension and is correspondingly prone to disruption and frequent dehydration. Here the technique is repeated several times by alternately directing the instrument cranially in the direction of the anterior superior iliac spine and cranio-dorsally in the direction of the fibers of gluteus maximus.

After the Rehydration Technique, the Pain Relief Technique is usually performed. Of course, it is also possible to start with this technique; however, beginning therapy with the gentle and rather pleasant Rehydration Technique has proven to be effective in the authors' opinion. The technique is, naturally, limited to the painful area(s). The most common painful area is typically where the iliotibial tract slides over the lateral epicondyle. Since this area of the iliotibial tract is not covered with much tissue, but rather is in direct contact with the bone or its periosteum, the pressure exerted with the instrument must be reduced. In order to achieve the greatest pain relief, the painful areas are provided with a high degree of mechanical stimulation through instrument scraping. The technique is performed directly over the painful areas with a progressive pressure (which should not increase the pain already present). This pressure is applied in both treatment directions: away from the treated area and then on the return. Extending the treated area in a cranial direction is recommended. More pressure can be applied there and thus more proprioceptive input given for increased pain reduction. If there are several pain points, they are treated consecutively.

The next technique applied is Regulation of Tone. Application is again dependent on the physiotherapeutic findings. The hypertonic muscles are identified on palpation and treated accordingly. In the case of iliotibial tract friction syndrome, the hypertonic muscles are usually located in the muscle belly of the tensor fasciae latae, particularly at the upper ventral edge. However, there are typically numerous hypertonic points along the entire iliotibial tract. Although the iliotibial tract has much fewer contractile properties than the muscular part, the authors' experience suggests that it is worthwhile applying this technique here as well. Once the therapist has located a hypertonic point, they place the instrument on it, apply vertical pressure to the tissue, and maintain this pressure until the tone subsides. The therapist may then have the impression that they can penetrate deeper into the tissue. At the new point of tension, the pressure is held again and the therapist waits for a new release. The technique can be completed by small movements of the instrument. In this case, the therapist moves the instrument back and forth on the spot or performs small, circular movements. Often, this "melting technique" brings an additional relaxing effect and thus increases the overall benefit.

The next technique applied is the Mobilization Technique. The superficial hypomobilities involve the fascia lata. It is treated according to the protocol previously described: first identified by the displacement test, then treated accordingly. The experienced therapist will have no difficulty locating the deeper hypomobile zones of the iliotibial tract.

Special attention should be paid to the direction of the tissue mobility limitation. This is not necessarily identical over the entire course of the same structure; moreover, several or even all directions can be affected. The limitation can be determined by a simple test of displacement using the therapist's hand or the instrument. In the authors' experience, there is seldom a single point, but the loss of mobility usually extends throughout the entire structure. There is often a particularly pronounced hypomobility both in the painful area at the lateral epicondyle and in the area of the greater trochanter. The important role of the iliotibial tract as a so-called "active ligament" (stabilization of the leg axis in the frontal plane during walking and running) requires a corresponding tensile strength in the longitudinal direction of the structure. However, the iliotibial tract is not very thick and is a relative thickening of the fascia lata; thus, it is often limited in its mobility in the posterior–anterior or anterior–posterior direction.

After the displacement test, the iliotibial tract is mobilized in the restricted direction. The instrument is selected depending on the size of the hypomobile area. Smaller areas are treated with the convexity of a curved or combination curve instrument; larger areas can be treated with the concavity of a curved or combination curve instrument. Sometimes, even after regulation of tone, the tension is so strong and the hypomobility so pronounced that the instrument is used with its short side because the lever arm is longer and allows better mobilization. These hypomobilities are often very painful. Alternating treatment with the Rehydration Technique and/or the Pain Relief Technique is recommended if this is the case. However, remember that it is important that the instrument always remains in contact with the same area. The instrument is not pushed over the skin, but the anatomical structure is mobilized in the restricted direction. The return movement is then performed without pressure and is described as returning to the starting position. The painful area over the lateral epicondyle is often chosen as a starting point for mobilization. The therapist can begin with the short side of the hook of an instrument, the advantage being that mobilization can be more selective and therefore more precise. Due to the flat nature of the short side of some instruments, the therapist sometimes slips over the structure; unfortunately, patients often find this unpleasant. The therapist then works along the iliotibial tract from hypomobility to hypomobility in the cranial direction.

The last technique applied in this standard treatment session is the Metabolization Technique. The therapist scrapes with the instrument over the area to be treated. The pressure is relatively high. It varies according to the volume of the tissue: the greater the volume (that is, the thicker the layer of tissue), the greater the pressure can be. The pressure is applied in one direction only and the speed of execution is relatively high; however, the pain already present must not be increased.

In addition to the "standard treatment" described above, various procedures can be performed. When the symptoms have been present for a long period of time, the painful area becomes larger and affects more structures. In the case of iliotibial tract friction syndrome, several other structures may have local hypertonicity and should be treated as described above. These structures are affected due to their proximity and also their functional interaction during the execution of movement. Regulation of Tone may be effective on the following structures: tibialis anterior, gluteus maximus and gluteus medius, quadriceps femoris (vastus lateralis, rectus femoris), and biceps femoris (short head).

The tendons of each of these muscles should be mobilized if necessary. Often, mobilization of the lateral patellar retinaculum and the lateral collateral ligament is indicated. The reader will find treatment of these areas in corresponding chapters; in addition to the table of contents, Figure I.1 in the Introduction is suitable for quickly finding the corresponding structures in the book. The treatment is virtually identical that already described. The therapist needs only to adapt the techniques to these structures or to the known conditions.

Myofascial Connected System (MCS) (Figure 11.1)

Schematic Representation of the Treatment

Diagnosis

Iliotibial tract friction syndrome (IT band syndrome, runner's knee).

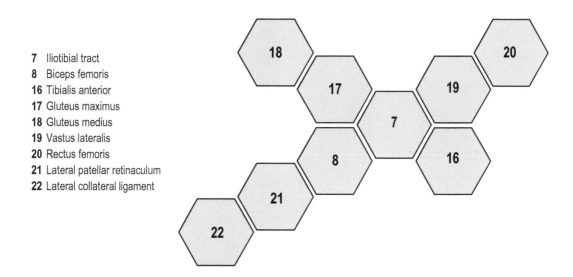

7   Iliotibial tract
8   Biceps femoris
16 Tibialis anterior
17 Gluteus maximus
18 Gluteus medius
19 Vastus lateralis
20 Rectus femoris
21 Lateral patellar retinaculum
22 Lateral collateral ligament

Figure 11.1 Iliotibial tract friction syndrome: representation of the MCS

Primary structures affected (Figure 11.2)
- Iliotibial tract (IT band).
- Tensor fasciae latae.

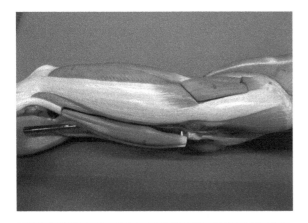

Figure 11.2 Iliotibial tract friction syndrome: primary structures affected

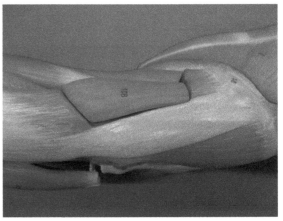

Figure 11.3 Iliotibial tract friction syndrome: secondary structures affected – cranial part of the IT band

Secondary structures frequently affected (Figures 11.3 and 11.4)
- Fascia lata and deep fascia of the leg (fascia cruris).
- Tibialis anterior.
- Gluteus maximus and gluteus medius.
- Quadriceps femoris (vastus lateralis, rectus femoris).
- Biceps femoris (short head).
- Lateral patellar retinaculum.
- Lateral collateral ligament.

Initial position
Lying supine.

Material
- Recommended: straight elongated instrument, curved instrument, straight short instrument.
- Optional: none.

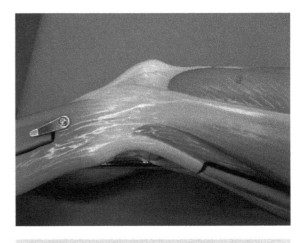

Figure 11.4 Iliotibial tract friction syndrome: secondary structures affected – caudal part of the IT band

Technique
- Recommended: Rehydration, Pain Relief, Regulation of Tone, Mobilization, Metabolization.
- Optional: none.

Table 11.1 Iliotibial tract friction syndrome: summary of recommended treatment protocol				
ReT	PRT	RoT	MoT	MeT
Iliotibial tract (and fascia lata)	Painful area	Tensor fasciae latae	Fascia lata	Portion of the iliotibial tract over the lateral epicondyle
Tensor fasciae latae		Iliotibial tract	Iliotibial tract	
			Tensor fasciae latae	

Recommended treatment protocol (Table 11.1)

Rehydration Technique (ReT)

- Iliotibial tract (and fascia lata).
- Tensor fasciae latae.

Pain Relief Technique (PRT)

- Iliotibial tract:
  ○ Portion of the iliotibial tract over the lateral epicondyle
  ○ Other painful points along the structure.

Regulation of Tone Technique (RoT)

- Tensor fasciae latae.
- Iliotibial tract.

Mobilization Technique (MoT)

- Fascia lata.
- Iliotibial tract.
- Tensor fasciae latae.

Metabolization Technique (MeT)

- Iliotibial tract: portion over the lateral epicondyle.

Optional treatment protocol (Table 11.2)

Regulation of Tone Technique (RoT)

- Tibialis anterior.
- Gluteus maximus and gluteus medius.
- Quadriceps femoris (vastus lateralis, rectus femoris).
- Biceps femoris (short head).

Mobilization Technique (MoT)

- Tibialis anterior.
- Gluteus maximus and gluteus medius.
- Quadriceps femoris (vastus lateralis, rectus femoris).
- Biceps femoris (caput breve).
- Lateral patellar retinaculum.
- Lateral collateral ligament.

Table 11.2 Iliotibial tract friction syndrome: summary of optional treatment protocol	
RoT	MoT
Tibialis anterior	Tibialis anterior
Gluteus maximus and gluteus medius	Gluteus maximus and gluteus medius
Quadriceps femoris (vastus lateralis, rectus femoris)	Quadriceps femoris (vastus lateralis, rectus femoris)
Biceps femoris (short head)	Biceps femoris (short head)
	Lateral patellar retinaculum
	Lateral collateral ligament

Visual Presentation of the Treatment Unit

Recommended treatment protocol

Rehydration Technique (ReT)

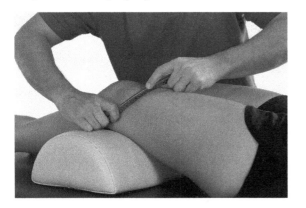

Figure 11.5 Iliotibial tract (and fascia lata)

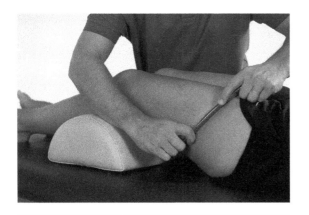

Figure 11.6 Tensor fasciae latae

Pain Relief Technique (PRT)

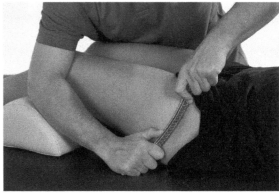

Figure 11.7 Tensor fasciae latae

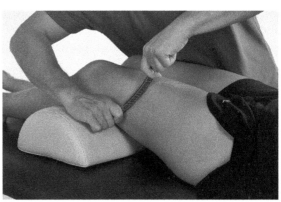

Figure 11.8 Iliotibial tract (and fascia lata)

Regulation of Tone Technique (RoT)

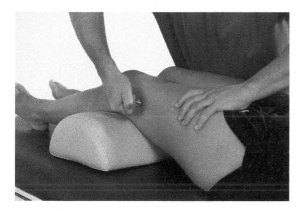

Figure 11.9 Tensor fasciae latae

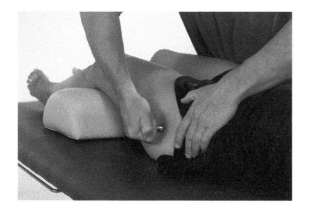

Figure 11.10 Iliotibial tract

Mobilization Technique (MoT)

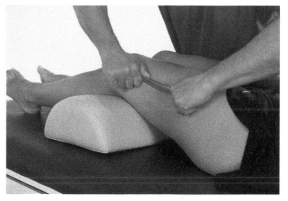

Figure 11.11 Iliotibial tract (and fascia lata)

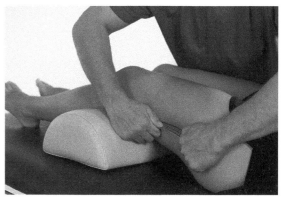

Figure 11.12 Tensor fasciae latae

Metabolization Technique (MeT)

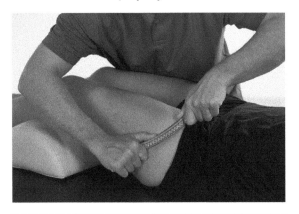

Figure 11.13 Iliotibial tract (and fascia lata)

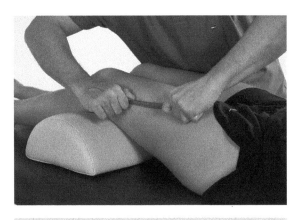

Figure 11.14 Tensor fasciae latae

Optional treatment protocol

Regulation of Tone Technique (RoT)

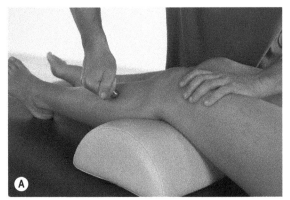

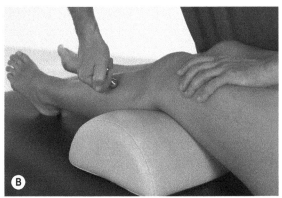

Figure 11.15 (A and B) Tibialis anterior

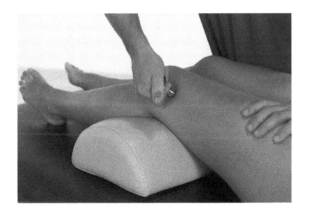

Figure 11.16 Vastus lateralis

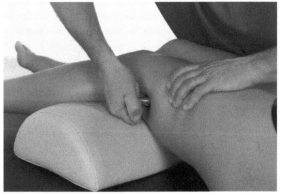

Figure 11.18 Biceps femoris

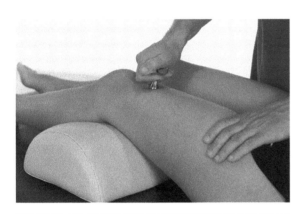

Figure 11.17 Rectus femoris

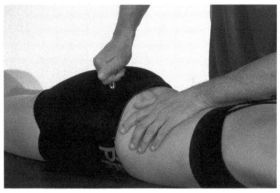

Figure 11.19 Gluteus maximus and medius

Mobilization Technique (MoT)

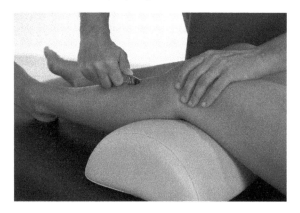

Figure 11.20 Tibialis anterior

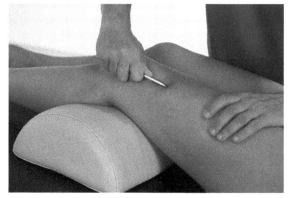

Figure 11.22 Quadriceps femoris (vastus lateralis, rectus femoris)

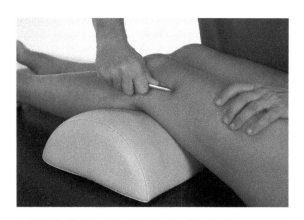

Figure 11.21 Gluteus maximus and gluteus medius

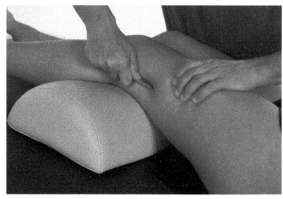

Figure 11.23 Biceps femoris (short head)

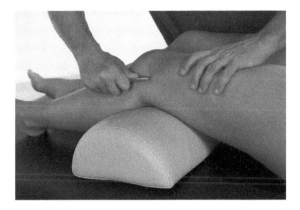

Figure 11.24 Lateral patellar retinaculum

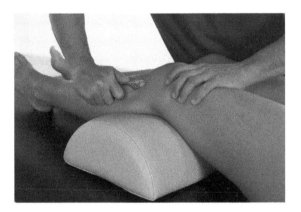

Figure 11.25 Lateral collateral ligament

Duration

Approximately 20 minutes.

Evaluation

- Numeric rating scale (NRS).
- Noble's test (pain provocation test: lying supine, knee extension from a flexed position with simultaneous pressure to the lateral femoral epicondyle (https://www.physio-pedia.com/Noble%27s_test)).
- Renne's test or Creak test (pain provocation test: one-leg standing position, knee flexion from an extended position (https://www.physio-pedia.com/Renne_test)).
- Analysis of run.
- Analysis of gait.

Exercise progression

- Tissue stretch: stretch starting position: lying on the side; hip extended and knee flexed to approximately 90 degrees.
- Progression: lying on the side; active movements of the hip (low-grade abduction–adduction) or active movements of the knee in flexion–extension between approximately 40 and 0 degrees (tissue dynamics).
- Tissue dynamics: resistive movement against elastic resistance.

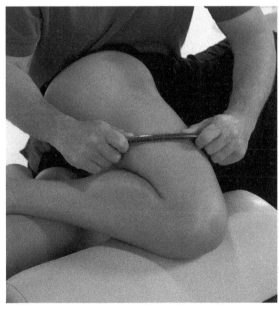

Figure 11.26 Tissue stretch: treatment in stretched position

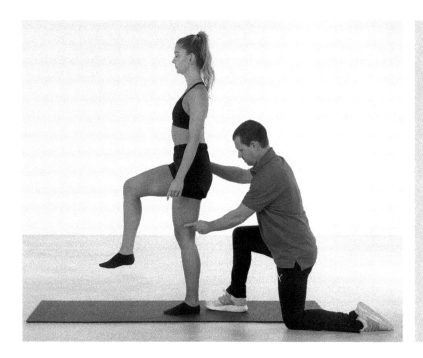

Figure 11.27 Tissue loading: treatment in functional position

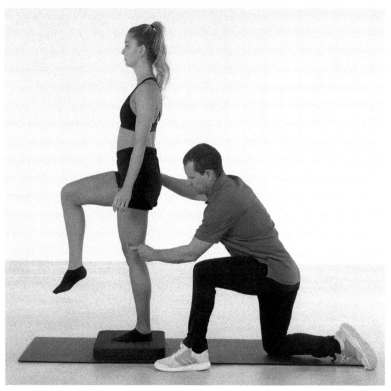

Figure 11.28 Tissue loading+: treatment on unstable surface

- Tissue loading: functionality of the starting position: e.g. standing.
- Tissue loading+: use of tools: e.g. bands, stability trainer.

Patellar Tendinopathy

Detailed Description of the Treatment

Tendinopathy of the patellar ligament (patellar tendinopathy, jumper's knee) affects the patellar tendon (including the lateral and medial patellofemoral ligaments) and the quadriceps femoris (including the medial and lateral patellar retinacula), as well as the adjacent structures: the fascia lata and deep fascia of the leg (fascia cruris), iliotibial tract, and the muscles of the pes anserinus superficialis (gracilis, semitendinosus, sartorius).

The patient lies supine with knee joints supported, or prone with the ankle joint supported (both for relaxation of the treated structure).

The therapy starts with the Rehydration Technique using large-area sliding of the entire quadriceps femoris. Starting from the patella, the technique is performed in a cranial direction up to the attachments of the different parts of the muscle (anterior inferior iliac spine, anterior and posterior surfaces of the femur). The pressure is proportional to the thickness of the soft tissue layers. The more tissue under the instrument, the higher the pressure can be; uniformity of the pressure is important. Treating the thigh in at least three parts is recommended (lateral, ventral, and medial), depending on the instrument and the circumference of the thigh. Each of these parts is treated several times. Then the painful area of the patellar tendon is addressed, from the tibial tuberosity cranially to the apex of the patella. Due to its narrow width, the tendon is best treated with the narrow edge of the hook of an instrument. Because of its anatomical proximity, the overlapping of insertions, and the resulting synergistic functioning, it is best to treat the patellar retinaculum, including the patellofemoral ligaments, as well. Even if the pain is mostly expressed at the patellar tendon, these structures are probably also affected. Although the pressure in this area should be low because the structures lie directly on the bone, it is advisable for the therapist to work with one hand and stabilize the patient's knee with the other hand.

After the Rehydration Technique, the Pain Relief Technique is usually performed. Of course, it is also possible to start with this technique; however, beginning therapy with the gentle and rather pleasant Rehydration Technique has proven beneficial, in the authors' opinion. The technique is, naturally, limited to the painful area(s). Usually, the most painful points of the patellar tendon are the tenoperiosteal junctions at the tibial tuberosity and/or at the patellar apex. The treatment can begin at either point.

In order to achieve the greatest pain relief, the painful areas are provided with a high degree of mechanical stimulation through scraping. The technique is performed directly over the painful areas with a progressive pressure (which should not increase the pain already present). This pressure is applied in both treatment directions: away from the treated area and then on the return. Due to the localization of the ligament directly over the bone and its well-innervated periosteum, the pressure is less than usual when scraping over thick tissue layers. If the therapist feels that this does not provide sufficient pain relief, the technique can also be applied further from the site of pain. In the localized area there are relatively thick muscle layers: quadriceps femoris proximally and tibialis anterior distally. Here, the technique is performed with correspondingly increased pressure. While the results of this indirect application may not be as effective as with a direct application, it should not be underestimated as an alternative in acute conditions or very painful cases.

The next technique applied is Regulation of Tone, dependent on the physiotherapeutic findings.

The hypertonic muscles are identified and treated accordingly. In the case of the patellar tendinopathy, the hypertonic areas are usually located in the muscle belly of quadriceps femoris, and in vastus medialis and lateralis. Nevertheless, all four parts of the quadriceps femoris muscle should be examined for local hypertonicity. Interestingly, there may be hypertonic points in the ligament itself, as well as in the medial and lateral retinacula. Although these structures do not have contractile properties, the authors' experience has shown that it is beneficial to use this technique here, possibly due to the summation of the individual small tonus reductions. Once the therapist has located a hypertonic area, they place the instrument on the point, apply vertical pressure to the tissue, and maintain this pressure until the tone subsides. The therapist may then have the impression that they can penetrate deeper into the tissue. At the new point of tension, the pressure is held again and the therapist waits for a new release. The technique can be completed by small movements of the instrument. In this case, the therapist moves the instrument back and forth on the spot or performs small circular movements. Often, this "melting technique" brings an additional relaxing effect and thus increases the overall benefit.

The next technique applied is the Mobilization Technique. The superficial hypomobilities involve the fascia lata. It is treated according to the protocol previously described: first identified by the displacement test, then treated accordingly. The experienced therapist will have no difficulty locating the deeper hypomobile zones of the patellar tendon, which usually involve the entire tendon. However, the hypomobility is not particularly pronounced in the vicinity of the bony insertions. The authors recommend the therapist to pay attention to these small areas and to mobilize them intensively.

Special attention should be paid to the direction of the tissue mobility limitation, which is not necessarily identical over the entire course of the same structure; moreover, several or even all directions can be affected. The limitation can be determined by a simple test of displacement using the therapist's hand or the instrument. In the authors' experience, there is seldom a single point, but the loss of mobility usually extends to the entire structure. Depending on the structure, the mobilization is carried out with the hook or the short, flat side of an instrument. It is important that the instrument always remains in contact with the same area. The instrument is not pushed over the skin, but the anatomical structure is moved in the restricted direction. The return movement is then done without pressure and is described as returning to the starting position. The tenoperiosteal junction at the tibial tuberosity is often chosen as a starting point for mobilization. Here, the therapist can work with the hook of an instrument, the advantage being that mobilization can be more selective and therefore more precise. The therapist then works along the patellar tendon from hypomobility to hypomobility further proximally.

In addition to the ligament itself, the medial and lateral patellofemoral ligaments should be mobilized. Since these structures are located below the retinacula, they are difficult to palpate precisely. Knowing the exact anatomy means that an indirect mobilization is possible. However, since these structures are not very deep and are found directly above the bone, global mobilization of the area of these ligaments and retinacula is an alternative. In practice, the therapist examines the areas for hypomobility in the usual manner (displacement test with hand or instrument) and mobilizes accordingly in all restricted directions (restrictions). The femoral region often shows a large number of hypomobilities, which may be mobilized:

- the insertions of the rectus femoris muscle at the patella and the anterior inferior iliac spine, as well as along its entire length

- the muscular septa
  - between vastus lateralis and tensor fasciae latae
  - between rectus femoris and vastus lateralis, and between rectus femoris and vastus medialis
  - between sartorius and rectus femoris, and between sartorius and vastus medialis
  - between vastus medialis and the adductors (medial intermuscular septum).

In order to treat these structures precisely and with the necessary pressure, it is advisable to use a longer curved instrument. Due to the longer lever arm, optimum pressure can be applied efficiently.

The final technique applied in this standard treatment session is the Metabolization Technique. The therapist scrapes with the instrument over the area to be treated. The pressure is relatively high but varies according to the volume of the tissue: the greater the volume (that is, the thicker the layer of tissue), the greater the pressure can be. The pressure is applied in one direction only and the speed of execution is also relatively high. The pain already present must not be increased.

In addition to the "standard treatment" described above, various procedures are performed. Because of the holistic nature of the myofascial system, such treatment is recommended. Particularly when the symptoms have been present for a long period of time, the lesion becomes larger and affects more structures. In the case of tendinopathy of the patellar tendon, the structures listed below often also have local hypertonicity that should be treated as described above. These structures are affected because of their spatial (anatomical) proximity and their functional interaction within the execution of movement. Regulation of Tone may be beneficial on the following: iliotibial tract (tensor fasciae latae) and the muscles of the pes anserinus superficialis (gracilis, semitendinosus, sartorius). The tendons of all these muscles should be mobilized if necessary. The reader will find treatment of these areas in corresponding chapters; in addition to the table of contents, Figure I.1 in the Introduction is suitable for quickly finding the corresponding structures in the book. Otherwise, the treatment is virtually identical to that already described. The therapist needs only to adapt the techniques to these structures or to the known anatomical conditions.

Myofascial Connected System (MCS) (Figure 11.29)

Schematic Representation of the Treatment

Diagnosis

Tendinopathy of the patellar ligament (patellar tendinopathy, jumper's knee).

Primary structures affected (Figure 11.30)

- Patellar tendon (including the patellofemoral ligaments, lateral and medial).
- Quadriceps femoris (including the lateral and medial patellar retinacula).

Secondary structures frequently affected (Figure 11.31)

- Fascia lata and deep fascia of the leg (fascia cruris).
- Iliotibial tract.
- Gracilis.
- Semitendinosus.
- Sartorius.

Initial position

Lying supine.

Material

- Recommended: straight elongated instrument, curved instrument.
- Optional: straight short instrument, combination curve instrument.

7   Iliotibial tract
16 Tibialis anterior
19 Vastus lateralis
20 Rectus femoris
21 Lateral patellar retinaculum
22 Lateral collateral ligament
23 Patellar ligament
24 Vastus medialis
25 Vastus intermedialis
26 Medial patellar retinaculum
27 Medial collateral ligament
33 Sartorius
36 Gracilis
37 Semitendinosus

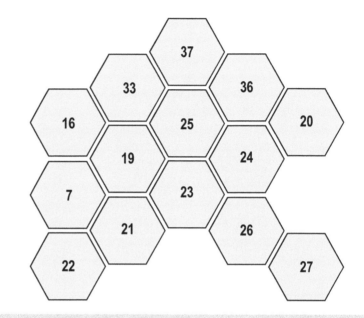

Figure 11.29 Patellar tendinopathy: representation of the MCS

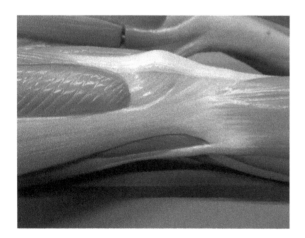

Figure 11.30 Patellar tendinopathy: primary structures affected

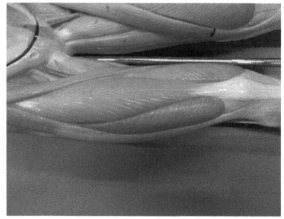

Figure 11.31 Patellar tendinopathy: secondary structures affected

Technique

- Recommended: Rehydration, Pain Relief, Regulation of Tone, Mobilization, Metabolization.
- Optional: none.

Recommended treatment protocol (Table 11.3)

Rehydration Technique (ReT)

- Quadriceps femoris (including the lateral and medial patellar retinacula).
- Patellar tendon (including the lateral and medial patellofemoral ligaments).

Pain Relief Technique (PRT)

- Patellar tendon: tenoperiosteal junctions:
  ○ at the tibial tuberosity and/or
  ○ at the patellar apex.
- Use an indirect technique if necessary.

Regulation of Tone Technique (RoT)

- Quadriceps femoris: vastus medialis and lateralis, rectus femoris, vastus intermedius.
- Patellar retinacula (lateral and medial).
- Patellar tendon.

Mobilization Technique (MoT)

- Fascia lata.
- Patellar tendon: vicinity of the bony insertions.
- Patellar retinacula and patellofemoral ligament (lateral and medial).
- Rectus femoris (insertions and along its entire length).
- Muscular septa
  ○ between vastus lateralis and tensor fasciae latae
  ○ between rectus femoris and vastus lateralis, and rectus femoris and vastus medialis

Table 11.3 Patellar tendinopathy: summary of recommended treatment protocol

ReT	PRT	RoT	MoT	MeT
Quadriceps femoris (including the lateral and medial patellar retinacula)	Painful area	Quadriceps femoris: vastus medialis and lateralis, rectus femoris, vastus intermedius	Fascia lata	Painful area
Patellar tendon (including the lateral and medial patellofemoral ligaments)		Patellar retinacula (lateral and medial)	Patellar tendon: vicinity of the bony insertions	
		Patellar tendon	Patellar retinacula and patellofemoral ligaments (lateral and medial)	
			Rectus femoris (insertions and along its entire length)	
			Muscular septa between • vastus lateralis and tensor fasciae latae • rectus femoris and vastus lateralis, and rectus femoris and vastus medialis • sartorius and rectus femoris, and sartorius and vastus medialis • vastus medialis and the adductors (medial intermuscular septum)	

○ between sartorius and rectus femoris, and between sartorius and vastus medialis

○ between vastus medialis and the adductors (medial intermuscular septum).

Metabolization Technique (MeT)

- Patellar ligament: tenoperiosteal junctions:
  ○ at the tibial tuberosity and/or
  ○ at the patellar apex.

Optional treatment protocol (Table 11.4)

Regulation of Tone Technique (RoT)

- Iliotibial tract.
- Gracilis.
- Semitendinosus.
- Sartorius.

Mobilization Technique (MoT)

- Iliotibial tract.
- Gracilis.
- Semitendinosus.
- Sartorius.

Table 11.4 Patellar tendinopathy: summary of optional treatment protocol

RoT	MoT
Iliotibial tract	Iliotibial tract
Gracilis	Gracilis
Semitendinosus	Semitendinosus
Sartorius	Sartorius

Visual Presentation of the Treatment Unit

Recommended treatment protocol

Rehydration Technique (ReT)

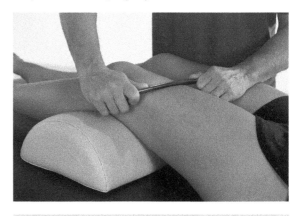

Figure 11.32 Quadriceps femoris

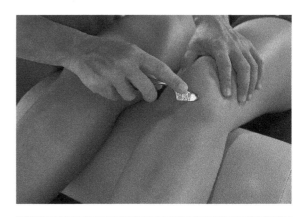

Figure 11.33 Patellar tendon

Pain Relief Technique (PRT)

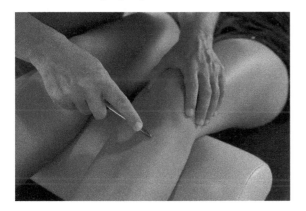

Figure 11.34 Patellar tendon: tenoperiosteal junctions at the tibial tuberosity

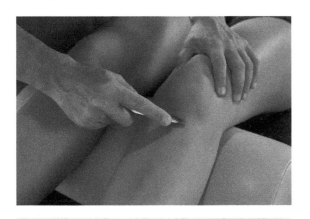

Figure 11.35 Patellar tendon: tenoperiosteal junctions at the patellar apex

Regulation of Tone Technique (RoT)

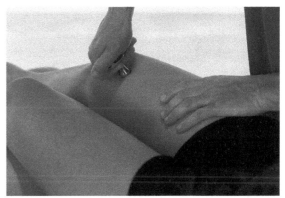

Figure 11.36 Quadriceps femoris: vastus medialis and lateralis

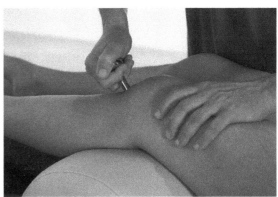

Figure 11.37 Patellar tendon

Mobilization Technique (MoT)

- Patellar tendon: vicinity of the bony insertions.
- Rectus femoris (insertion at base of patella).
- Muscular septa
  - between vastus lateralis and tensor fasciae latae
  - between rectus femoris and vastus lateralis, and between rectus femoris and vastus medialis
  - between sartorius and rectus femoris, and between sartorius and vastus medialis, respectively
  - between vastus medialis and the adductors (medial intermuscular septum).

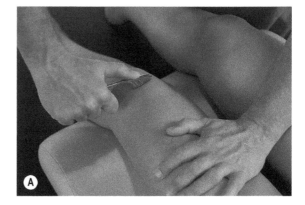

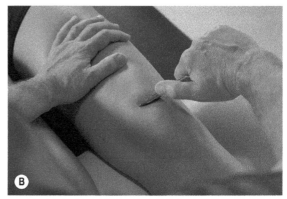

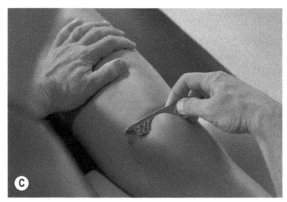

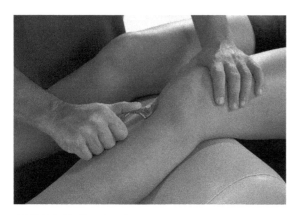

Figure 11.38 Patellar tendon

Figure 11.39 (A–C) Rectus femoris

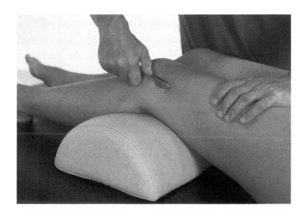

Figure 11.40 Septum between vastus lateralis and IT band

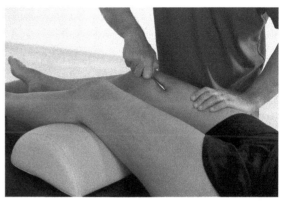

Figure 11.42 Septum between rectus femoris and vastus medialis

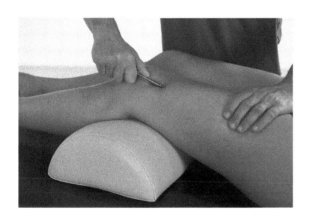

Figure 11.41 Septum between rectus femoris and vastus lateralis

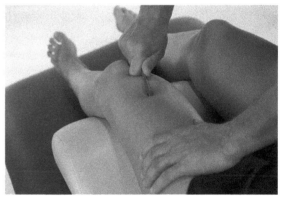

Figure 11.43 Septum between sartorius and vastus medialis

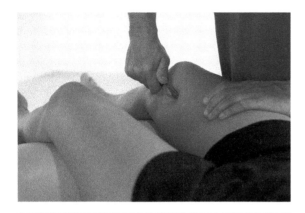

Figure 11.44 Septum between vastus medialis and the adductors

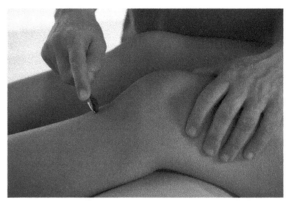

Figure 11.46 Patellar tendon: tenoperiosteal junctions at the patellar apex

Metabolization Technique (MeT)

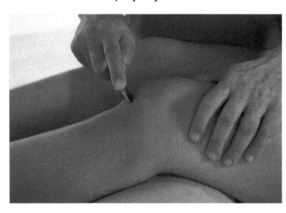

Figure 11.45 Patellar tendon: tenoperiosteal junctions at the tibial tuberosity

Optional treatment protocol
See Figures 11.5–11.24 on pages 188–193.

Regulation of Tone (RoT)

- Iliotibial tract.
- Gracilis.
- Semitendinosus.
- Sartorius.

Mobilization Technique (MoT)

- Iliotibial tract.
- Gracilis.
- Semitendinosus.
- Sartorius.

Duration
Approximately 20 minutes.

Evaluation
- Numeric rating scale (NRS).
- Pain provocation test in lying (knee extension against resistance).
- Pain provocation by jump.
- Analysis of jump (landing phase).
- Analysis of gait.

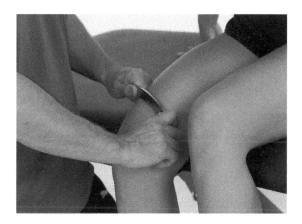

Figure 11.47 Tissue stretch: treatment in stretched position

Exercise progression

- Tissue stretch: stretch starting position: lying supine; knee bent in 90 degrees, then fully bent (knee to buttock) (tissue stress).
- Tissue dynamics: sitting position; active movements of the knee (flexion–extension).
- Tissue dynamics+: sitting position; active movements of the knee (flexion–extension) against elastic resistance.
- Tissue loading: functionality of the starting position: e.g. standing.
- Tissue loading+: use of tools: e.g. bands, stability trainer.

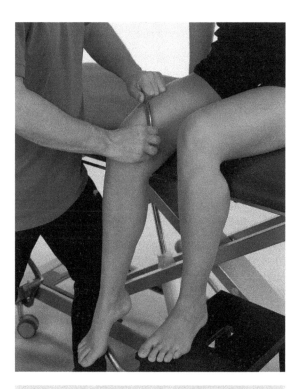

Figure 11.48 Tissue dynamics: treatment in active movement (starting position in flexion)

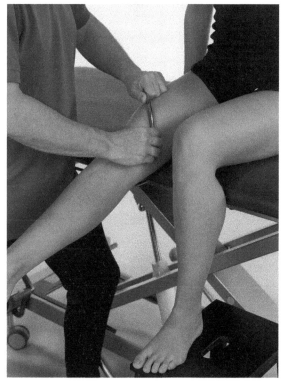

Figure 11.49 Tissue dynamics: treatment in active movement (end position in extension)

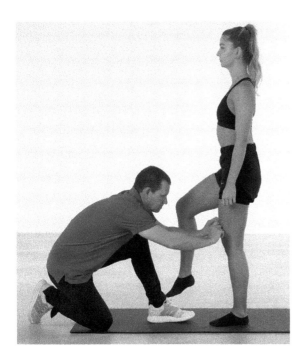

Figure 11.50 Tissue loading: treatment in a functional position

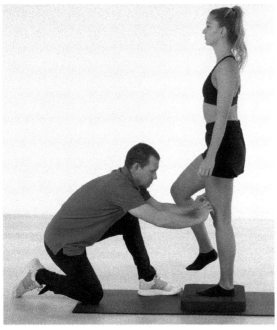

Figure 11.51 Tissue loading+: treatment using an unstable surface (stability trainer)

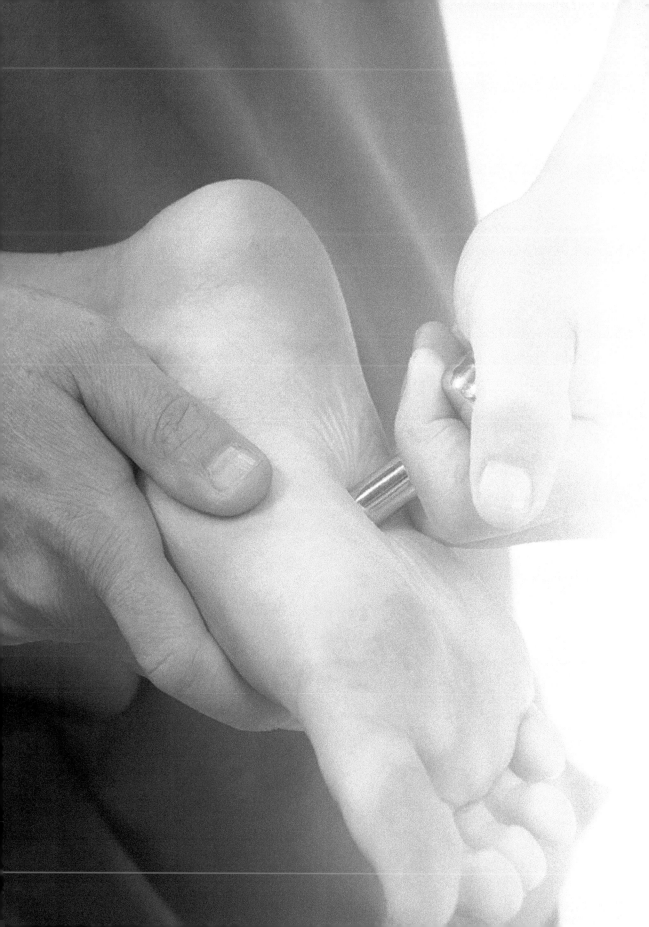

Two common diagnoses are presented for the ankle and foot region: Achilles tendinopathy and plantar fasciitis. These diagnoses are representative of the entire range of musculoskeletal pathologies in the ankle and foot; treatment is adapted according to the symptoms and the suspected causes.

Achilles Tendinopathy

Detailed Description of the Treatment

As an exemplary diagnosis, Achilles tendinopathy is assumed here. The affected structures are the Achilles tendon and the triceps surae muscle, and also the adjacent structures: the deep fascia of the leg (fascia cruris), popliteus, flexor digitorum longus, flexor hallucis longus, and tibialis posterior, as well as peroneus longus and brevis.

The patient lies prone, with ankle joints supported (relaxation of the treated structure) or feet in overhang. The Rehydration Technique starts with large-area sliding of the entire triceps surae. Starting from the musculotendinous transition, the technique is performed in a proximal direction up to the attachment of the two heads of the gastrocnemius muscle to the femoral condyles. The pressure is proportional to the actual thickness of the soft tissue layers: the more tissue under the instrument, the higher the pressure can be. Treating the lower leg in two or three parts is recommended, depending on the instrument and the circumference of the lower leg. Each of these parts is treated several times.

The Achilles tendon area is treated from the calcaneal tuberosity (tenoperiosteal transition) proximally to the musculotendinous transition. The insertion at the tuberosity is broad and does not taper towards the opening into the tendon. It is best to use a relatively short part of the instrument

for treatment. Although the pressure in this area should be low because the tendon runs directly on the bone, it is advisable for the therapist to work with one hand and stabilize the patient's foot with the other hand. The Achilles tendon is often affected in both the easily accessible dorsal area and in the much more difficult to reach ventral area. Therefore, the therapist should rehydrate with the narrow edge of a straight, short instrument.

Then, after the Rehydration Technique, the Pain Relief Technique is usually performed. Beginning therapy with the gentle and rather pleasant Rehydration Technique has proven to be effective clinically. The technique is, naturally, limited to the painful area(s). Experience has shown that the most common areas are the transition between the calcaneus and the tendon (tenoperiosteal transition), and the transition between the tendon and the muscle (musculotendinous transition). The treatment can begin at either point. In order to achieve the greatest pain relief, the painful areas are provided with a high degree of mechanical stimulation through scraping. The technique is performed directly over the painful areas with a progressive pressure (which should not increase the pain already present). This pressure is applied in both treatment directions: away from the treated area and then on the return. If there are several pain points, they are treated consecutively.

The next technique applied is Regulation of Tone. Application is again dependent on the physiotherapeutic findings. The hypertonic structures are identified through palpation and treated accordingly. In the area of the calf, these are usually located in the two heads of the gastrocnemius muscle and in the deeper-lying soleus. Therefore, all three parts of the triceps surae muscle should be examined for local hypertonicity. Once the therapist has located a hypertonic point, they place the straight, short instrument on it, apply vertical pressure to the tissue, and maintain this pressure until the tone subsides. The therapist may then have the impression that they can penetrate deeper into the tissue. At the new point of tension, the pressure is held again and the therapist waits for a new release. The technique can be completed by small movements of the instrument. In this case, the therapist moves the instrument back and forth on the spot or performs small, circular movements. Often, this "melting technique" brings an additional relaxing effect and thus increases the overall benefit.

The next technique applied is the Mobilization Technique. The experienced therapist will have no difficulty locating the hypomobile zones of the Achilles tendon. The superficial hypomobilities often involve the deep fascia of the leg (fascia cruris). They are treated according to the protocol already described: first sensed by the displacement test, then treated accordingly.

Special attention should be paid to the direction of the tissue mobility limitation. This is not necessarily identical over the entire course of the same structure; moreover, several or even all directions can be affected. The limitation can be determined by a simple test of displacement using the therapist's hand or the instrument. In our experience, there is seldom a single point, but the loss of mobility usually extends to the entire structure. The characteristics vary from one patient to another. Depending on the structure, the mobilization is carried out with the hook or the short, flat side of the instrument. It is important that the instrument always remains in contact with the same area. The instrument is not pushed over the skin, but the anatomical structure is moved in the restricted direction. The return movement is then done without pressure and is described as returning to the starting position.

The tenoperiosteal junction at the calcaneus is often chosen as a starting point for mobilization. Here one can work with the short side of an instrument, the advantage being that mobilization can be more selective and therefore more precise. Furthermore, due to the flat nature of the short side of an appropriate instrument, the therapist sometimes tends to slip over the structure. Patients often find this unpleasant. The therapist then works along the Achilles tendon from hypomobility to hypomobility further proximally. In addition to the tendon itself, the musculotendinous transition (gastrocnemius and Achilles tendon) and the transitions between the gastrocnemius and soleus muscles and between soleus and the peroneal muscles (posterior intermuscular septum of the leg) are also affected. In order to treat these structures precisely and with the necessary pressure, it is advisable to use a curved instrument. Due to the longer lever arm, optimum pressure can be applied more efficiently.

The last technique applied in this standard treatment session is the Metabolization Technique. The therapist scrapes with the instrument over the area to be treated. The pressure is relatively high. It varies according to the volume of the tissue: the greater the volume (that is, the thicker the layer of tissue), the greater the pressure can be. The pressure is applied in one direction only and the speed of execution is also relatively high. The pain already present must not be increased.

In addition to the "standard treatment" described above, various procedures can be performed. Because of the holistic nature of the myofascial system, additional treatment is often recommended. For chronic conditions where symptoms have existed for a long period of time, the lesion becomes larger and affects more structures. In the case of Achilles tendinopathy, the following structures often also have local hypertonicity, which should be treated as described above. These structures are often affected because of both their anatomical proximity and their functional interaction during movement. Regulation of Tone Technique may be beneficial for the following structures: popliteus, flexor digitorum longus, flexor hallucis longus, and tibialis posterior, as well as peroneus longus and brevis. The tendons of these muscles should also be mobilized if necessary. Often, mobilization of the chiasma crurale (the fascial intersection of the tibialis posterior and flexor digitorum longus tendons above the ankle) and the fascia between the deep compartment and lateral compartment boundaries is also indicated. The treatment is virtually identical to that already described. The therapist only needs to adapt the techniques to these structures or to the known anatomical conditions.

Myofascial Connected System (MCS) (Figure 12.1)

Schematic Representation of the Treatment

Diagnosis
Achilles tendinopathy.

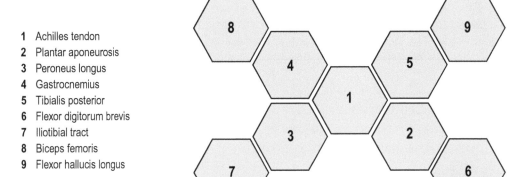

1   Achilles tendon
2   Plantar aponeurosis
3   Peroneus longus
4   Gastrocnemius
5   Tibialis posterior
6   Flexor digitorum brevis
7   Iliotibial tract
8   Biceps femoris
9   Flexor hallucis longus

Figure 12.1 Achilles tendinopathy: representation of the MCS

Primary structures affected (Figure 12.2)
- Achilles tendon.
- Triceps surae.

Secondary structures frequently affected (Figures 12.3 and 12.4)
- Deep fascia of the leg (fascia cruris).
- Popliteus.
- Flexor digitorum longus.
- Flexor hallucis longus.
- Tibialis posterior.
- Peroneus longus and brevis.

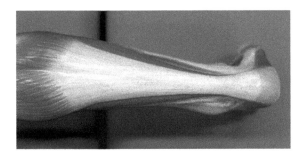

Figure 12.2 Achilles tendinopathy: primary structures affected

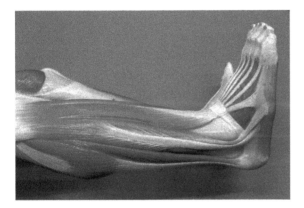

Figure 12.3 Achilles tendinopathy: secondary structures affected (lateral view)

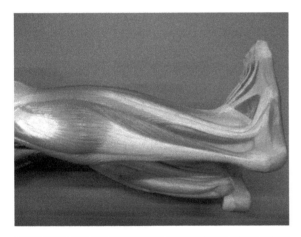

Figure 12.4 Achilles tendinopathy: secondary structures affected (dorsolateral view)

Initial position

Lying prone, with a cushion underlying ankle joints (relaxation of the treated structure) or feet in overhang.

Material

- Recommended: straight, elongated instrument, a combination curve instrument or a straight short instrument.

- Optional: curved instrument.

Technique

- Recommended: Rehydration, Pain Relief, Regulation of Tone, Mobilization, Metabolization.
- Optional: none.

Recommended treatment protocol (Table 12.1)

Rehydration Technique (ReT)

- Deep fascia of the leg: medial, dorsal, and lateral sides of the calf.
- Achilles tendon.

Pain Relief Technique (PRT)

- Tenoperiosteal transition between the calcaneus and the Achilles tendon.
- Musculotendinous transition between gastrocnemius and the Achilles tendon.

Regulation of Tone Technique (RoT)

- Gastrocnemius.
- Soleus.

Mobilization Technique (MoT)

- Deep fascia of the leg.
- Tenoperiosteal transition (calcaneus and Achilles tendon).
- Musculotendinous transition of gastrocnemius and Achilles tendon.
- Transition of gastrocnemius and soleus.
- Transition of soleus and the peronei (fibularis) muscles (posterior intermuscular septum of the leg).
- Achilles tendon.

Metabolization Technique (MeT)

- Tenoperiosteal transition between the calcaneus and the Achilles tendon.
- Musculotendinous transition between gastrocnemius and the Achilles tendon.

Table 12.1 Achilles tendinopathy: summary of recommended treatment protocol

ReT	PRT	RoT	MoT	MeT
Calf	Painful area	Gastrocnemius	Deep fascia of the leg (fascia cruris)	Painful area
Achilles tendon		Soleus	Tenoperiosteal transition	
			Musculotendinous transition	
			Transition of gastrocnemius and soleus	
			Transition of soleus and the peronei muscles	
			Achilles tendon	

Optional treatment protocol (Table 12.2)

Regulation of Tone Technique (RoT)

- Popliteus.
- Flexor digitorum longus.
- Flexor hallucis longus.
- Tibialis posterior.
- Peroneus longus and brevis.

Mobilization Technique (MoT)

- Chiasma crurale (the fascial intersection of the tibialis posterior and flexor digitorum longus tendons above the ankle).

Table 12.2 Achilles tendinopathy: summary of recommended treatment protocol

RoT	MoT
Popliteus	Chiasma crurale
Flexor digitorum longus	Tendon of flexor digitorum longus
Flexor hallucis longus	Tendon of hallucis longus
Tibialis posterior	Tendon of tibialis posterior
Peroneus longus and brevis	Tendon of peroneus longus and brevis
	Transition of deep compartment and lateral compartment boundaries

- Fascia between the deep compartment and lateral compartment boundaries.

Visual Presentation of the Treatment Unit

Recommended treatment protocol

Rehydration Technique (ReT)

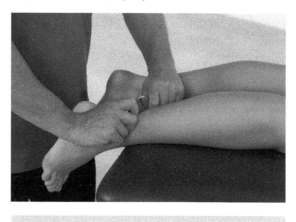

Figure 12.5 Lateral–central part of the calf

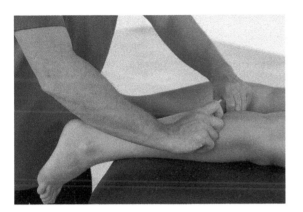

Figure 12.6 Medial–lateral part of the calf

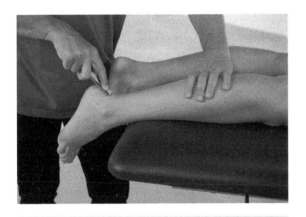

Figure 12.7 Rehydration of the dorsal part of the Achilles tendon

Pain Relief Technique (PRT)

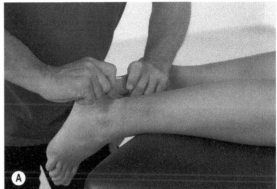

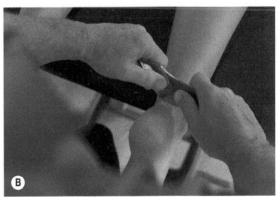

Figure 12.8 (A and B) PRT Achilles tendon

Regulation of Tone Technique (RoT)

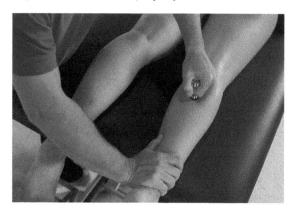

Figure 12.9 Tone regulation of gastrocnemius

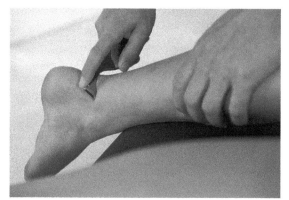

Figure 12.11 Mobilization of the Achilles tendon

Mobilization Technique (MoT)

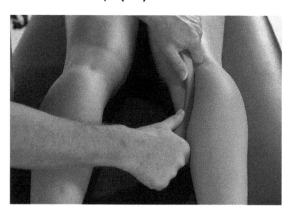

Figure 12.10 Mobilization of gastrocnemius

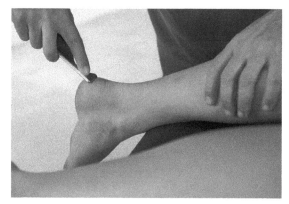

Figure 12.12 Mobilization of calcaneal tuberosity

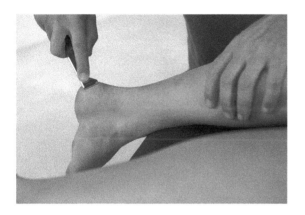

Figure 12.13 Mobilization of intermuscular septum

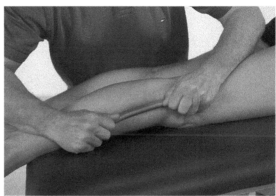

Figure 12.15 Mobilization gastrocnemius (lateral head)

Metabolization Technique (MeT)

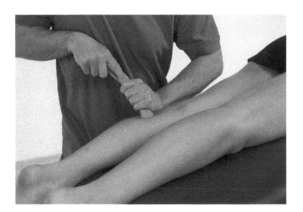

Figure 12.14 Mobilization posterior intermuscular septum: transition of soleus and the peronei muscles

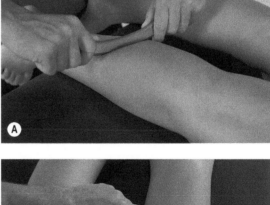

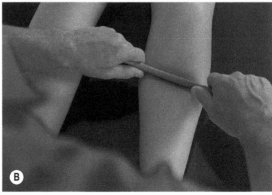

Figure 12.16 (A and B) Metabolization of the calf

Optional treatment protocol

Regulation of Tone Technique (RoT)

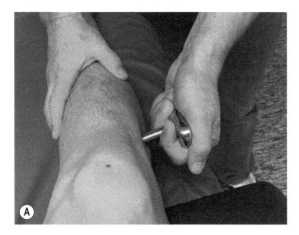

(A)

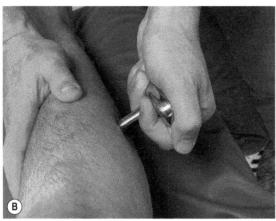

(B)

Figure 12.17 (A and B) Regulation of tone peroneus longus

Mobilization Technique (MoT)

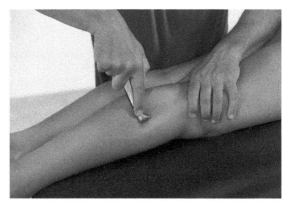

Figure 12.18 Mobilization of peroneus longus: muscle belly

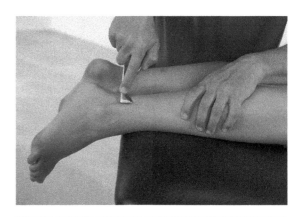

Figure 12.19 Mobilization of peroneus longus: tendon

Duration
Approximately 20 minutes.

Evaluation
- Numeric rating scale (NRS).
- ROM ankle joint.
- End-feel dorsiflexion.
- Knee to wall test.
- Heel seat with stretched toes.
- Analysis of standing position.
- Analysis of gait.
- Tiptoe test.

Exercise progression
- Tissue stretch: stretch starting position in dorsiflexion.
- Tissue dynamics: active movements of the ankle.
- Tissue dynamics+: resistive movement against elastic resistance.
- Tissue loading: functionality of the starting position: e.g. standing.
- Tissue loading+: use of tools: e.g. bands, stability trainer.

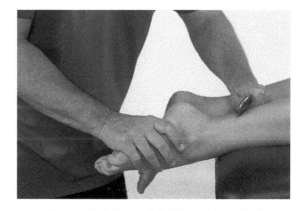

Figure 12.21 Tissue dynamics: dorsiflexion

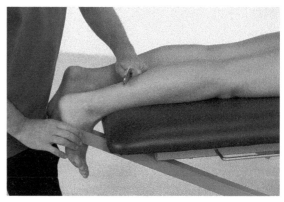

Figure 12.22 Tissue dynamics+: resistive movement against elastic resistance

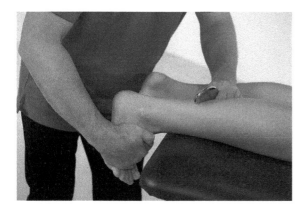

Figure 12.20 Tissue dynamics: plantar flexion

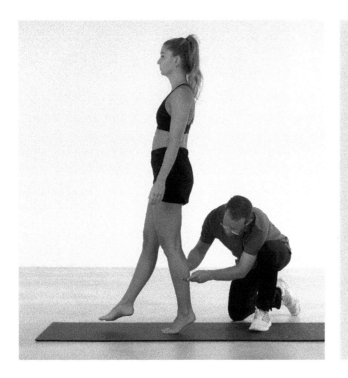

Figure 12.23 Tissue loading: treatment in functional position

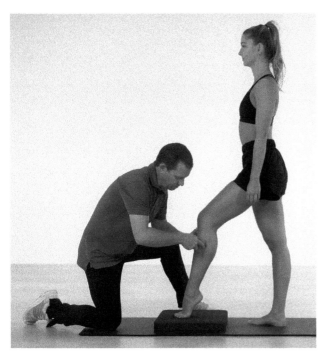

Figure 12.24 Tissue loading+: treatment using unstable surface (stability trainer)

Plantar Fasciitis

Detailed Description of the Treatment

Plantar fasciitis affects the plantar aponeurosis (including the transverse and longitudinal fibers), as well as the short intrinsic muscles of the toes and metatarsals (abductor hallucis, adductor hallucis, abductor digiti minimi, flexor digitorum brevis, quadratus plantae (flexor accessorius), plantar interossei and the lumbrical muscles)), as well as the deep fascia of the leg (fascia cruris).

The patient lies prone, with ankle joints supported (relaxation of the treated structure) or the feet in overhang. Treatment in the supine position is also possible but usually not very comfortable for the therapist.

On the foot, the use of a lubricant is highly recommended; quite a few people are sensitive there. Without lubricant, adequate treatment is usually not possible, and patients flinch as the pressure is felt to be "ticklish."

The Rehydration Technique starts with large-area sliding of the entire foot sole. Starting from the calcaneal tuberosity, the technique is performed in a distal direction toward the heads of the metatarsals. The pressure is proportional to the thickness of the soft tissue layers. The more tissue under the instrument, the higher the pressure can be. Usually, the entire sole of the foot can be treated simultaneously. If an area of the sole of the foot is particularly affected, it can be treated separately with the short edge of an instrument. The Rehydration Technique is performed several times. Next, the insertion of the plantar aponeurosis around at the calcaneal tuberosity is treated separately because this area often has a particularly poor tissue quality. The insertion is rather narrow and widens significantly distally. It is best to use a relatively short part of the instrument for treatment. Although the pressure in this area is low because the aponeurosis runs directly on the bone, it is advisable for the therapist to work with

one hand and stabilize the patient's heel with the other hand.

After Rehydration, the Pain Relief Technique is usually performed. Of course, it is also possible to start with this technique; however, beginning therapy with the gentle and rather pleasant Rehydration Technique has proven to be very effective clinically in recent years. The technique is, naturally, limited to the painful area(s). Experience has shown that the most common painful areas are located between the rear and the middle third of the sole of the foot. This area coincides with the myotendinous transition of the flexor digitorum brevis and the quadratus plantae (flexor accessorius). In this case, it is best to start the treatment at this point. If another area is more painful (the myotendinous transition of abductor hallucis), treatment can begin there. In principle, all painful points are treated consecutively. In order to achieve the greatest pain relief, the painful areas are provided with a high degree of mechanical stimulation through scraping. The technique is performed directly over the painful areas with a progressive pressure (which should not increase the pain already present). This pressure is applied in both treatment directions: away from the painful area and then on return. If there are several pain points, they are treated consecutively.

The next technique applied is Regulation of Tone. Application is dependent on the physiotherapeutic findings. The hypertonic muscles are identified on palpation and treated accordingly. In the sole of the foot, hypertonicity is usually located in the belly of the digitorum brevis, quadratus plantae, and abductor hallucis muscles, or, more rarely, in adductor hallucis (oblique fibers). Nevertheless, all parts of the sole of the foot should be examined for local hypertension. Once the therapist has located a hypertonic point, they place the instrument on it, apply vertical pressure to the tissue, and maintain this pressure until the tone subsides. The therapist then has the impression that they can penetrate deeper into the tissue. At the new point of tension, the pressure is held again and the therapist waits for a new release. The technique can be completed by small movements of the instrument. In this case, the therapist moves the instrument back and forth on the spot or performs small, circular movements. Often, this "melting technique" brings an additional relaxing effect and thus increases the overall benefit.

The next technique applied is the Mobilization Technique. The experienced therapist will have no difficulty locating the superficial hypomobile zones of the foot sole. The superficial hypomobilities involve the plantar aponeurosis. They are treated according to the protocol already described: first sensed by the displacement test, then treated accordingly.

Special attention should be paid to the direction of the tissue mobility limitation. This is not necessarily identical over the entire course of the same structure; moreover, several or even all directions can be affected. The limitation can be determined by a simple test of displacement using the therapist's hand or the instrument. In the authors' experience, there is seldom a single point, but the loss of mobility usually extends to the entire structure. The characteristics vary from one patient to another. Depending on the structure, the mobilization is carried out with the hook or the short, flat side of the instrument. It is important that the instrument always remains in contact with the same area. The instrument is not pushed over the skin, but the anatomical structure is moved in the restricted direction. The return movement is then done without pressure and is described as returning to the starting position.

The deeper hypomobilities are usually located at the tenoperiosteal junction at the calcaneus. This is often chosen as a starting point for mobilization. Here the therapist can work with the short side of an instrument, the advantage being that mobilization can be a little more selective

and therefore more precise. Furthermore, due to the flat nature of the short side of the instrument, the therapist sometimes tends to slip over the structure. Patients often find this unpleasant. The therapist then works along the plantar aponeurosis from hypomobility to hypomobility in the direction of the toes. In addition to the aponeurosis itself, including its transverse and longitudinal fascial excursions, the musculotendinous transitions of flexor digitorum brevis and quadratus plantae are also affected. In order to treat these structures precisely and with the necessary pressure, it is advisable to use a straight, elongated instrument, a combination curve instrument, or a straight, short instrument.

The last technique applied in this standard treatment session is the Metabolization Technique. The therapist scrapes with the instrument over the area to be treated. The pressure is relatively high. It varies according to the volume of the tissue: the greater the volume (that is, the thicker the layer of tissue), the greater the pressure can be. The pressure is applied in one direction only and the speed of execution is relatively high. The pain already present must not be increased.

In addition to the "standard treatment" described above, various procedures can be performed. In terms of the holistic nature of the myofascial system, such treatment is even recommended. When the symptoms have existed for a long period of time, the lesion becomes larger and affects more structures. In the case of plantar fasciitis, the following structures also have local hypertonicity, which should be treated as described above. These structures are typically affected because of their anatomical proximity and the functional interaction during movement. Regulation of Tone may be beneficial on the following structures:

- muscles of the fifth toe (opponens, flexor, and abductor digiti minimi)

- muscles of the calf (triceps surae, tibialis posterior, flexor digitorum longus, and flexor hallucis longus)
- lateral muscles of the lower leg (peroneus longus and peroneus brevis)
- ventral muscles of the lower leg (tibialis anterior, extensor digitorum longus, and extensor hallucis longus).

The tendons of these muscles – especially the long, so-called "gliding" tendons – should be mobilized if necessary. A detailed description of the treatment can be found earlier in this chapter; in addition to the table of contents, Figure I.1 in the Introduction is suitable for quickly finding the corresponding structures in the book. The treatment is virtually identical to that already described. The therapist needs only to adapt the techniques to these structures or to the known anatomical conditions.

Myofascial Connected System (MCS) (Figure 12.25)

Schematic Representation of the Treatment

Diagnosis
Plantar fasciitis.

Primary structure affected (Figure 12.26)
- Plantar aponeurosis (including transverse and longitudinal fibers).

Secondary structures frequently affected
- Flexor digitorum brevis.
- Quadratus plantae (flexor accessorius).
- Abductor and adductor hallucis.
- Abductor digiti minimi.
- Plantar interossei.
- Lumbrical muscles.
- Deep fascia of the leg (fascia cruris).

Initial position
Lying prone, with ankle joints supported (relaxation of the treated structure) or feet in overhang.

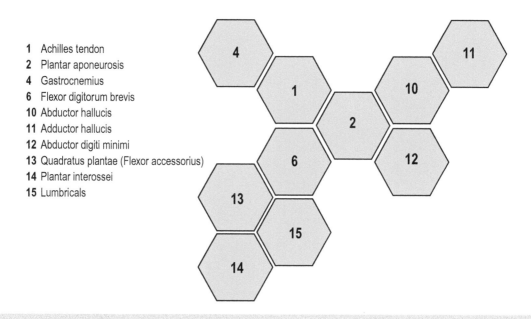

1 Achilles tendon
2 Plantar aponeurosis
4 Gastrocnemius
6 Flexor digitorum brevis
10 Abductor hallucis
11 Adductor hallucis
12 Abductor digiti minimi
13 Quadratus plantae (Flexor accessorius)
14 Plantar interossei
15 Lumbricals

Figure 12.25 Plantar fasciitis: representation of the MCS

Material

- Recommended: straight, elongated instrument, a combination curve instrument, or a straight short instrument.
- Optional: none.

Technique

- Recommended: Rehydration, Pain Relief, Regulation of Tone, Mobilization, Metabolization.
- Optional: none.

Recommended treatment protocol (Table 12.3)

Rehydration Technique (ReT)

- Entire sole of the foot (plantar aponeurosis, including transverse and longitudinal fibers).

Pain Relief Technique (PRT)

- Myotendinous transition of flexor digitorum brevis.
- Myotendinous transition of quadratus plantae (flexor accessorius).
- Myotendinous transition of abductor hallucis.
- Adductor hallucis (oblique fibers).

Regulation of Tone Technique (RoT)

- Flexor digitorum brevis.
- Quadratus plantae (flexor accessorius).
- Abductor hallucis.
- Adductor hallucis (oblique fibers).

Mobilization Technique (MoT)

- Plantar aponeurosis: tenoperiosteal junction at the calcaneus.
- Plantar aponeurosis: entire structure, including the transverse and longitudinal fibers.
- Musculotendinous transition of flexor digitorum brevis.
- Musculotendinous transition of quadratus plantae (flexor accessorius).

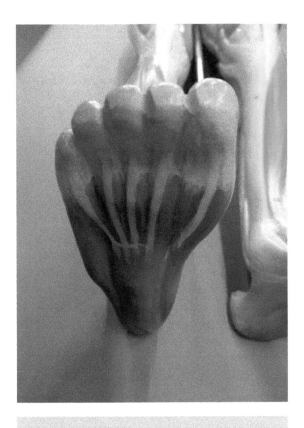

Figure 12.26 Plantar fasciitis: primary structure affected

Metabolization Technique (MeT)

- Myotendinous transition of flexor digitorum brevis.
- Myotendinous transition of quadratus plantae (flexor accessorius).
- Myotendinous transition of abductor hallucis.
- Adductor hallucis (oblique fibers).

Optional treatment protocol (Table 12.4)

Regulation of Tone Technique (RoT)

- Muscles of the fifth toe (opponens, flexor, and abductor digiti minimi).
- Muscles of the calf (triceps surae, tibialis posterior, flexor digitorum longus, and flexor hallucis longus).

- Lateral muscles of the lower leg (peroneus longus and peroneus brevis).
- Ventral muscles of the lower leg (tibialis anterior, extensor digitorum longus, and extensor hallucis longus).

Mobilization Technique (MoT)

- Muscles of the fifth toe (opponens, flexor, and abductor digiti minimi).
- Muscles of the calf (triceps surae, tibialis posterior, flexor digitorum longus, and flexor hallucis longus).
- Lateral muscles of the lower leg (peroneus longus and peroneus brevis).

- Ventral muscles of the lower leg (tibialis anterior, extensor digitorum longus, and extensor hallucis longus).
- Chiasma plantae.
- Deep fascia of the leg (fascia cruris).

Visual Presentation of the Treatment Unit

Recommended treatment protocol

Rehydration Technique (ReT)

Pain Relief Technique (PRT)

Regulation of Tone (RoT)

Table 12.3 Plantar fasciitis: summary of recommended treatment protocol					
ReT	**PRT**	**RoT**	**MoT**	**MeT**	
Entire sole of the foot	Painful area	Flexor digitorum brevis	Plantar aponeurosis	Painful area	
		Quadratus plantae (flexor accessorius)	Musculotendinous transition of flexor digitorum brevis		
		Abductor hallucis	Musculotendinous transition of quadratus plantae (flexor accessorius)		
		Adductor hallucis (oblique fibers)			

Table 12.4 Plantar fasciitis: summary of optional treatment protocol	
RoT	**MoT**
Muscles of the fifth toe (opponens, flexor, and abductor digiti minimi)	Muscles of the calf (triceps surae, tibialis posterior, flexor digitorum longus, and flexor hallucis longus)
Muscles of the calf (triceps surae, tibialis posterior, flexor digitorum longus and flexor hallucis longus)	Muscles of the fifth toe (opponens, flexor, and abductor digiti minimi)
Lateral muscles of the lower leg (peroneus longus and peroneus brevis)	Lateral muscles of the lower leg (peroneus longus and peroneus brevis)
Ventral muscles of the lower leg (tibialis anterior, extensor digitorum longus and extensor hallucis longus)	Ventral muscles of the lower leg (tibialis anterior, extensor digitorum longus, and extensor hallucis longus)
	Chiasma plantae
	Deep fascia of the leg (fascia cruris)

Mobilization Technique (MoT)

Metabolization Technique (MeT)

Optional treatment protocol

Regulation of Tone Technique (RoT)

Mobilization Technique (MoT)

Duration
Approximately 10 minutes.

Evaluation
- Numeric rating scale (NRS).
- ROM ankle joint.
- End-feel dorsiflexion.
- Knee to wall test.
- Heel seat with stretched toes.
- Analysis of standing position.
- Analysis of gait.
- Tiptoe test.

Exercise progression
- Tissue stretch: stretch starting position in dorsiflexion and toe extension.

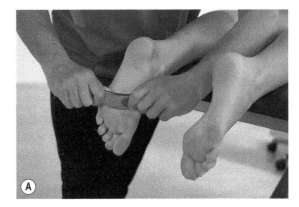

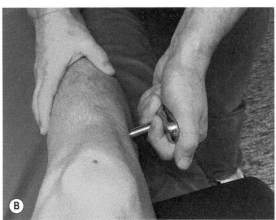

Figure 12.27 (A and B) Entire sole of the foot

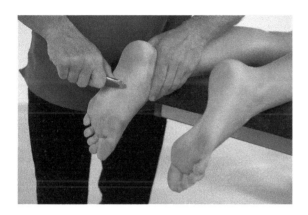

Figure 12.28 Myotendinous transition of flexor digitorum brevis

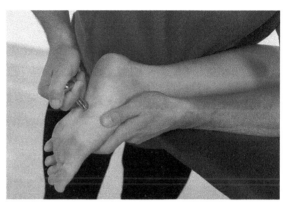

Figure 12.30 Flexor digitorum brevis

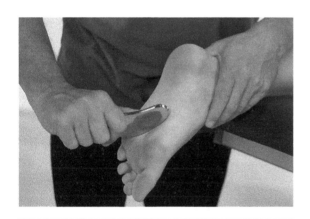

Figure 12.29 Adductor hallucis (oblique fibers)

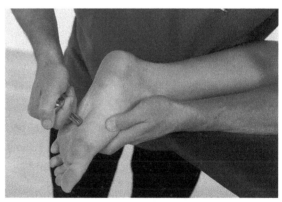

Figure 12.31 Adductor hallucis (oblique fibers)

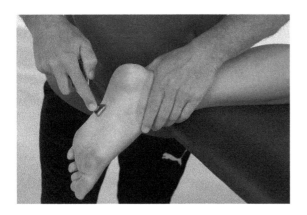

Figure 12.32 Plantar aponeurosis: tenoperiosteal junction at the calcaneus

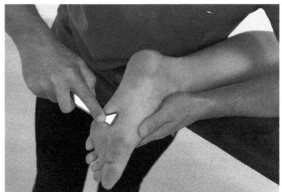

Figure 12.34 Musculotendinous transition of flexor digitorum brevis

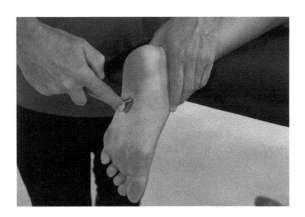

Figure 12.33 Plantar aponeurosis: entire structure, including transverse and longitudinal fibers

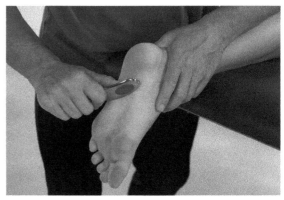

Figure 12.35 Myotendinous transition of quadratus plantae (flexor accessorius)

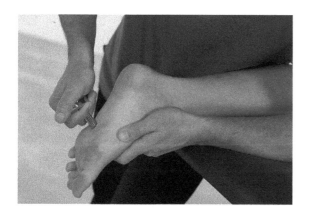

Figure 12.36 Opponens digiti minimi

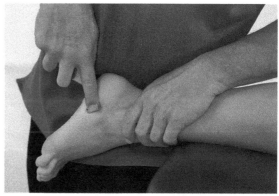

Figure 12.38 Chiasma plantae

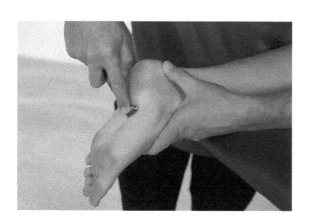

Figure 12.37 Tendon of peroneus longus

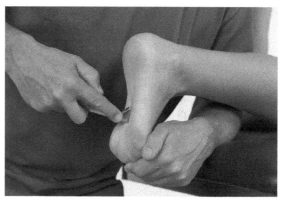

Figure 12.39 Tissue stretch: treatment in stretched starting position

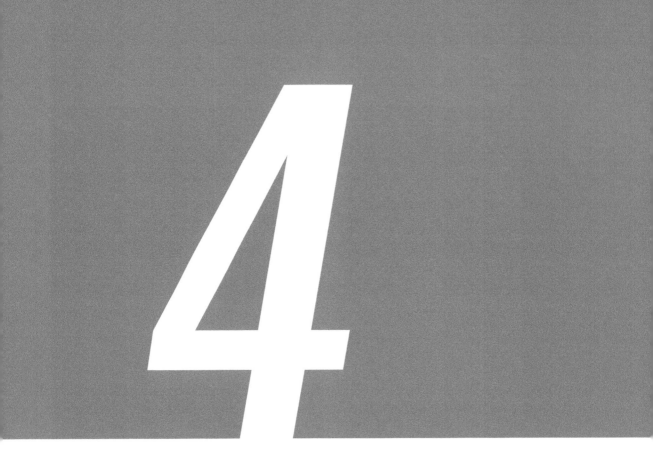

4

Clinical Applications of IAMT: Scars and Osteoarthrosis

As in the previous two sections, the chapters in Part 4 deal with the clinical application of the instruments on the patient: IAMT in daily practice. Treatment for scars in the deep and superficial fascia and osteoarthrosis is described here. We continue to strive for good readability and high relevance to everyday practice, and follow the same structure, which allows the reader to tackle each chapter separately and still be able to apply the corresponding therapy directly.

A detailed description of the treatment is given first, followed by a schematic representation of the treatment with numerous illustrations, for immediate and optimal implementation of the therapy in the reader's practice. A treatment protocol is provided, which has proven itself in practice. Of course, it can and should always be adapted to the patient or the condition. Sometimes not all steps are necessary; sometimes a certain part of the treatment must be carried out more intensively. However, especially when the therapist is still gaining experience with IAMT, it is advisable to follow the protocols; they lend a certain structure and often give the therapist a corresponding sense of security. They also increase comparability between patients.

A visual representation of the treatment is also provided, for quick reference. Finally, the authors give information on the possible duration of the therapy, suggest evaluation tests, and present possibilities for progression as well as pre- and post-treatment techniques. In the latter case, reference should always made to Chapter 4 since these techniques are almost always identical.

Clinical Applications of IAMT: Scars and Osteoarthrosis

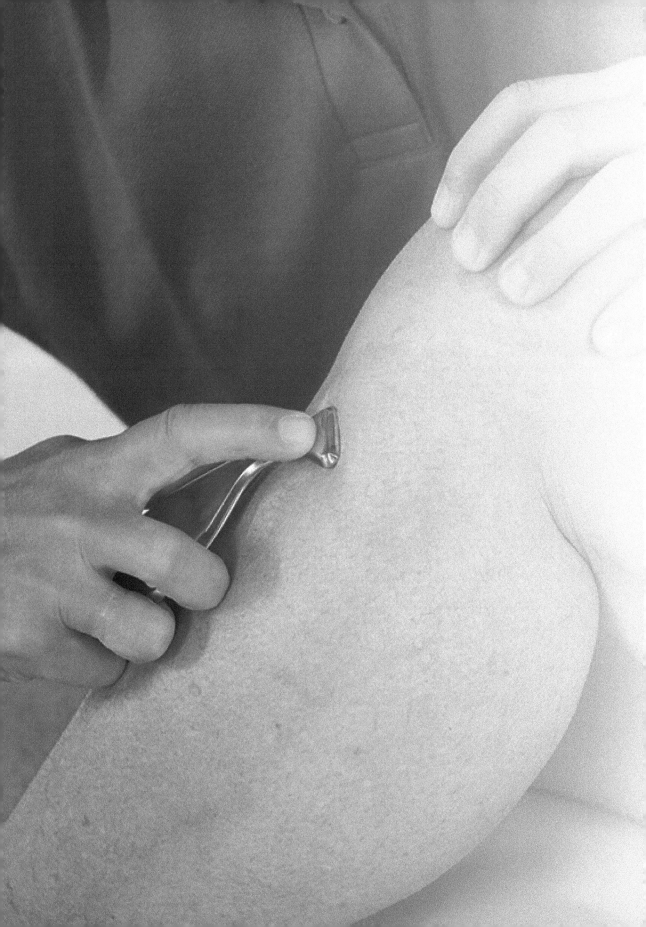

This chapter presents IAMT treatment for superficial scars. Superficial scars may be caused by surgery or other injuries. Superficial fascial structures have generally lower tissue density and a rather irregular orientation of the fibers. Both deeper visceral fascia and the intramuscular fascia share these characteristics as well.

The treatment presented here does not concern a physiological scar, which is very close to the original tissue in terms of elasticity and function. Physiological scars result from injury and undergo primary wound healing. They are generally asymptomatic and characterized by a lack of physical and/or psychological suffering.

Instead, this chapter will cover symptomatic superficial scars, including sclerotic scars, hypertrophic scars, and keloids. Obviously, wound healing must be completed for the therapy to be implemented. Frequently, scars with a poor-quality structure are formed. This type of wound healing is sometimes described as secondary wound healing. These scars are characterized by impaired function due to new tissue formation and wound contracture, and may pose a cosmetic problem with consequent psychological suffering.

After an injury, immobilization for healing, pain, or orthosis can form a scar that is stressed in one direction only. If this scar is exercised in a typically normal manner (functionally, with three-dimensional movement), recurrent damage can occur. This may result in symptomatology that is often expressed by a unidirectional "adhesive character" and resulting disturbances in displacement of the different tissue layers involved; the latter, in turn, presents itself clinically with limitations in joint mobility. If this cause–consequence symptomatology is local, there is no difficulty in diagnosing and treating it; however, things become more problematic when this reaction is located throughout the myofascial chains.

At first glance, the scar and the movement restriction (and/or pain) may be unrelated. The age of the scar or the time between scar formation and the appearance of symptoms is often considerable. The scar as a structure and as a disturbance to movement is generally permanent; thus, the reaction (the restriction of movement) is also permanent. In the authors' opinion, this suggests that scars (especially older ones) should always be considered when myofascial symptoms are present.

In order to present this important chapter adequately, the authors have decided to describe the techniques for any given scar (in this case, a scar on the lateral knee joint) first and then to illustrate a detailed treatment using the example of a very common scar that is not always easy to treat: the scar after osteosynthesis of a distal radius fracture.

Description of the Treatment Techniques

The therapy goals are pain relief (if pain is present) and improvement of function. Techniques that aim for rehydration, tone regulation in the surrounding tissue, and mobilization are beneficial. Since dysfunctional scars are usually accompanied by some form of excess new tissue formation, the Pain Relief Technique and the Metabolization Technique are not used locally; however, they may be applied at a distance. While these effects may be "indirect," clinical experience suggests that this approach can help with stubborn "scarring pain." In the case of "classic" movement restrictions due to scarring, the outcomes are often worse; pain relief in this case is also achieved indirectly. In addition to the cosmetic aspect, these non-physiological or dysfunctional scars usually have an influence on movement(s). Some are painful only in certain positions or during certain movements; therefore, exercise progressions are very important for these scars after soft tissue mobilization.

Rehydration Technique (ReT)

This superficial shoving ("gliding") consists of continuous pushing of the instrument (mostly a straight, elongated instrument, a curved instrument, or a combination curve instrument) with pressure (like the bow of a boat through a wave) around and over the scar; the return to the starting point is pressure-free. The pressure in this case is low because the scar is superficial. Continuous pressure should be applied in all directions since

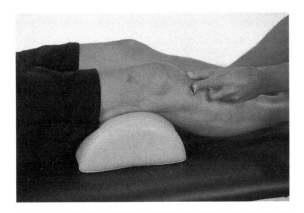

Figure 13.1 ReT: start position

tissues are not always organized in parallel structures. However, if swelling or edema is visible, a retrograde (proximal/cranial) direction seems more prudent.

Regulation of Tone (RoT)

The technique consists of vertical pressing at the desired point (mostly with a straight, short instrument) to the tissue around and over the scar until an initial "end-feel" is perceived. The pressure is held until the tone noticeably decreases. The technique can then be repeated on a new "end-feel."

Mobilization Technique (MoT)

This technique consists in rubbing or frictioning applied to the restriction to be treated. First the instrument (any of the instruments presented) is moved with pressure in the direction of the restriction of the scar or the surrounding tissue until the displaceability of the tissue is at a maximum. Now, without pressure (but also without loss of contact), either the instrument is returned to the starting position or the final position is held for some time (approximately 20 seconds) before it is returned. The instrument does not slide over the skin at all, but moves in solidarity with the

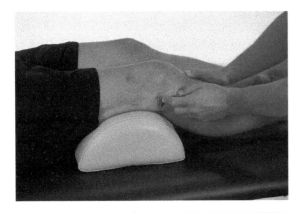

Figure 13.2 ReT: end position

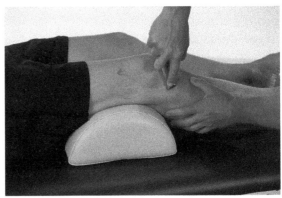

Figure 13.3 Anterior to posterior

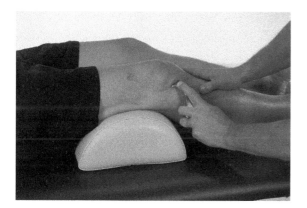

Figure 13.4 Posterior to anterior

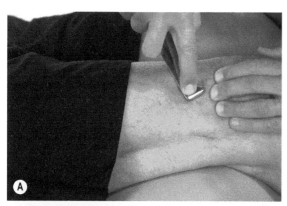

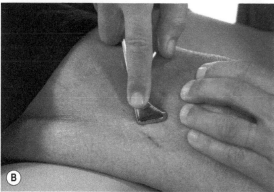

Figure 13.5 (A and B) MoT: superficial treatment in different directions

mobilized structure; therefore, the use of a lubricant is not necessary.

The superficial fasciae are not arranged in one direction only, but built in a looser and less structured architecture. Therefore, the technique should always be performed in different directions. The therapist tests all directions of the scar and treats accordingly. Depending on the restriction, the pressure is always applied away from the restriction in order to mobilize the fibers; the return is always without pressure.

After one restriction is treated, the therapist applies the instrument to a new restriction. It is very rare that only one direction is restricted; usually there are several. Most importantly, the direction of the restriction can be different at each location on the scar. This means that treatment of the scar is very complex and must be very detailed. Accordingly, it is costly but the experience of the authors shows it is well worth spending time and effort on it! As already mentioned, some restrictions are apparent only at the end of the movement and so must also be treated in this position.

Detailed Description of the Treatment of a Scar after Osteosynthesis of a Distal Radius Fracture

The treatment for superficial scars will be described in this chapter taking a common pathology as an example that can be applied to scars anywhere on the body. A distal radius fracture is one of the most common fractures; it is often treated surgically and results in a post-operative scar on the palmar aspect of the distal forearm.

The patient sits next to the treatment table; the entire forearm lies relaxed and supinated, and is best supported distally with a cushion. The elbow is slightly bent.

The therapy starts with sliding of the area around the scar with the Rehydration Technique. In this case, this is best done with the edge of the

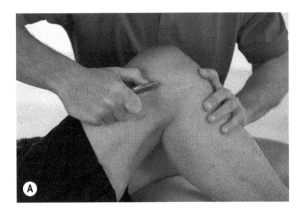

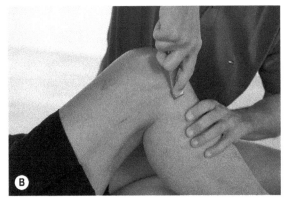

Figure 13.6 (A and B) MoT: treatment in stretched position

hook of an instrument. The therapist pushes the instrument very slowly around the entire scar in a variety of directions. It is important that the technique addresses all sides of the scar. Thus, the treatment starts at the wrist: the therapist pushes the instrument proximally to the end of the scar, circles it in the opposite direction, and then pushes the instrument distally towards the wrist and circles the scar again. Of course, individual areas that are particularly affected can also be treated intensively and repeatedly. The direction of scraping should be varied and repeated as much as possible to increase the local effect; the next pass starts from the wrist in the opposite direction.

It is also possible to treat each side of the scar separately; the radial side first, then the ulnar side, and finally both ends of the scar are treated. In both directions, the therapist does not start directly on the scar but at a short distance, getting closer to the scar during the treatment. At the end, the scar itself is treated if the patient tolerates it.

It is important to note that the technique is not always carried out parallel to the scar because the direction of the superficial tissue fibers is irregularly organized. The therapist therefore pushes the instrument perpendicularly and diagonally to the scar. The pressure is proportional to the actual thickness of the soft tissue layers. The more tissue under the instrument, the higher the pressure can be; however, the uniformity of pressure is important. It is advisable for the therapist to work with one hand and stabilize the patient's hand and forearm with the other hand.

Neurophysiologically, wounds are protected using musculature; the corresponding musculature is typically hypertonic. This is a vital protective mechanism that is controlled subcortically and thus is unconscious. After the wound has healed and a scar remains as an end-product of wound healing, the protective hypertonicity should theoretically disappear because it is no longer needed for protection. While this process is typical of physiological scars, the hypertonic protection remains in the case of non-physiological scars because the scar is not sufficiently mobile.

After successful treatment of the scar, experience suggests that the therapist must also address the hypertonic areas. Therefore, the next technique applied is Regulation of Tone. Application is again dependent on the physiotherapeutic findings. The hypertonic area is identified on palpation and treated accordingly. In the case of a post-operative scar on the palmar side of the wrist, hypertonic areas are usually located in the antebrachial fascia, the palmar aponeurosis, and the flexors of the wrist and the fingers (flexor digitorum superficialis, flexor digitorum profundus, flexor carpi radialis, flexor carpi ulnaris, palmaris longus), as well as in the pronators (pronator teres and quadratus). Nevertheless, all the wrist and finger flexors should be examined for local hypertension.

Once the therapist has located a hypertensive point, they place the straight, short instrument on it, apply vertical pressure to the tissue, and maintain this pressure until the tone subsides. The therapist may then feel they can penetrate deeper into the tissue. At the new point of tension, the pressure is held again, and the therapist waits for a new release. The technique can be completed by small movements of the instrument. In this case, the therapist moves the instrument back and forth on the spot or performs small, circular movements. Often, this "melting technique" brings an additional relaxing effect and thus increases the overall benefit.

The last technique applied in this standard treatment is the Mobilization Technique. The experienced therapist will have no difficulty locating the hypomobile zones around the scar. The superficial hypomobilities involve the antebrachial fascia, palmaris longus, and the palmar aponeurosis. They are treated according to the protocol previously described: first sensed by the displacement test, then treated accordingly.

The importance of treating superficial hypomobilities is often underestimated; in the case of superficial wrist scar treatment, this technique is crucial because the tissue layer is not very thick. If the therapist treats deeper scars, such as in the abdominal area, the Mobilization Technique is used to prepare the superficial tissue to enable deeper treatment. In the opinion of the authors, treating the deep layers significantly influences the treatment outcomes.

Special attention should be paid to the direction of the tissue mobility limitation; this is not necessarily identical over the entire scar, and several or even all directions can be affected. The limitation can be determined by a simple test of displacement using the therapist's hand or the instrument. In the case of scars, there is rarely a single point of hypomobility; the loss of mobility usually extends to the entire area around the scar. These characteristics obviously vary from one patient to another. Depending on the structure, the mobilization is carried out with the edge of the hook or the short, flat side of the instrument. It is important that the instrument always remains in contact with the same area. The instrument is not pushed over the skin, but the anatomical structure is moved in a restricted direction. Very often, the entire scar is affected by hypomobility, although not uniformly; some areas are severely affected. In these areas, it is advisable to hold the final position of the instrument for several (20–30) seconds. The return movement is then done without pressure and is described as returning to the starting position. The authors recommend starting with relatively well-moving or pain-free areas and then treating the difficult zones.

Duration
Approximately 10 minutes.

Evaluation
- ROM wrist.
- End-feel wrist extension.
- Barrier phenomenon (instead of slowly increasing, springy resistance, a suddenly appearing, firm barrier, possibly with pain, stinging, and possibly radiations).
- Scar scale: Vancouver, Manchester, Stony Brook.

Exercise progression
- Tissue stretch: stretch starting position in wrist extension.
- Tissue dynamics: active movements of the wrist (flexion–extension).

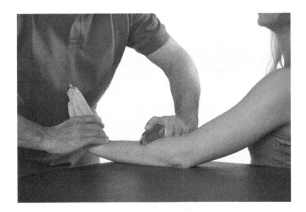

Figure 13.7 Tissue stretch: treatment in stretched position

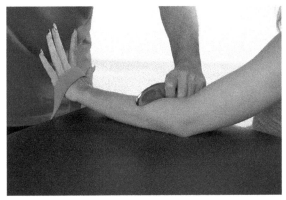

Figure 13.9 Tissue dynamics+: treatment with movements against elastic resistance

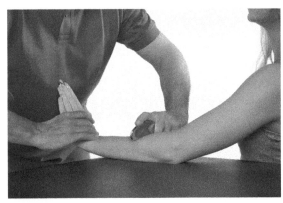

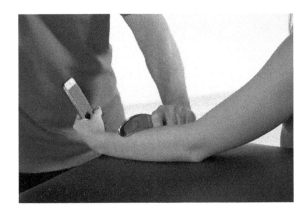

Figure 13.10 Tissue loading+: treatment during activities of daily living

- Tissue dynamics+: resistive movement against elastic resistance.
- Tissue loading+: use of tools: e.g. PC, smartphone.

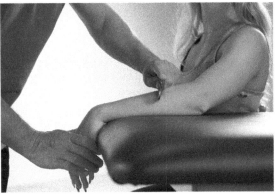

Figure 13.8 Tissue dynamics: treatment with active movements. (A) Flexion. (B) Extension.

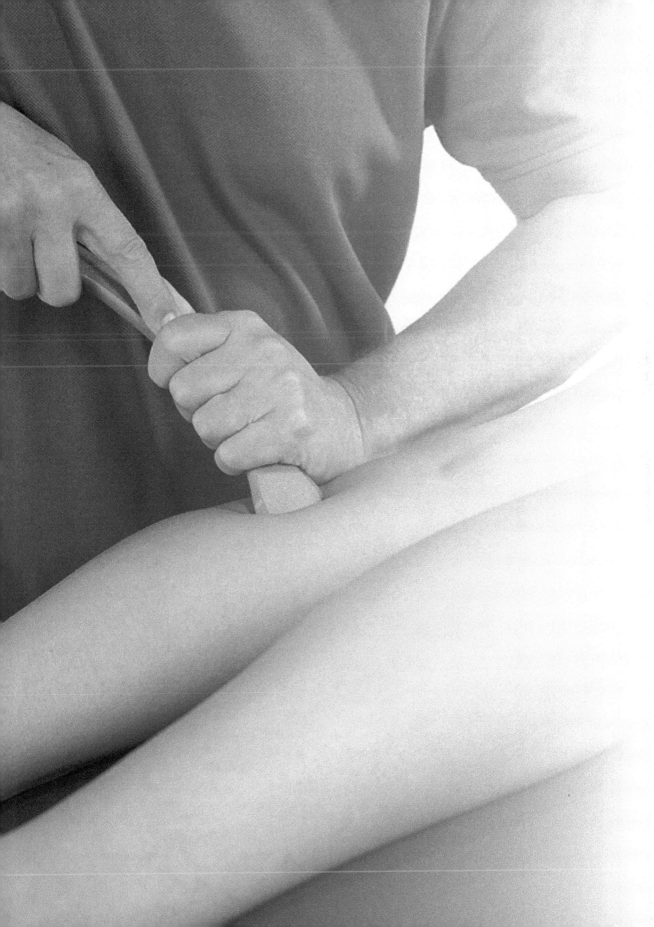

This second chapter on the treatment of scars will focus on deep scars of the fascia. The fascial structures have a higher tissue density and a more regular orientation of the fibers compared to superficial fascial structures. These aspects are found in tendons, ligaments, and joint capsules, as well as in the deeper fascia and the aponeurosis. Deeper scars may be caused by injuries like ligament sprains and muscles strains or surgical intervention in these areas.

The treatment presented here does not concern a physiological scar, which is very close to the original tissue in terms of elasticity and function. Physiological scars result from injury and undergo primary wound healing. They are generally asymptomatic and characterized by a lack of physical and/or psychological suffering.

Instead, this chapter will cover symptomatic superficial scars, including sclerotic scars, hypertrophic scars, and keloids. Obviously, wound healing must be completed for the therapy to be implemented. Frequently, scars with a poor-quality structure are formed. This type of wound healing is sometimes described as secondary wound healing. These scars are characterized by impaired function due to new tissue formation and wound contracture, and may pose a cosmetic problem with psychological suffering.

After an injury, immobilization for healing, pain, or orthosis can form a scar that is stressed in one direction only. If this scar is exercised in a typically normal manner (functionally with three-dimensional movement), recurrent damage can occur. This can result in symptomatology that is often expressed by a unidirectional "adhesive character" and the resulting disturbances in displacement of the different tissue layers involved; the latter, in turn, presents itself clinically with limitations in joint mobility. If this cause–consequence symptomatology is local, there is no difficulty in diagnosing and treating it; however, things become more problematic when this reaction is located throughout the myofascial chains. At first glance, the scar and the movement restriction (and/or pain) may be unrelated. The age of the scar or the time between scar formation and the appearance of symptoms is often considerable. The scar as a structure and as a disturbance to movement is generally permanent; thus, the reaction (the restriction of movement) is also permanent. In the authors' opinion, this suggests that scars (especially older scars) should always be considered when myofascial symptoms are present.

The therapy goals are pain relief (if pain is present) and improvement of function. Techniques that aim for rehydration, tone regulation in the surrounding tissue, and mobilization are beneficial. Since dysfunctional scars are usually accompanied by some form of excess new tissue formation, the Pain Relief Technique and the Metabolization Technique are not used locally; however, they may be applied at a distance. While these effects may be "indirect," clinical experience suggests this approach can help stubborn "scarring pain." In the case of "classic" movement restrictions due to scarring, the outcomes are often worse; pain relief in this case is also achieved indirectly. In addition to the cosmetic aspect, these non-physiological or dysfunctional scars usually have an influence on movement(s). Some are painful only in certain positions or during certain movements; therefore, exercise progressions are very important for these scars after soft tissue mobilization.

The treatment for deep fascial scars given in this chapter will be described using a common pathology as an example that can be applied to deep scars anywhere in the body. The ankle is one of the most commonly injured joints in the body. While these injuries do not generally require formal physical therapy, sprains of ankle ligaments will heal with typical "scarring" of these deeper structures. Immobilization is often recommended after an ankle sprain, which limits exposure of the healing ligament to the functional loads required for collagen alignment. This may lead to pain and reduced function because of immobilization rather than ligamentous laxity. In addition, compensatory motions in the joints below and above the ankle may lead to inter-related pain and dysfunction in the foot, knee, hip, and spine through the MCS. When coupled with the fact that ankle re-injuries are extremely common, early treatment of the ankle and related joints, in addition to balance exercise, is warranted.

Detailed Description of the Treatment

To demonstrate deep fascial scar treatment, IAMT after an acute ankle sprain is presented here. Due to the most common inversion mechanism of injury (a combination of supination and plantar flexion), the collateral fibular ligament complex is affected within its three parts: the anterior talofibular ligament is most commonly affected, while the posterior talofibular ligament and the calcaneofibular ligament are less affected. In the authors' experience, other structures are involved yet are rarely considered: the syndesmotic ligaments (tibiofibular ligament), the ligaments of Chopart's joint line (dorsal calcaneocuboid and bifurcate ligaments), the peroneal muscles (peroneus longus and brevis), and – last but not least – the deep fascia of the leg (fascia cruris) and the plantar aponeurosis. In this chapter, only the local treatment of the ligaments of the (upper) ankle joint and the syndesmosis is presented. Treatment of the other structures is also important but has been described in previous chapters.

The patient lies supine, with knee joints supported, or lies prone with the ankle joint supported (both for relaxation of the treated structure).

The therapy starts with the Rehydration Technique, using sliding of the area around the lateral side of the ankle; this is best done with the edge of the hook of an instrument. The therapist pushes the instrument very slowly around the ankle. The direction is not important but it is crucial that the technique addresses all parts of the ligaments concerned. Thus, the treatment starts ventrally at the distal tibia (insertion of the anterior syndesmotic ligament) and rotates around the entire joint to the dorsal distal tibia (insertion of the posterior syndesmotic ligament). The technique is repeated several times and each time the therapist starts moving the instrument a little more distally so that all structures are treated.

The direction of pushing should be varied as much as possible to increase the local effect. The technique should be repeated several times, starting with the next pass from the dorsal side in the opposite direction. Individual areas that are particularly affected (the anterior talofibular ligament) should be treated intensively and repeatedly. The instrument is pushed over each band individually several times in all directions: parallel to the fiber course, perpendicular, and diagonally. The pressure is proportional to the thickness of the soft tissue layers. The more tissue under the instrument, the higher the pressure can be. However, as previously described, uniformity of the pressure is important. It is recommended that the therapist works with one hand and stabilizes the patient's foot with the other hand.

The peroneal musculature should be addressed, as it may have been damaged by the mechanism of injury, having contracted to protect the joint. Neurophysiologically, injuries are often subconsciously protected using muscle tension, resulting in hypertonic musculature. After the injury has healed and scar tissue is formed, the protective hypertonicity should disappear, as it is no longer necessary with physiological scarring. In the case of non-physiological scars, the subconscious muscular protection remains because the scar lacks the necessary mobility. Muscles providing dynamic joint stabilization are often hypertonic (and thus limited in function) for an extended period; therefore, the next technique applied is Regulation of Tone. Application is dependent on the physiotherapeutic findings. The hypertonic areas are identified and treated accordingly. After an ankle sprain, these are usually located in peroneus longus and peroneus brevis. Nevertheless, all the ankle-stabilizing muscles should be examined for local hypertonicity. Once the therapist has located a hypertonic point, they place the straight, short instrument on it, apply vertical pressure to the tissue, and maintain this pressure until the tone subsides. The therapist may then have the impression that they can penetrate deeper into the tissue. At the new point of tension, the pressure is held again, and the therapist waits for a new release. The technique can be completed by small movements of the instrument. In this case, the therapist moves the instrument back and forth on the spot or performs small, circular movements. Often, this "melting technique" brings an additional relaxing effect and thus increases the overall benefit.

The final technique applied in this standard treatment is the Mobilization Technique. The experienced therapist will have no difficulty locating the hypomobile zones. The hypomobilities often involve the deep fascia of the leg (fascia cruris) and the plantar aponeurosis after ankle sprains. They are treated according to the protocol already described: first sensed by the displacement test, then treated accordingly. In the case of ankle sprain treatment, this technique is particularly important because the tissue layer is relatively thin.

Special attention should be paid to the direction of the tissue mobility limitation. This is not necessarily identical over the entire course of the scar; moreover, several or even all directions can be affected. The limitation can be determined by a simple test of displacement using the therapist's hand or the instrument. In the case of scars, there is rarely a single point, but the loss of mobility usually extends to the entire area around the scar. Depending on the structure, the mobilization is carried out with the edge of the hook or the short flat side of the instrument. It is important that the instrument always remains in contact with the same area. The instrument is not pushed over the skin, but the anatomical structure is moved in the restricted direction.

Often, the entire ligament is affected by hypomobility, but some areas are more affected than others. At these hypomobile points, it is advisable to hold the final position of the instrument for several (20–30) seconds. The return movement is then performed without pressure and is described as returning to the starting position. The authors recommend starting with relatively well-moving or pain-free areas and then treating the more difficult zones.

Duration
Approximately 10 minutes.

Evaluation
- ROM ankle joint.
- End-feel ankle supination (and plantar flexion).
- Standing and walking on the outside edge of the foot.
- Analysis of normal standing position.
- Analysis of gait.

Progression

- Tissue stretch: stretch starting position in plantar flexion.

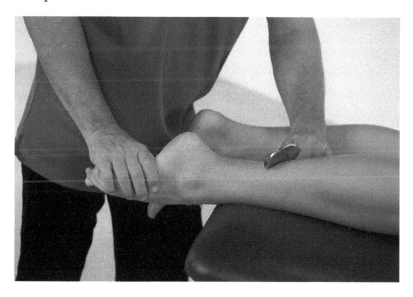

Figure 14.1 Treatment in stretch starting position: plantar flexion

- Tissue dynamics: active movements of the ankle.

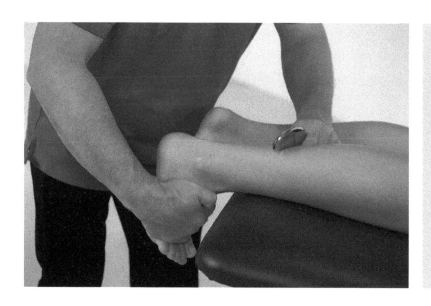

Figure 14.2 Tissue dynamics: plantar flexion

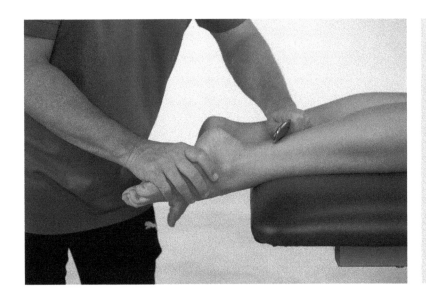

Figure 14.3 Tissue dynamics: dorsiflexion

- Tissue dynamics+: resistive movement against elastic resistance.

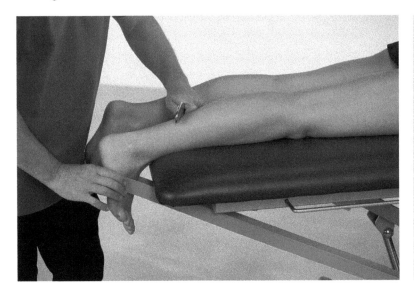

Figure 14.4 Resistive movement against elastic resistance

- Tissue loading: functionality of the starting position: e.g. standing.

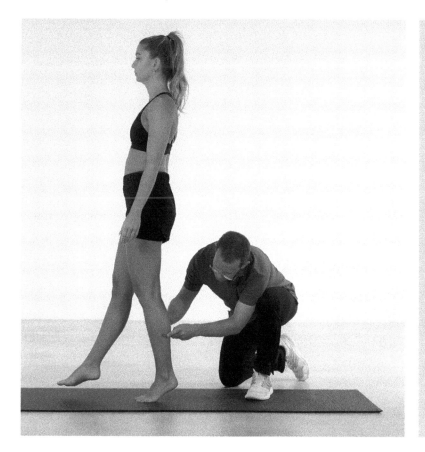

Figure 14.5 Tissue loading: treatment in functional position

- Tissue loading+: use of tools: e.g. bands, stability trainer.

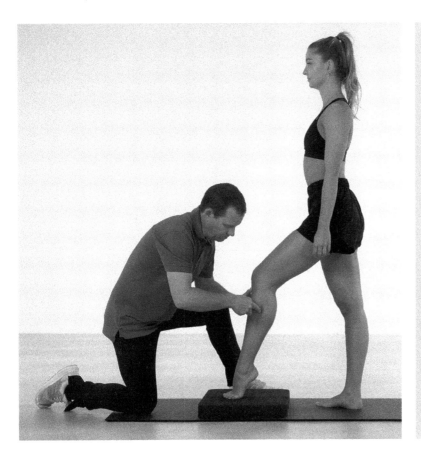

Figure 14.6 Tissue loading+: treatment using unstable surface (stability trainer)

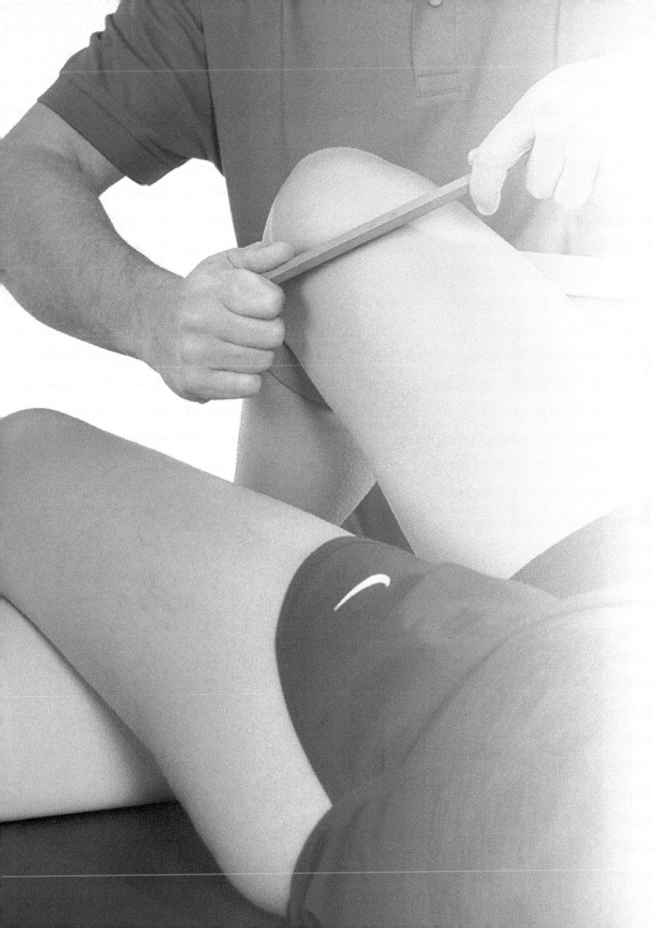

Osteoarthritis (OA) is one of the most common diseases of the musculoskeletal system and is one of the conditions most frequently encountered by the therapist in practice. All areas of the body can be affected, although some are more involved than others. In the authors' opinion, IAMT can make an important contribution to the treatment of OA, thus requiring special attention as a chapter in this book.

OA is a degenerative joint disease that often leads to chronic musculoskeletal pain in other areas of the body. Because it is a degenerative condition, the treatment of OA is important, in that it should be performed consistently on a regular basis over a long period of time. Thus, the therapist can treat the involved structures gradually; the goal should be improvement of the condition and function of these structures as the pain decreases, while limiting degenerative changes. The techniques of Rehydration, Pain Relief, Regulation of Tone, Mobilization, and Metabolization are used for OA. The treatment is both symptom- and function-oriented. Patient-specific adjustments are necessary and important due to the heterogeneity of OA. Of course, the instrument-assisted treatment of OA is not a stand-alone therapy; further measures are essential, particularly therapeutic exercises and regular physical activity.

In order to allow the therapist to individualize the treatment of OA patients and to integrate this into practice, three areas of treatment are described here: local, regional, and global. Each treatment can be used separately and at different times; they can also be applied consecutively in one session. This approach has proved clinically effective for the authors, particularly in long-term patients, varying the therapy as needed. OA affects the joints, muscles, and the MCS through regional interdependence.

Local treatment of the structures around the affected joint is described first as a starting point for therapy. Second, regional treatment of the structures of the functional unit of the affected joint (in this case, the lumbar–pelvic–hip region) is described. This regional treatment can be helpful after the acute symptoms have subsided. Finally, a treatment with a more global approach is described, which integrates the entire myofascial chain or muscle sling/loop. While the local treatment uses all IAMT techniques, the regional and global treatments apply Tone Regulation and Mobilization only. Beyond the local treatment, the other techniques are either not useful (Pain Relief Technique and Metabolization) or not practical (Rehydration).

A primary change in muscle tone due to excessive and constant use (postures and movements) will lead to hypomobilities, then pain, and later dehydration, and eventually degeneration of the structures. These adaptations will lead to a vicious cycle, in that both the cause and the consequence come to need treatment.

Swiss neurologist Alois Brügger MD described this mechanism as the "arthro-tendo-myotic reaction" in 1958 (Brügger 1958). By using this term, he wanted to signal that the whole system is involved in a protective mechanism: muscle, tendon, and joint. Today, this is referred to as the Myofascial Connected System (MCS). It is important for the therapist to determine whether this reaction is a primary dysfunction or protective of underlying dysfunction.

The theoretical foundation for a global (or body-wide) treatment is the assumption that the MCS is a continuum. The structures of this system are not grouped by their type of tissue; rather, the MCS is formed of synergistic myofascial connections. These connections have been characterized as muscle chains or loops or slings by various authors, whose opinions sometimes differ. These myofascial connections are highly functional;

their goal is enabling whole-body movement such as running, throwing, or jumping. In the authors' experience, treating these connections can significantly increase the success of treatment, particularly in the absence of a clearly injured structure such as a fracture. The clinical manifestations of this overload–compensation–pain cascade are familiar complaints from everyday therapeutic practice. The treatment procedure is basically the same as the treatment described in previous chapters; however, this approach extends beyond the painful area into causal mechanisms. Thus, treatment does not begin at the site of pain, but where the therapist assumes the cause of the problem to be.

As an example of treating chronic arthritic conditions, IAMT of hip OA is presented here. In this example, the *local* muscle function groups of the hip flexors, adductors, and external rotators are treated with Rehydration, Regulation of Tone, and Mobilization. From clinical experience, these are often tight and hypertonic. *Regionally*, the multijoint muscles are treated, as they play a major role in the transmission of restrictions: rectus femoris, iliotibial tract (IT band), the muscles of the pes anserinus superficialis, and the hamstring muscles. *Globally*, the anti-gravity erector muscles (the functional extensor chain) are treated, as clinical experience suggests that these exhibit dysfunction in patients with hip OA, specifically through the "superficial back line" described by Myers (2013: 79–99). These structures include the plantar fascia, short and long flexors of the foot and toes, triceps surae muscle, hamstring muscles, sacrotuberous ligament, erector spinae muscle, the epicranius (occipitofrontalis) muscle, and the epicranial aponeurosis. The reader will find the treatment of these structures in the corresponding chapters.

In addition, all these structures should be treated with loading (stretching and strengthening) and neuromuscular integration (stabilization and synchronization). Of course, the exercises that specifically involve the lower quarter, and especially the hips and the knees, are preferred. The patient should regularly perform the exercise program at home and document progress; in this way, a continuous and progressive treatment can be maintained.

Local Treatment

Schematic Representation of the Treatment

Diagnosis

Osteoarthritis of the hip.

Locally affected structures (Figures 15.1 and 15.2)

- Hip flexors (iliopsoas, sartorius, rectus femoris).
- Hip adductors (pectineus, adductor longus, adductor brevis, adductor magnus, gracilis, gluteus maximus).
- Hip external rotators (especially gemellus superior, obturator internus, gemellus inferior, quadratus femoris).

Initial position

First lying supine (ventral and medial structures), then lying prone (dorsal structures).

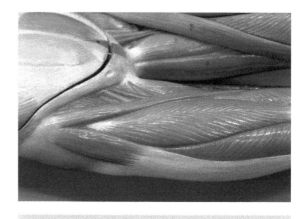

Figure 15.1 Locally affected anterior structures

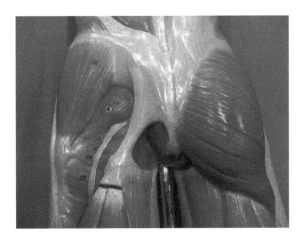

Figure 15.2 Locally affected posterior structures

Material

- Recommended: straight elongated instrument or combination curve instrument, straight short instrument.
- Optional: curved instrument.

Technique

- Recommended: Rehydration, Pain Relief, Regulation of Tone, Mobilization, Metabolization.
- Optional: none.

Recommended treatment protocol (Table 15.1)

Rehydration Technique (ReT)

- Fascia lata and gluteal fascia (entire area of the hip).

Pain Relief Technique (PRT)

- Painful area in the buttocks, groin, or thigh.

Regulation of Tone Technique (RoT)

- Iliopsoas, sartorius, rectus femoris.
- Pectineus, adductor longus, adductor brevis, adductor magnus, gracilis, gluteus maximus.
- Gemellus superior, obturator internus, gemellus inferior, quadratus femoris.

Mobilization Technique (MoT)

- Tenoperiosteal transition of iliopsoas, sartorius, rectus femoris.
- Tenoperiosteal transition of pectineus, adductor longus, adductor brevis, adductor magnus, gracilis, gluteus maximus.
- Tenoperiosteal transition of gemellus superior, obturator internus, gemellus inferior, quadratus femoris.

Metabolization Technique (MeT)

- Painful area in the buttocks, groin, or thigh.

Table 15.1 Osteoarthritis: summary of recommended treatment protocol (local)

ReT	PRT	RoT	MoT	MeT
Fascia lata and gluteal fascia (entire area of the hip)	Painful area in the buttocks, groin, or thigh	Iliopsoas, sartorius, rectus femoris	Tenoperiosteal transition of iliopsoas, sartorius, rectus femoris	Painful area in the buttocks, groin, or thigh
		Pectineus, adductor longus, adductor brevis, adductor magnus, gracilis, gluteus maximus	Tenoperiosteal transition of pectineus, adductor longus, adductor brevis, adductor magnus, gracilis, gluteus maximus	
		Gemellus superior, obturator internus, gemellus inferior, quadratus femoris	Tenoperiosteal transition of gemellus superior, obturator internus, gemellus inferior, quadratus femoris	

Visual Presentation of the Treatment Unit

Rehydration Technique (ReT)

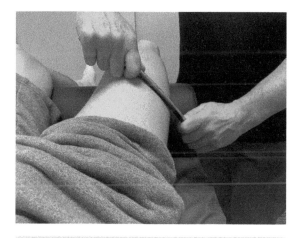

Figure 15.3 Lateral thigh

Regulation of Tone Technique (RoT)

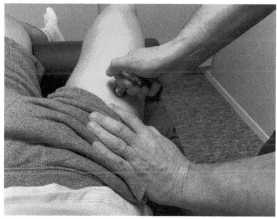

Figure 15.5 Rectus femoris

Pain Relief Technique (PRT)

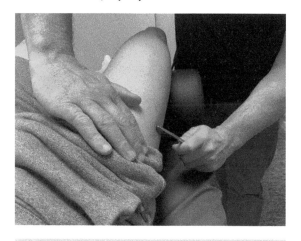

Figure 15.4 Painful area in the (lateral) thigh

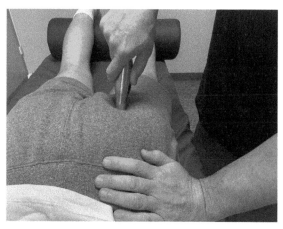

Figure 15.6 Quadratus femoris

Mobilization Technique (MoT)

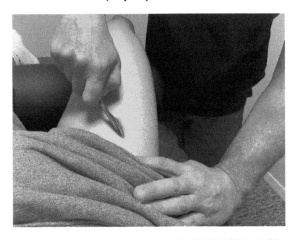

Figure 15.7 Tenoperiosteal transition: sartorius

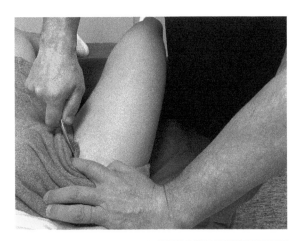

Figure 15.8 Tenoperiosteal transition: pectineus

Metabolization Technique (MeT)

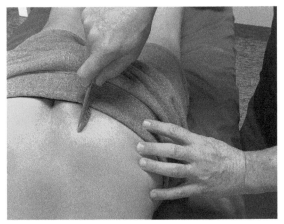

Figure 15.9 Painful area in the buttocks

Duration
Approximately 20 minutes.

Evaluation
- Numeric rating scale (NRS).
- ROM and end-feel hip and knee.
- Straight leg raise or extension of the knee in flexed position of the hip.
- Analysis of standing position, analysis of gait.
- Tiptoe test.

Regional Treatment

Schematic Representation of the Treatment

Diagnosis
Osteoarthritis of the hip.

Regionally affected structures
(Figures 15.10 and 15.11)
- Rectus femoris.
- Iliotibial tract (IT band) and tensor fasciae latae.

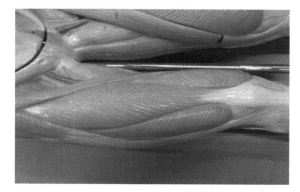

Figure 15.10 Regionally affected anterior structures

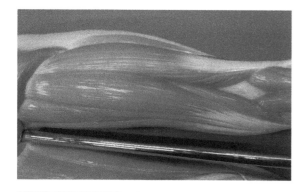

Figure 15.11 Regionally affected posterior structures

- Muscles of the pes anserinus superficialis (sartorius, gracilis, semitendinosus).
- Hamstring muscles.

Initial position

First lying supine (ventral and lateral structures), then lying prone (dorsal structures).

Material

- Recommended: straight elongated instrument or combination curve instrument, straight short instrument.
- Optional: curved instrument.

Technique

- Recommended: Regulation of Tone, Mobilization.
- Optional: Rehydration.

Recommended treatment protocol (Table 15.2)

Regulation of Tone Technique (RoT)

- Rectus femoris.
- Iliotibial tract (IT band) and tensor fasciae latae.
- Muscles of the pes anserinus superficialis.
- Hamstring muscles.

Mobilization Technique (MoT)

- Rectus femoris.
- Iliotibial tract (IT band) and tensor fasciae latae.
- Muscles of the pes anserinus superficialis.
- Hamstring muscles.

Table 15.2 Osteoarthritis: summary of recommended treatment protocol (regional)

ReT	PRT	RoT	MoT	MeT
		Rectus femoris	Rectus femoris	
		Iliotibial tract (IT band) and tensor fasciae latae	Iliotibial tract (IT band) and tensor fasciae latae	
		Muscles of the pes anserinus superficialis	Muscles of the pes anserinus superficialis	
		Hamstring muscles	Hamstring muscles	

Visual Presentation of the Treatment Unit

Regulation of Tone Technique (RoT)

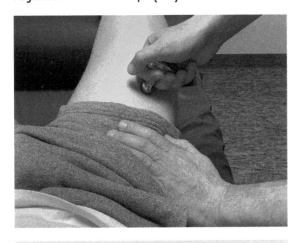

Figure 15.12 Rectus femoris

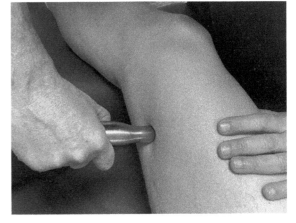

Figure 15.14 Course of the muscles of the pes anserinus (e.g. gracilis)

Mobilization Technique (MoT)

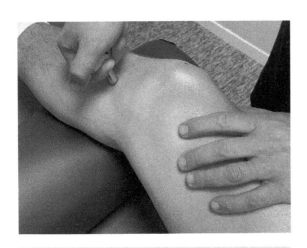

Figure 15.13 Insertion of the muscles of the pes anserinus superficialis

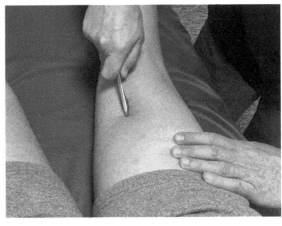

Figure 15.15 Hamstring muscles

Duration

Approximately 15 minutes.

Evaluation

- Numeric rating scale (NRS).
- ROM and end-feel hip and knee.
- Straight leg raise or extension of the knee in flexed position of the hip.
- Analysis of standing position, analysis of gait.
- Tiptoe test.

Global Treatment

From a global perspective, structures are treated based on the "superficial back line" (SBL) of Myers (2013) (see the schematic treatment below) and the "great diagonal muscle loop" (GDML) of Brügger (1986) (see the schematic treatment on page 256); according to Brügger, the GDML is an important muscle loop in human locomotion. The first treatment (SBL) is described as an example of treatment in a lying position. The second treatment (GDML) is described as an example for treatment in a more functional starting position (standing or stepping position). Due to the duration of the treatment, often only the Regulation of Tone Technique is used; however, as described in the progressions, almost all techniques are possible or useful in different starting positions. In the MCS, the combinations are almost infinite.

Schematic Representation of the Treatment: SBL

Diagnosis

Osteoarthritis of the hip.

Globally affected structures (Figures 15.16–15.20)

- Plantar fascia.
- Short and long flexors of the foot and toes.
- Triceps surae.
- Hamstring muscles.

- Sacrotuberous ligament.
- Erector spinae.
- Epicranius.
- Epicranial aponeurosis.

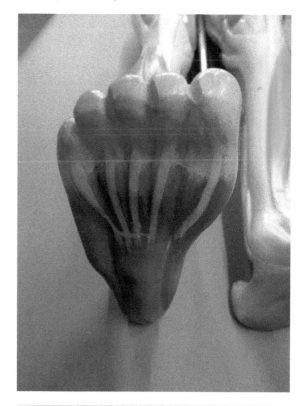

Figure 15.16 Plantar structures of the foot

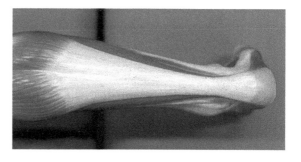

Figure 15.17 Dorsal structures of the leg

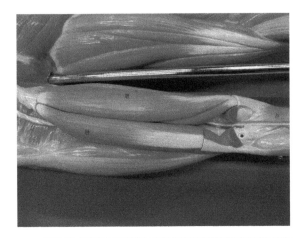

Figure 15.18 Dorsal structures of the thigh (deeper layer)

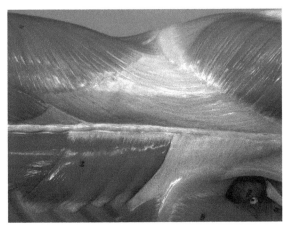

Figure 15.20 Dorsal structures of the (lumbar) spine

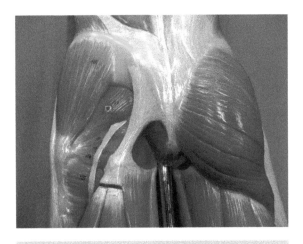

Figure 15.19 Dorsal structures of the pelvis

Initial position

Lying prone, with ankle joints supported (relaxation of the treated structure) or feet in overhang.

Material

- Recommended: straight, short instrument.
- Optional: none.

Technique

- Recommended: Regulation of Tone.
- Optional: none.

Recommended treatment protocol (Table 15.3)

Regulation of Tone Technique (RoT)

- Short and long flexors of the foot and toes.
- Triceps surae.
- Hamstring muscles.
- Erector spinae.
- Epicranius.

Table 15.3 Osteoarthritis: summary of recommended treatment protocol (SBL)

ReT	PRT	RoT	MoT	MeT
		Short and long flexors of the foot and toes		
		Triceps surae		
		Hamstring muscles		
		Erector spinae		
		Epicranius		

Visual Presentation of the Treatment Unit

Regulation of Tone Technique (RoT)

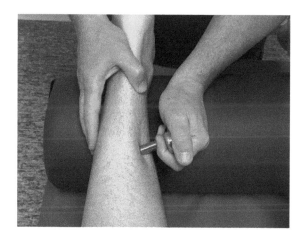

Figure 15.22 Long flexors of the toes: flexor hallucis longus

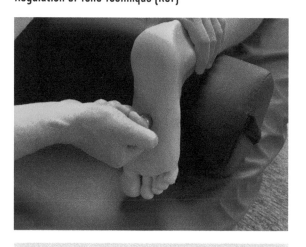

Figure 15.21 Short flexors of the foot: digitorum brevis

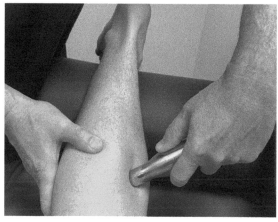

Figure 15.23 Triceps surae, medial head

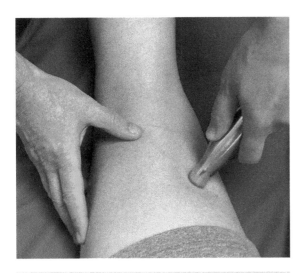

Figure 15.24 Semitendinosus (hamstring muscles)

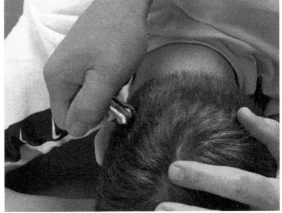

Figure 15.26 Epicranius

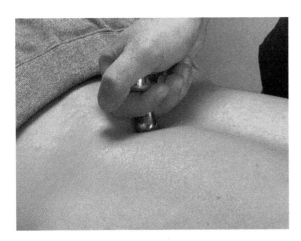

Figure 15.25 Erector spinae

Duration

Approximately 20 minutes.

Evaluation

- Numeric rating scale (NRS).
- Analysis of gait.
- Analysis of activities of daily living.

Schematic Representation of the Treatment: GDML

Diagnosis

Osteoarthritis of the hip.

Globally affected structures

- Tibialis anterior and posterior.
- Peroneus longus and brevis.
- Iliotibial tract (IT band).
- Tensor fasciae latae.
- Sartorius.
- Internal and external obliques (opposite side of the body).
- Erector spinae (via ribs).
- Trapezius, ascending/lower part (via scapulae).
- Pectoralis major.

Initial position
Standing or stepping position.

Material
- Recommended: straight short instrument.
- Optional: none.

Technique
- Recommended: Regulation of Tone.
- Optional: none.

Recommended treatment protocol (Table 15.4)

Regulation of Tone Technique (RoT)

- Tibialis anterior and posterior.
- Peroneus longus and brevis.
- Iliotibial tract (IT band) and tensor fasciae latae.
- Sartorius.
- Internal and external obliques.
- Erector spinae.
- Trapezius (ascending/lower part).
- Pectoralis major.

Table 15.4 Osteoarthritis: summary of recommended treatment protocol (GDML)				
ReT	PRT	RoT	MoT	MeT
		Tibialis anterior and posterior		
		Peroneus longus and brevis		
		Iliotibial tract (IT band) and tensor fasciae latae		
		Sartorius		
		Internal and external obliques		
		Erector spinae		
		Trapezius (ascending/lower part)		
		Pectoralis major		

Visual Presentation of the Treatment Unit

Regulation of Tone Technique (RoT)

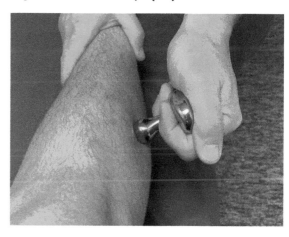

Figure 15.27 Tibialis anterior

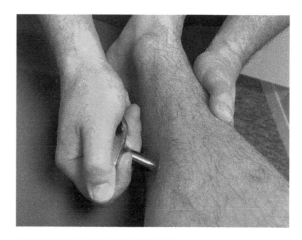

Figure 15.28 Tibialis posterior

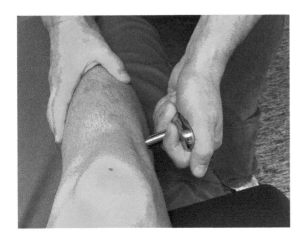

Figure 15.29 Peroneus longus

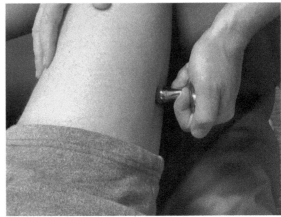

Figure 15.31 Iliotibial tract (IT band)

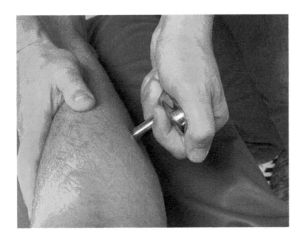

Figure 15.30 Peroneus brevis

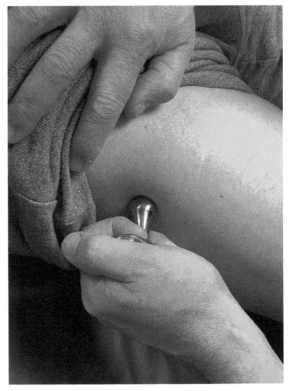

Figure 15.32 Tensor fasciae latae

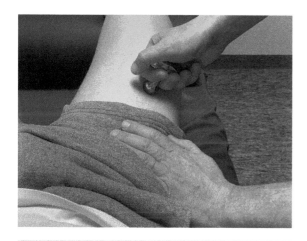

Figure 15.33 Sartorius

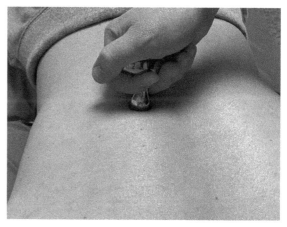

Figure 15.35 Erector spinae

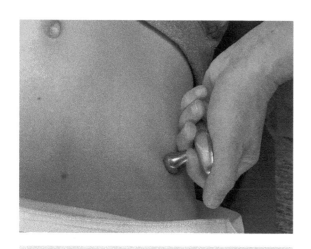

Figure 15.34 Internal and external obliques

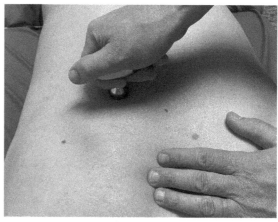

Figure 15.36 Trapezius (ascending/lower part)

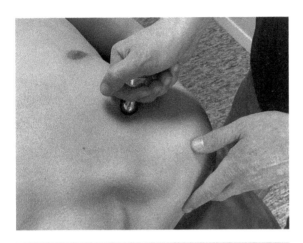

Figure 15.37 Pectoralis major

Duration
Approximately 15 minutes.

Evaluation
- Numeric rating scale (NRS).
- Analysis of gait.
- Analysis of activities of daily living.

References

Brügger A (1958) Über die Tendomyose. Dtsch. med. Wschr 83:1048.

Myers TW (2013) Anatomy Trains E-Book: Myofascial Meridians for Manual and Movement Therapists. Philadelphia: Elsevier Health Sciences.

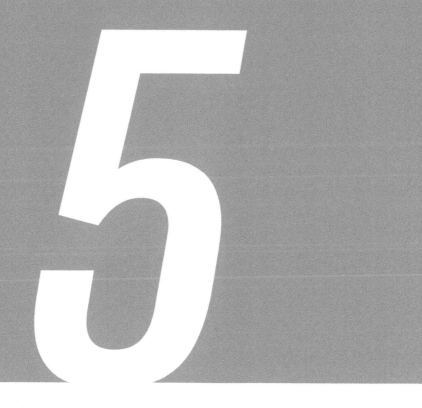

5

Case Studies and Treatment Protocols/
Algorithms

The following part of the book deals with a selection of case studies and treatment protocols, to give the reader some real clinical examples of work in IAMT. In physical therapy, an account of treatments from practice not only is common, but also has very high value. In science, of course, the situation is somewhat different but, for the purposes of this book, the authors felt that these chapters were very enriching. The special thing is that they have been written by really well-known colleagues. Even if that means that the writing style and mode of expression deviate somewhat, it seemed to the authors both more authentic and more purposeful not only to accept that, but even to promote it! The result is a real treasure trove for the practitioner. The explanations are very stimulating and deal not only with the large joints of the extremities such as the shoulder and hip, but also with the spine (cervical and lumbar). The chapters are also illustrated and clearly structured but avoid overly detailed structural descriptions, so the reader is free to appreciate not only the authors' enthusiasm but also their experience and expertise.

Case Studies and Treatment Protocols/Algorithms

When Instrument-assisted Soft Tissue Mobilization (IASTM) is applied to the shoulder region, a proper diagnosis is necessary for better selection of technique. While all soft tissue treatment has a neurologic component that attempts to reset the tone of tissue, tendon injuries or capsular restriction will utilize pro-inflammatory applications and bursitis will utilize anti-inflammatory applications.

Some of the most common disorders associated with the shoulder are related to impingement. The most common impairments associated with impingement include scapular dyskinesia, anterior laxity, posterior capsule contractures, rotator cuff injury or imbalances, and acromioclavicular outlet issues (congenital or acquired). For the purposes of this chapter, we will also address acromioclavicular/sternoclavicular (AC/SC) sprains and bursitis. However, we will not consider the conditions that may create increased mechanical strain on internal derangement issues, such as labral or SLAP tears (superior labral tears from anterior to posterior), as well as arthrosis. For these conditions, the clinician must address the imbalances that create greater strain on the internal structures. The imbalances will be considered in terms of the causes of impingement listed above.

When applying IASTM for a particular diagnosis, the clinician first needs to understand the state of the soft tissue they are treating. Is it in an acute phase, such as following a fall or single-event injury? Is it a chronic condition stemming from a postural disorder or chronic degeneration? The pressure/duration applied with IASTM will affect the way the body reacts to it. The heavier the pressure, the greater the fibroblastic proliferation and the greater the inflammatory response. The lighter the pressure, the more the treatment orients to a neurologic response and superficial vascular changes.

In this chapter, different shoulder impairments associated with common impingement will be presented using a standardized approach. First, a provocation technique is applied to elicit symptoms before treatment and is repeated after treatment to measure effectiveness. Next, the treatment region is identified. The treatment is then described, often involving active or resisted movement, along with the types of IASTM stroke, pressure, and duration. Finally, the goals of the treatment are established. Common impairments include scapular dyskinesia, rotator cuff imbalance, capsular imbalance, AC outlet issues, and bursitis.

Scapular Dyskinesia

This is one of the most common disorders of the shoulder (Box 16.1). It is rare for there to be ideal scapular movements in any impingement or shoulder injury. In order to treat dyskinesia with IASTM, the entire upper quadrant must be addressed. The scapula is a coordinated "ballet" of muscular movements. If there is any imbalance, the scapula will no longer move correctly, which will create much greater strain on all shoulder structures. IASTM is most effective when it is utilized to neurologically rebalance the firing pattern of these muscles. This can be accomplished with soft tissue treatment to all muscles that attach to the scapula, with some extra neurologic stimulation of movement (Figure 16.1).

Box 16.1

IASTM treatment protocol for scapular dyskinesia

Provocation assessment: Scapular mobility is most easily tested watching for symmetry during shoulder abduction

Treatment: Shoulder abduction is most commonly used but all motions can be helpful

Region: The upper quadrant of the involved side. All muscles that attach to the scapula either directly or indirectly through joint attachments in the upper quadrant

Type of stroke: Broad, longer strokes about 10 cm (4 inches) in length with overlapping strokes

Application/pressure: Neurosensory/weight of instrument to slightly deeper at a 30–60-degree angle

Duration: Until a hyperemia is created; then reassess. No more than three reassessments in a treatment

Goal: Always start initial treatment assessment by having the patient note their pain level during provocation as "10" before treatment. The clinician should hope to reduce symptoms to 5 or below by post-assessment.

Rotator Cuff Imbalances

Rotator cuff injuries or imbalances can be due to repetitive strain or acute trauma. The cause will determine the type of IASTM treatment. Since most tendinopathies involve chronic degenerative tissue from repetitive injury, the clinician will use a pro-inflammatory approach. In the case of a single-event injury, an anti-inflammatory approach can be adopted. The most commonly involved rotator cuff tendon is that of supraspinatus, followed by that of infraspinatus. Two separate sites should always be considered when treating rotator cuff injuries: the myotendinous junction and the insertion of the tendon. The tendons involved should be determined through manual muscle testing of the suspected tissue. While this section focuses on the rotator cuff, it is important to include biceps tendinopathy here as well. As pro-inflammatory applications are designed to boost fibroblastic proliferation, and eccentric loading

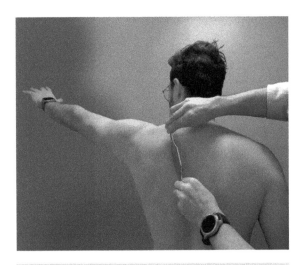

Figure 16.1 IASTM to the medial scapular border during shoulder abduction for scapular dyskinesia

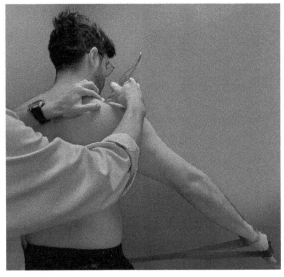

Figure 16.2 Applying IASTM with eccentric shoulder abduction using an elastic band for supraspinatus tendinopathy

on injured tendons greatly increases the amount of collagen produced, the clinician will combine both eccentric loading and heavier pressure (pro-inflammatory) (Figures 16.2 and 16.3; Box 16.2).

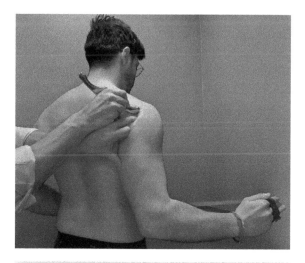

Figure 16.3 Applying IASTM with eccentric shoulder external rotation using an elastic band for posterior rotator cuff tendinopathy

Box 16.2

IASTM treatment protocol for rotator cuff imbalances

Provocation assessment: Muscle test that reproduces the pain of the involved tendon or tendons

Treatment: Eccentric loading of the involved tendon with a pro-inflammatory application using an elastic band

Region: Tissues and tendons associated with the positive muscle test

Type of stroke: Broad, longer strokes about 10 cm (4 inches) in length with overlapping strokes over the involved muscle. Shorter strokes of 1.25–2.50 cm (½–1 inch) at the myotendinous junction and/or the tendon attachment sites

Application/pressure: Neurosensory/weight of instrument to slightly deeper over the muscle region at a 30–60-degree angle. Pro-inflammatory application over the myotendinous junction and/or tendon attachment sites at an angle closer to 90 degrees

Duration: Pro-inflammatory tendon treatments should not last more than 10–15 seconds. No more than three reassessments in a treatment.

Goal: Always start initial treatment assessment as 10 on provocation. The clinician should hope to reduce symptoms to 5 or below by last assessment. It is important to understand that part of the reduction in pain is a contact anesthesia. It is also critical to inform the patient that the pain will return as the "anesthetic effect" wears off and that soreness from the pro-inflammatory treatment, while normal, will start within 2 hours of the treatment and may continue for 24–48 hours. Any longer than this should cause the clinician to reduce the intensity on the next visit.

Capsular Imbalance

The shoulder requires a joint capsule that provides both mobility and stability through a wide range of motion. Anterior laxity is not generally treated with IASTM, but much like scapular dyskinesia, the goal for the clinician is to balance the structures that assist in creating anterior translation, while "waking up" the tissues that assist in keeping the humerus in the glenoid. In this situation, the clinician will treat capsular imbalance very similarly to scapular dyskinesia (Box 16.3). The only exception will be if there is a posterior capsule contracture to accompany it. The easiest way to determine if anterior laxity is present is a positive relocation test during supine external rotation (ER). The easiest way to determine if there is a posterior capsule contracture is by testing for passive internal rotation (IR) while the patient is supine.

Box 16.3

IASTM treatment protocol for capsular imbalance

Provocation assessment: Relocation test for anterior laxity, passive IR for posterior capsule contracture

Treatment: Motion or activity that reproduces the anterior laxity, active IR from 90 degrees of abduction and full ER position for the posterior capsule

Region: Tissues associated with the upper quadrant for the anterior laxity and the posterior capsule

Type of stroke: Broad, longer strokes about 10 cm (4 inches) in length with overlapping strokes at a 30–60-degree angle for the anterior laxity and a "pin and stretch" technique on the posterior capsule at an angle closer to 90 degrees

Application/pressure: Neurosensory/weight of instrument to slightly deeper until hyperemia for anterior laxity and pro-inflammatory heavy pressure on the posterior capsule

Duration: Until a hyperemia is created; then reassess for anterior laxity. For the posterior capsule, three passes from the ER position in abduction to IR. No more than three reassessments in a treatment

Goal: Always start initial treatment assessment as 10 on provocation. The clinician should hope to reduce symptoms to 5 or below by last assessment. Following the posterior capsule treatment, 50 percent reduction in symptoms and reduced anterior translation of the head of the humerus in passive IR.

Acromioclavicular Outlet Issues

With AC outlet issues associated with either congenital or arthritic (acquired) acromion process shaping that reduces the supraspinatus outlet, the goal is to improve scapular mechanics to increase the amount of space created as the arm is going through elevation; however, the coracoacromial ligament may also thicken. IASTM can help in reducing fibrosis of the ligament, allowing for reduced compression in impingement zones. In this section, we will discuss injuries that are more applicable to the AC region, such as AC sprains. AC sprains are one of the injuries that are most successfully treated with IASTM. The ligaments are so superficial that, even in a pro-inflammatory situation like this, the amount of pressure needed is minimal to achieve great results. As fibroblastic proliferation tends to occur over lines of strain, the clinician should try to accomplish the same goal with AC ligaments. Since different tensions are placed on the ligaments in different positions, several can be used to accomplish this goal. Depression, elevation, or activities such as a push-up can accomplish this strain as the ligament is treated in a pro-inflammatory application. If the AC sprain took place over a very short period of time, very little pressure needs to be applied, as inflammation in the ligament has already occurred and the

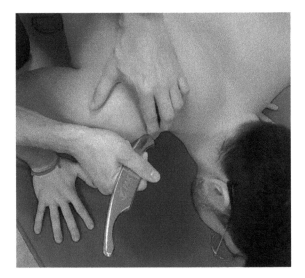

Figure 16.4 Applying IASTM to the AC ligament during a push-up

clinician will simply assist in the remodeling of the ligament. In an injury that took place over a few days, slightly heavier pressure will be used. The same is true for the SC ligaments (Figure 16.4; Box 16.4).

in an anti-inflammatory process, injection may be avoidable. Treatment can be performed daily over 4 days or in a varying schedule of every other day, or twice a week, depending on the severity of symptoms. The key is an extremely light pressure over the inflamed bursal area. The patient should move within their capabilities, such as moving from IR to ER while the arm is at the side, or simply supination and pronation with the arm at the side and advancing into elevation maneuvers (Box 16.5).

Box 16.4

IASTM treatment protocol for AC outlet issues

Provocation assessment: Is there a position, motion, or activity that reproduces the pain?

Treatment: In the position, motion or activity that reproduces the pain

Type of stroke: Broad, longer strokes about 10 cm (4 inches) in length with overlapping strokes on the muscles attaching to the clavicle or acromion at an angle of 30–60 degrees. Short strokes of 1.25 cm (½ inch) over the ligaments at an angle closer to 90 degrees

Application/pressure: Neurosensory/weight of instrument over the muscles attaching to the clavicle or acromion. Pro-inflammatory application (still light due to the superficial position of the ligaments) over the AC or SC ligaments

Region: Associated tissues that attach to the clavicle or acromion. AC ligaments, coracoacromial ligaments, SC ligaments

Duration: Until a hyperemia is created over the muscles; then reassess. Over the ligaments no more than 10–15 seconds at a time. No more than three reassessments in a treatment

Goal: Always start initial treatment assessment as 10 on provocation. The clinician should hope to reduce symptoms to 5 or below by last assessment. ROM should also drastically improve following treatment in elevation.

Box 16.5

IASTM treatment protocol for shoulder bursitis

Provocation assessment: All shoulder testing is positive during bursitis evaluation. It gives a "muddled" appearance

Treatment: In the position, motion, or activity that reproduces very minimal pain

Region: Over the inflamed bursa

Type of stroke: Broad, longer strokes about 10 cm (4 inches) in length with overlapping strokes at an angle of 30–60 degrees, closer to 30 degrees to minimize the amount of pressure

Application/pressure: Anti-inflammatory, not even the weight of the instrument

Duration: Until a very light hyperemia is created; then reassess. No more than three reassessments in a treatment

Goal: While achieving a 50 percent reduction in a treatment is highly unlikely, the goal with bursitis is from treatment to treatment with reduction in pain, improved ROM, and better sleep. Bursitis should be eliminated after four visits. If not, refer for injection

---

Bursitis

Shoulder bursitis is most commonly treated with cortisone injections; however, if IASTM is applied

A Critical Link to Daily Occupations

The elbow is a critical link to our daily occupations and our surrounding world. It provides load transfer of forces and stability in a variety of closed and open chain activities. These important occupations range from self-feeding, grooming, independent living skills, employment, and engagement in leisure activities. Injury to the elbow and surrounding tissue often leads to significant limitations in activities that are essential for function and may have lasting undesirable effects (Vincent et al. 2021).

The elbow is not a simple hinge joint. It is a complex system that is an essential link to the performance of both distal and proximal structures. The elbow complex is comprised of three joints: active/passive stabilizers and the joint capsule. It is a conduit for the median, radial, and ulnar nerves, providing neuromuscular, sensory, and proprioceptive input for the distal motor units. These closely packed and congruent structures allow for a variety of movements such as pronation/supination for forearm rotation, along with elbow flexion and extension (Lockard 2006). Functional motions of the elbow allowing for engagement in daily activities such as answering a telephone, using utensils, opening a door, and typing on a keyboard have been shown to range from 130 to 23 degrees of elbow flexion/extension and 65 to 77 degrees of forearm pronation/supination (Sardelli et al. 2011).

It has been demonstrated that immobilization of the elbow can lead to flexion/extension contractures, as well as having a negative impact on brain neural plasticity and alterations in the somatosensory cortex (Langer et al. 2012; Moisello et al. 2008). Limitations in superficial fascial glide where the integument requires mobility mean that the elbow is unable to respond efficiently to tactile input via mechanoreceptors such as Meissner's, Ruffini, and Pacinian corpuscles, and Merkel's disks, which impacts afferent sensory input and efferent motor output (Purves et al. 2001). Deeper fascial adhesions in the skeletal muscle unit at the level of the epimysium and perimysium negatively impact smooth controlled motor unit activation forces, leading to abnormal movement patterns in the system as a whole via the concept of regional interdependence (Sueki et al. 2013).

The Elbow and Instrument-assisted Soft Tissue Mobilization (IASTM)

IASTM has been shown to have a positive impact on soft tissue flexibility, musculoskeletal pain management, proprioception, and tactile discrimination (Kim et al. 2017; Bitra and Sudhan 2019; Cheatham et al. 2019). To date, there is no formal evidence-based research-driven protocol related to dosage and application for IASTM. A thorough clinical examination of the involved region to be treated should precede IASTM intervention and should include:

- a history of previous/present dysfunction
- active/passive range of motion (ROM)
- strength testing, integument
- sensory and pain assessments
- provocative testing.

After a thorough differential diagnosis of elbow pathology has been completed and the location of dysfunction has been identified, IASTM can proceed.

Common conditions of the elbow that have been treated with IASTM include, but are not limited to, all of the following:

- elbow flexion contractures
- medial/lateral tendinopathy
- distal biceps/triceps injuries

- lateral and medial collateral ligament injuries
- post-surgical scarring.

Limitations in ROM due to soft tissue shortening and adhesions caused by injury have been documented to develop over a short period. The anterior/posterior capsule of the elbow has been noted to increase in density as much as 3–4 mm (⅛ inch) within days of injury (Dávila and Johnston-Jones 2006). A comprehensive understanding of bone, ligament, tendon, nerve, and integument healing is essential prior to administering IASTM in a safe and efficacious manner.

Application of IASTM at the elbow must first begin with a process of scanning selected soft tissue compartments/regions from cephalad and caudal to the involved structures. This can be done with a single-bevel convex instrument so as to create a more focal intense edge to identify soft tissue limitations. These areas should include, but are not limited to:

- posterior/anterior shoulder girdle
- quadrangular spaces
- biceps brachii
- antecubital fossa
- bicipital aponeurosis
- triceps brachii
- supracondylar ridge
- proximal flexor/pronator mass
- proximal extensor wad
- supinator
- anconeus.

The scanning of the previously stated regions on the ipsilateral extremity is to establish a baseline of soft tissue quality compared to the contralateral limb. The clinician assesses for tissue reactivity, soft tissue rigidity, granular, gritty restriction, shortening of motor units, myofascial trigger points, and any tissue hypomobility that may be associated with the suspected pathology (Figure 17.1A).

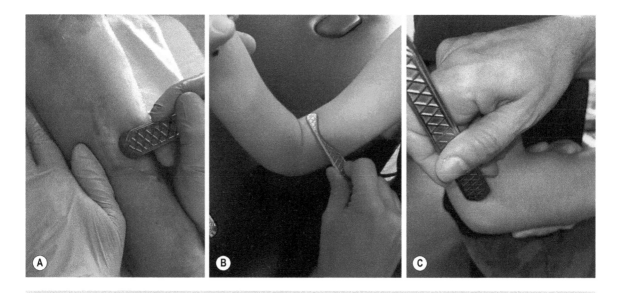

Figure 17.1 (A) Scar nudging for differential soft tissue mobilization. (B) Sweeping the brachioradialis and extensor wad. (C) Cross-friction/strumming along the lateral epicondyle of the humerus.

Techniques

A sensible algorithm for intervention regarding lateral epicondylosis initially involves treating the triceps and lateral triceps fascia along the supracondylar ridge, proximal extensor wad, and anconeus. This approach can have positive inhibitory effects on surrounding hypomobile tissue before engaging the hyperirritable common extensor origin at the lateral condyle of the distal humerus. The elbow can be flexed to shorten the biceps in a forearm-pronated position and the soft tissue structures pinned underneath the instrument performing the "pin and stretch" technique for fascial lengthening (Figure 17.1B). As the elbow is actively or passively extended and the forearm pronated or supinated, the instrument glides to mobilize the engaged tissue. Instrument dosage is based on the patient's sensitivity, tissue reactivity, and response to applied intervention using a test–retest approach. At the lateral elbow epicondyle, a 60–90-degree small oscillation strumming technique with a single-bevel edge can be utilized in one direction; this is comparable to Dr James Cyriax's transverse friction massage to decrease soft tissue ischemia and promote fibroblastic proliferation, which has been shown to mitigate pain (Kharabian et al. 2014) (Figure 17.1C). As with any intervention after manual therapy, a new cortical motor pattern must be established. The incorporation of exercise and activity in a functional multiplanar movement program is paramount to engaging the newly lengthened soft tissue structures for greater neuromuscular control. The case study in Box 17.1 gives light to the complete therapeutic intervention process from evaluation and treatment planning, to layering of multiple treatment modalities in conjunction with IASTM for a holistic integration approach.

Box 17.1

Case example

A 37-year-old right-handed male presented with slow insidious onset of right lateral elbow pain which is self-limiting. This individual came to clinic approximately 18 weeks from onset of pain with no previous physiotherapy or conservative interventions being administered. The patient's occupational profile revealed a sedentary administrative position held for 30–50 hours per week performing computer typing, telephone meetings, and writing skills. The patient reported subjective pain as 6/10, and mechanical pain only focally at the lateral epicondyle, greatest with elbow extension, forearm pronation, wrist extension, and with gripping and forearm rotation.

Formal evaluation demonstrated full active ROM throughout both upper extremities equally, with bilateral manual muscle testing revealing 4/5 strength with general complaints of proximal muscle fatigue and generalized diminished posterior cuff muscle tone. A negative cervical screen was determined for radiculopathy or thoracic outlet syndrome. Positive provocative testing for lateral epicondylitis included a (+) Cozen's test, (+) middle finger extension test, (+) resisted supination, Mill's test, and pain with palpation at the superior portion of the lateral epicondyle.

Intervention was multimodal and began with a home program that included workstation ergonomics, levator scapulae/upper trapezius/scalene stretch, posterior resisted rotator cuff/periscapular conditioning exercises, soft tissue mobility, and transverse friction massage. In-clinic treatment began with focal ultrasound for soft tissue heat, and instrument-assisted soft tissue mobility with progression of progressive resistive exercises from isometric to concentric to eccentric exercise. Short-term pain was mitigated with the use of kinesiology tape and topical analgesics.

The Quick Disabilities of Arm, Shoulder, and Hand (DASH) outcome measure was documented as 0.0 with 90 percent reduction in mechanical pain at time of discharge in a total of eight visits. The patient reported that greatest relief stemmed from IASTM and use of progressive resistive exercises.

IASTM plays an important role in the management of many chronic and acute elbow conditions. A thorough assessment of the osseous and soft tissue structures via identification of the restrictions that limit function is essential before any treatment should be initiated. Incorporating a test–retest approach, monitoring dosage of intervention, and incorporating movement to establish neuromuscular control into the IASTM program are essential to the intervention's success.

References

Bitra M, Sudhan SG (2019) Instrument assisted soft tissue mobilisation in the management of musculoskeletal pain: a literature review with implications for clinical practice guidelines. J Clin Diagn Res 13(12).

Cheatham SW, Kreiswirth E, Baker R (2019) Does a light pressure instrument assisted soft tissue mobilization technique modulate tactile discrimination and perceived pain in healthy individuals with DOMS? J Can Chiropr Assoc 63(1):18.

Dávila SA, Johnston-Jones K (2006) Managing the stiff elbow: operative, nonoperative, and postoperative techniques. J Hand Ther 19(2):268–281.

Kharabian S, Mazaherinejad A, Angorani H et al. (2014) The comparison of effectiveness of Cyriax deep transverse friction massage with ultrasound therapy in lateral epicondylitis of humerus: a randomized clinical trial. Razi J Med Sci 20(116):56–65.

Kim J, Sung DJ, Lee J (2017) Therapeutic effectiveness of instrument-assisted soft tissue mobilization for soft tissue injury: mechanisms and practical application. J Exerc Rehab 13(1):12.

Langer N, Hänggi J, Müller NA et al. (2012) Effects of limb immobilization on brain plasticity. Neurology 78(3):182–188.

Lockard M (2006) Clinical biomechanics of the elbow. J Hand Ther 19(2):72–81.

Moisello C, Bove M, Huber R et al. (2008) Short-term limb immobilization affects motor performance. J Mot Behav 40(2):165–176.

Purves D, Augustine GJ, Fitzpatrick D et al. (2001) Mechanoreceptors specialized to receive tactile information. In: Neuroscience, 2nd edn. Sunderland, MA: Sinauer Associates.

Sardelli M, Tashjian RZ, MacWilliams BA (2011) Functional elbow range of motion for contemporary tasks. J Bone Joint Surg Am 93(5):471–477.

Sueki DG, Cleland JA, Wainner RS (2013) A regional interdependence model of musculoskeletal dysfunction: research, mechanisms, and clinical implications. J Man Manip Ther 21(2):90–102.

Vincent JI, MacDermid JC, King GJ et al. (2021) The Patient-Rated Elbow Evaluation and The American Shoulder and Elbow Surgeons–Elbow form capture aspects of functioning that are important to patients with elbow injuries. J Hand Ther 34(3):415–422.

The Use of IASTM in Non-Arthritic Hip Pathologies to Improve Function

Hip pain is the second most common cause of lower limb musculoskeletal pain and is commonly seen in active individuals (Kemp et al. 2019). Non-arthritic, intra-articular hip pathologies are becoming better understood and are more frequently identified in the orthopedic realm. In fact, a recent study reported a prevalence of radiographic findings consistent with femoroacetabular impingement (FAI) in 60.5 percent of patients with hip pain (Zhou et al. 2020; Hale et al. 2021). Using a variety of treatment interventions, including Instrument-assisted Soft Tissue Mobilization (IASTM), is very helpful in addressing pain, range of motion (ROM) loss, soft tissue restrictions, and muscle inhibition.

Intra-articular pathologies such as FAI syndrome, labral tears, synovitis, ligamentum teres damage, and generalized micro-instability can result in extra-articular soft tissue pain and dysfunction involving the anterior hip musculature,

adductors (particularly adductor longus), lateral musculature, and the posterior hip. The IASTM techniques can be implemented with other manual interventions, neuromuscular re-education, and therapeutic exercise to assist in normalizing the joint mechanics and decreasing the stress on the hip joint and intra-articular structures (Figure 18.1).

A complete and comprehensive evaluation of the patient should precede IASTM intervention around the hip. Once movement dysfunctions are identified, mobility and stability impairments can be addressed accordingly. Initial scanning of all tissues through IASTM should be part of the assessment process before and after treatment to determine changes in tissue quality, tone, and subjective pain reports.

Anterior Hip Techniques

The most common restrictions of the anterior hip are noted in the iliopsoas and rectus femoris muscles. Frequently, these are areas of guarding more than truly tight structures; however, the pain and

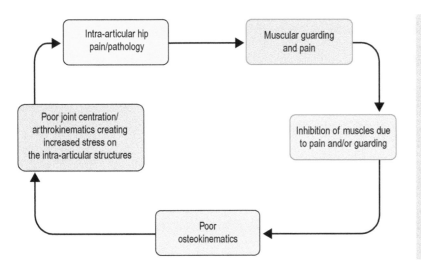

Figure 18.1 Hip pathology pain cycle: boxes outlined in orange highlight the areas where IASTM can be helpful in the rehabilitation process

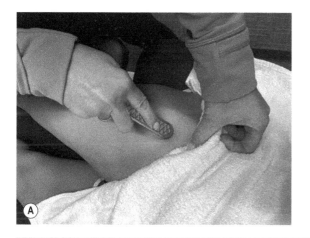
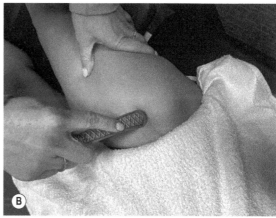

Figure 18.2 (A) Brushing over the anterior hip musculature including rectus femoris and iliopsoas. (B) Strumming across the longitudinal tissues of the anterior hip.

increased tone make them less active and create poor overall mechanisms, as noted in Figure 18.1. Use of light to moderate brushing and strumming techniques can assist in relaxation of the anterior musculature and improve tolerance to soft tissue mobilization and/or hip flexion stabilization exercises without pain (Figure 18.2). Starting with the hip in a slightly flexed position to place the muscle on slack and progressing to neutral or even slightly extended positions is advised as the muscle relaxes. In cases where the hip flexors are adaptively shortened, these techniques are followed by appropriate hip flexor stretching.

Medial Hip Techniques

Adductor longus is traditionally the most affected muscle in patients with intra-articular hip pathology. Individuals with complaints of groin pain may have pain from both intra-articular sources, as well as proximal adductor irritability. It is important to assess muscular imbalances related to the adductors and abductors to help in determining how they may be affecting each other. The

techniques described for the anterior hip may be used here as well; however, an effective strategy for relaxing the adductors is a "pin and stretch" variety with a broad edge. Utilizing light pressure and a concave treatment edge on the convex tissue, start with passive abduction in mid-range and progress ROM followed by active abduction (Figure 18.3).

Lateral Hip Techniques

On the lateral aspect of the hip, the bursa often gets the blame; however, gluteal tendinopathy is more common in these patients. The use of strumming, as described in the anterior hip section (Figure 18.2B), near the musculotendinous junction, just posterior to the greater trochanter, can be a particularly helpful technique. In addition, the use of fanning to globally address the muscle mass is useful and can often assist in relaxation and decrease pain to improve the ability to contract and control the lateral stability of the pelvis (Figure 18.4). Positioning of the hip into varying amounts of hip flexion and adduction can add stretch to the tissues and vary the intensity of the treatment.

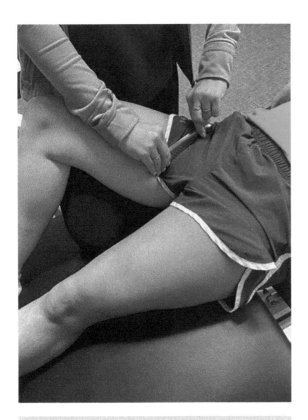

Figure 18.3 "Pin and stretch" release of the proximal adductor musculature: placing the hip in a slightly flexed position and moving the leg passively and actively through abduction/adduction with the concave surface on the tissues

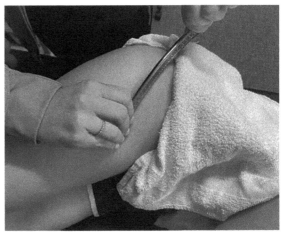

Figure 18.4 In the side lying position, the use of fanning across the gluteal musculature is performed with a single-bevel edge

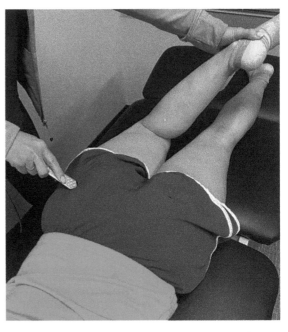

Figure 18.5 Light to moderate pressure applied to piriformis with a smaller treatment edge and passive rotational motion of the affected hip

Posterior Hip Techniques

Although less common than anterior pain, posterior hip pain can result from intra-articular pathology. More commonly, the posterior structures of the hip, such as piriformis, quadratus femoris, and proximal hamstrings, are the source of pain. Utilization of a comprehensive physical examination can assist in making this distinction. Often, posterior pain with sitting is labeled as piriformis syndrome without examination findings to support this diagnosis. In the case of true restriction, trigger points, or shortening in piriformis, the use of IASTM directly in this region with passive internal and external rotation can create relaxation of the muscle. This should be applied with light to moderate pressure, allowing the instrument and tension of the muscle to do most of the work (Figure 18.5).

A case example for hip flexor strain is given in Box 18.1.

Box 18.1

Case example: hip flexor strain

A 17-year-old female dancer presents with complaints of left hip and groin pain for 6 months. Pain is progressively worsening and limiting activity participation. She was modifying dance but is now having pain with activities of daily living, such as prolonged walking, prolonged sitting, and stair climbing. She presents to clinic after previous physical therapy for 4 weeks at initial onset of pain, with the diagnosis from her primary care provider of a hip flexor strain. She reports no change or worsening of pain with interventions, which included hip flexor stretching and gluteal strengthening, as well as ice and electrical stimulation.

Evaluation reveals increased lordosis in standing and walking with avoidance of terminal hip extension and increased lumbar spine extension. Active straight leg raise (SLR) is limited and painful at 60 degrees; however, pain is abolished with cues for neutral pelvis and ROM increased to 80 degrees. Passive SLR is 95 degrees and hip flexion passive ROM is 130 degrees bilaterally with end-range pain on the left. Hip internal rotation is 30 degrees bilaterally with end-range pain on the left and external rotation 70 degrees bilaterally and pain-free. Left hip abduction strength is 4/5 with anterior compensations from tensor fasciae latae and hip flexors; adduction 4/5 with pain on resistance; extension 3–/5; internal rotation 4/5; external rotation 3–/5 with spine compensations. Right

hip strength is 5/5 throughout. Palpation of the left hip flexors and proximal adductors is painful and tone is increased compared to the right. Left hip abductors are tender compared to the right. Flexion/adduction/internal rotation (FADIR) is positive with painful catching, and flexion/abduction/external rotation (FABER) is positive for anterior hip pain with limited ROM.

Intervention includes a multimodal approach with in-clinic use of high-powered laser for decreased pain and improved tolerance to manual therapy, postural awareness and education for neutral pelvic position in standing and walking, and IASTM to the anterior, medial, and lateral hip, followed by corrective exercises focused on neuromuscular control to engage the deep rotator group, adductors, and transversus abdominis. Exercise progresses to weight-bearing and multiplanar stabilization to create improved hip and pelvis control within the demands of activities of daily living and dance-specific activity.

The patient reports a decrease in resting visual analog scale for pain from 6/10 to 0/10 in four sessions, and from 8/10 with dance-related activity to 2/10 in the same time period. She demonstrates normal, 5/5 hip strength without pain after four treatment sessions. She is able to return unrestricted to dance without pain after sixteen treatment sessions over the course of 8 weeks.

Although commonly used for muscular strains around the hip and pelvis, IASTM can be a useful treatment modality in the care of patients with non-arthritic, intra-articular hip pathology. Incorporating a thorough evaluation of movement patterns and determining impairments is the key to proper treatment selection.

References

Hale RF, Melugin HP, Zhou J et al. (2021) Incidence of femoroacetabular impingement and surgical management trends over time. Am J Sports Med 49(1):35–41. doi:10.1177/0363546520970914.

Kemp J, Grimaldi A, Heerey J et al. (2019) Current trends in sport and exercise hip conditions: intra-articular and extra-articular hip pain, with detailed focus on femoroacetabular impingement (FAI) syndrome. Best Pract Res Clin Rheumatol 33(1):66–87. doi:10.1016/j.berh.2019.02.006.

Zhou J, Melugin HP, Hale RF et al. (2020) The prevalence of radiographic findings of structural hip deformities for femoroacetabular impingement in patients with hip pain. Am J Sports Med 48(3):647–653. doi:10.1177/0363546519896355.

Instrument-assisted Soft Tissue Mobilization (IASTM) in the treatment of musculoskeletal disorders can bring added value to the therapist's clinical practice. In this chapter we explore the utilization of IASTM in the treatment of common knee disorders.

Most musculoskeletal knee complaints that we will treat utilizing IASTM comprise extra-articular pathologies; these can include, but are not limited to, tendonitis, tendinopathies, ligamentous injuries, muscle strain and/or tears, diffuse myofascial pain, patellar femoral syndrome (PFS), bursitis, and even inflammation of the knee retinaculum. Additionally, patients with pre- and post-surgical conditions might have IASTM incorporated in their plan of care.

IASTM is applied keeping two key points in mind: depth of application and tone of the underlying tissue. In managing "depth," we teach students to err on the conservative side following the guideline of superficial to deeper application, based on patient response. By starting superficially, we limit a patient's negative correlation to IASTM by approaching them gently. Tone, which all muscles have to some degree, can change according to neurological input from the patient. A patient sitting on a plinth table, with their knee bent and leg hanging, has a degree of "resting tone" to which IASTM can be applied. The clinician applying IASTM to the anterior knee can decrease this tone and thus the effects of IASTM, by considering changes effected via contraction of a local antagonist: in this case, the hamstrings pulling the knee into flexion. Tone could also be increased on the basis of contracting an agonist within the target area: in this case, the quadriceps muscle, which can be treated through a progression of isometric to concentric to eccentric to weight-bearing (Box 19.1).

Box 19.1

IASTM algorithm for treatment of the knee

Type of stroke: Utilizing a medium-size or broad beveled edge, start with linear (sweeping) and curvilinear (fanning) strokes through the larger muscles of the knee (e.g. quadriceps and/or hamstrings)

Starting position: Patients could be seated with the leg off the table or lying prone or supine in our entry-level approach

Angle: Application of the instrument starts at 45 degrees plus or minus 15 degrees (30–60-degree angle), with the force applied through the beveled edge in the direction of the stroke. The more "vertically" you apply the instrument (that is, at 60 degrees), the more aggressive the treatment will generally be for the patient, whereas the "lower" you keep the angle (30 degrees), the less aggressive the treatment

Application/pressure: Application strokes will be in continual contact with the skin (in order to avoid excessive afferent or noxious stimuli from repeated lifting and repositioning of the instrument). The pressure is applied mainly in the direction of the beveled edge, whether pushing or pulling. Strokes are small in amplitude (5–10 cm/2–4 inches), then glided back with only skin contact before pushing or pulling again, akin to taking two steps forward, one step back, slowly working through the desired region of the area being treated

Grip: Instruments can be held with a single hand-hold grip or with a two-handed approach. The advantage of the single-hand technique is the ability to keep the non-instrumented hand free to contact the skin and manually alter the tissue, approximating to the instrument application. The therapist could pull or press said tissues, making the application under the instrument more effective. The trade-off with using one hand rather than two is losing some level of control of the instrument. This process generally improves over time as clinicians add more technique hours to their practice

Tissue feel/response: Make mental notes of any variances in tissue feel and/or response during this process, as certain areas may be more fibrotic, sensitive, or just "different." It may be necessary to split the larger muscles of the leg into two or three different regions in order to treat with shorter strokes, thus making it more comfortable for the person receiving treatment

Duration: Treatment should not exceed 2–3 minutes in any one locale, although it is possible to utilize IASTM up to 10-15 minutes in total if treating multiple areas and structures around the knee. Be cognizant of skin hyperemia and/or petechiae as signs of potential tissue response. Though ideally avoided, these are not considered a restriction on IASTM, but a possible by-product within reason.

Progression

Once through the aforementioned process, the clinician utilizing IASTM can progress in a number of ways: they can repeat the technique over the same area with larger or smaller instrument(s), change the treatment edge (bevel or shape), and/or change the depth of force (more aggressive). A therapist can also change the length and/or tone of the underlying tissue by treating the knee in different positions. Putting the knee into greater or lesser flexion or reducing or adding tone to the area by use of muscle contractions are examples. A clinician could also progress by changing the location of their treatments: for example, by moving from the larger muscles to the smaller region of the knee joint line, various tendon(s) crossing the knee, and their attachments distally.

I will typically switch to smaller instruments and begin "framing" the patella, joint lines, and tibial tubercle while making a note of any areas that either reproduce the current symptoms or feel as if they could be contributing to the current symptoms (there is some artful practice here). I will then begin tilting the patella with my non-instrumented hand in an attempt to apply IASTM under the patellar borders. In the same way as attempting to reach the smaller regions, I will apply IASTM utilizing small edges and/or hooks to the joint line space and parapatellar tendon while constantly receiving feedback from the client. I may passively rotate the tibia in order to change the opening at the joint line, thus allowing a small instrument edge improved access to this area (for example, the coronary ligaments attach to the meniscus at this locale). From here, I may add agonist or antagonist muscle contractions on subsequent visits while striving to progress to weight-bearing and more functional positions.

Further Considerations

There are some additional considerations when applying IASTM to the knee. Larger muscle groups can be treated by both superficial and deeper strokes; thus, in addition to the linear and curvilinear strokes, the therapist might choose to use "J-strokes" or deeper "pin and stretch" strokes to effect the change they are looking for. Consider this when treating the quadriceps, hamstring muscle bellies, and the proximal gastrocnemius/calf complex. In areas around the tibiofemoral joint, patella, tibial tubercle, hamstring (tendon) insertions, and pes anserinus, the tissue is very shallow, and thus superficial techniques (sweeping and fanning) work best. If it is desirable to go "deeper," it often works best to shorten the tissue being treated (either passively or actively).

It is important to remember that the knee is simply one joint in the overall lower quarter. Although IASTM can be applied directly to the knee and surrounding structures, there are times where knee symptoms may be referred from areas proximal or distal to the primary complaint. A proper evaluation should draw attention to these areas. As an example, oftentimes knee complaints will occur concurrently with issues affecting the muscles of the pelvis. I find the gluteus medius muscle to be a key area for performing IASTM, as we often discover this is sensitive and weak. In practice, a few minutes of local treatment to gluteus medius while the patient is in side lying can result in measurable changes to hip strength, leading many to speculate on the potential neurologic effects of IASTM. Regardless of the root causes, treating areas above and below the knee can bring real-time changes for the patient, which in turn may improve their ability to perform other aspects of their rehabilitation program (stretching and strengthening).

We should also remember that IASTM is used to facilitate changes in the soft tissue of the patient, whether these are a result of the therapy's neurologic effect, changes in fluid dynamics, local mechanical changes, or more global myofascial alterations; research and collective opinions are still being gathered. Ultimately, the key goal of IASTM is to effect change in the soft tissue of a properly diagnosed condition, which, once that condition is treated, results in improved symptoms and function. As mentioned in earlier sections of this book, we assess, treat, reassess, and treat again – multiple times in a session – while looking for significant positive changes as reported by the person being treated. Once these are achieved, we will then move to other aspects of our treatment model (stretching, strengthening and so on). As a general rule of practice, if a condition is not changing (for either the better or the worse) after three sessions of IASTM, re-evaluation of the condition and plan of care is recommended.

Instrument-assisted Soft Tissue Mobilization (IASTM) in the treatment of musculoskeletal disorders can bring added value to the therapist's clinical practice. In this chapter we explore the utilization of IASTM in the treatment of common ankle disorders.

Most musculoskeletal ankle/foot complaints that we will treat utilizing IASTM comprise extra-articular pathologies; these can include, but are not limited to, tendonitis, tendinopathies, ligamentous injuries, retinacular injuries, muscle strain and/or tears, diffuse myofascial pain, plantar fasciitis, bursitis, and even inflammation of free nerve endings (as in Morton's neuroma). Additionally, patients with pre- and post-surgical conditions, post-fracture, and/or post-immobilization (cast or brace use) might have IASTM incorporated in their plan of care.

IASTM is applied keeping two key points in mind: depth of application and tone of the underlying tissue. In managing "depth," we teach students to err on the conservative side, following the guideline of superficial to deeper application, based on patient response. By starting superficially, we limit a patient's negative correlation to IASTM by approaching them gently. Tone, which all muscles have to some degree, can change according to neurological input from the patient. A patient lying on a plinth table, with their foot elevated, has a degree of "resting tone" to which IASTM can be applied. The clinician applying IASTM to the anterior shin, dorsal retinaculum, and common foot dorsiflexors can decrease this tone, and thus the effects of IASTM, by considering changes effected via contraction of local antagonist(s): in this case, gentle plantar flexion (pushing the toes down or the foot into plantar flexion). Tone could also be increased on the basis of contracting an agonist within the target area: in this case, encouraging dorsiflexion, which can

be treated through a progression of isometric to concentric to eccentric to weight-bearing. In most cases, IASTM should be a precursor to any tissue lengthening (stretching) and stability strengthening (rehabilitation).

The following ankle/foot treatments utilizing IASTM constitute a basic entry-level approach to the lower quarter (Box 20.1). A skilled clinician utilizing these techniques and progressing them on the basis of information gained from other parts of this book should be able to move their specific treatments forward. (It is assumed that a basic understanding of the use of emollients, hand holds, instrument positioning, beveled edges, their shape(s), and force ramifications has been acquired prior to application of IASTM.)

Box 20.1

IASTM algorithm for treatment of the ankle

Type of stroke: Utilizing a medium- to smaller-size beveled edge, start with linear (sweeping) and curvilinear (fanning) strokes through the larger muscles of the lower leg (e.g. gastrocnemius, soleus, and/or tibialis anterior)

Starting position: Patients could be lying prone or supine in our entry-level approach

Angle: Application of the instrument starts at 45 degrees plus or minus 15 degrees (30–60-degree angle), with the force applied through the beveled edge in the direction of the stroke. The more "vertically" you apply the instrument (that is, at 60 degrees), the more aggressive the treatment will generally be for the patient, whereas the "lower" the angle (30 degrees), the less aggressive the treatment

Application/pressure: Application strokes will be in continual contact with the skin (in order to avoid excessive afferent or noxious stimuli from repeated lifting and repositioning of the instrument). The pressure is applied mainly in the direction of the beveled edge, whether pushing or pulling. Strokes are small in amplitude (5–10 cm/2–4 inches), then glided back with only skin contact before pushing or pulling again, akin to taking two steps forward, one step back, slowly working through the desired region of the area being treated

Grip: Instruments can be held with a single hand-hold grip or with a two-handed approach. The advantage of the single-hand technique is the ability to keep the non-instrumented hand free to contact the skin and manually alter the tissue, approximating to the instrument application. The therapist could pull or press said tissues, making the application under the instrument more effective. The trade-off with using one hand rather than two is losing some level of control of the instrument. This process generally improves over time as clinicians add more technique hours to their practice

Tissue feel/response: Make mental notes of any variances in tissue feel and/or response during this process, as certain areas may be more fibrotic, sensitive, or just "different." It may be necessary to split the larger muscles of the lower leg into two or three different regions in order to treat with shorter strokes, thus making it more comfortable for the person receiving treatment

Additional treatment: Following treatment of the larger muscles, there is a transition to smaller instruments to "frame" around one malleolus or both malleoli, taking into consideration the diagnosis and, more specifically, the focus of the treatment, whether this is muscle, tendon, and/or ligaments. Depending on the condition, additional treatment could include a focus on tissues such as the Achilles tendon, plantar fascia, and the inter-tarsal joints, extending into one or more toes.

Duration: Treatment should not exceed 2–3 minutes in any one locale, although it is possible to employ IASTM for up to 10–15 minutes in total if treating multiple areas and structures around the

foot or ankle. Be cognizant of skin hyperemia and/or petechiae as signs of potential tissue response. Though ideally avoided, these are not considered a restriction on IASTM, but a possible by-product within reason.

Progression

Once through the aforementioned process, the clinician utilizing IASTM can progress in a number of ways: they can repeat the technique over the same area with larger or smaller instrument(s), change the treatment edge (bevel or shape), and/or alter the depth of force (more aggressive). A therapist can also change the length and/or tone of the underlying tissue by treating the ankle or foot in different positions. Putting the ankle into greater or lesser flexion, changing the degree of inversion or eversion, or reducing or adding tone to the area by use of muscle contractions are examples. A clinician could also progress by changing the location of the treatments: for example, by moving proximally into the larger muscles of the lower leg or smaller regions of the ankle or foot's various joints, various tendon(s) crossing the ankle, and their attachments distally.

I will typically switch to smaller instruments and begin "framing" the smaller joints affected. I will apply IASTM to joint lines and the multiple smaller ligaments and retinacula while making a note of any areas that either reproduce the current symptoms or feel as if they could be contributing to the current symptoms (there is some artful practice here). I will then begin tilting or rotating the subtalar joint with my non-instrumented hand in an attempt to apply IASTM to the smaller joint spaces. In trying to access these smaller regions, I will apply small edges and/or hooks into the joint line space, while constantly receiving feedback from the client. I may passively rotate the forefoot in order to change the opening at the joint line, thus allowing a small instrument edge improved access to this area. From here, I may add agonist or antagonist muscle contractions on subsequent visits while striving to progress to weight-bearing and more functional positions.

Further Considerations

There are some additional considerations when applying IASTM to the ankle or foot. Larger muscle groups can be treated by both superficial and deeper strokes; thus, in addition to the linear and curvilinear strokes, the therapist might choose to use "J-strokes" or deeper "pin and stretch" strokes to effect the change they are looking for. If it is desirable to go "deeper," it often works best to shorten the tissue being treated (either passively or actively). Consider this when treating the proximal and middle gastrocnemius/calf complex, which is easier to access with the patient in prone and the knee passively brought into flexion. In other areas, such as around the malleolus, distal Achilles tendon, and dorsal retinaculum, the tissue is very shallow and thus superficial techniques (sweeping and fanning) work best. Another consideration that is unique to the ankle/foot region arises when dorsiflexion is limited more by soft tissue compression (anterior dysfunction) than tightness or restriction of tissues on the posterior side. I have seen many attempts to perform IASTM on the calf complex in hopes of "stretching" or improving

dorsiflexion, only to achieve limited results, yet when IASTM was applied to the dorsal retinacula and general soft tissue of the anterior ankle, subsequent dorsiflexion improved. This was likely the result of loosening soft tissue that was previously compressed during attempts to put the ankle into end-range dorsiflexion.

It is important to remember that the ankle/foot is simply one area in the overall lower quarter. Although IASTM can be applied directly to the ankle and surrounding structures, there are times when ankle symptoms may be referred from areas arising proximal or distal to the primary complaint. A proper evaluation should draw attention to these areas. As an example, oftentimes ankle complaints will occur concurrently with issues affecting the muscles in the opposite lower leg compartment. I find the tibialis anterior muscle to be a key area for performing IASTM in persons with primary complaints within their posterior compartment, and vice versa. To take another example, we often find that persons with primary plantar fascia complaints may also present with reduced mobility of their first ray extension (hallux rigidus) and in other cases have additional restrictions further proximally up the lower quarter. We often find these areas to be sensitive, hypomobile, and often weak; a few minutes of IASTM can be an effective technique as a precursor to other components of the plan of care (stretching and strengthening).

When Instrument-assisted Soft Tissue Mobilization (IASTM) is applied to the cervical spine region, a proper diagnosis is necessary for better selection of technique. IASTM is largely a neurologic process that attempts to reset the tone of tissue; however, there are times when it will be anti-inflammatory and rare times when it will be pro-inflammatory.

Some of the most common disorders associated with the cervical spine include cervicogenic headaches, whiplash, myofascial pain, upper crossed syndrome, cervical disc herniation with or without radiculopathy, cervical stenosis with or without radiculopathy, and facet joint disorders. If choosing IASTM is an important part of treatment, the clinician should select the diagnosis that offers the greatest benefit. In general, cervical disc herniation and stenosis with or without radiculopathy are better treated with other interventions; therefore, they are not discussed here.

When applying IASTM for a particular diagnosis, the clinician first needs to determine the state of the soft tissue they are treating. Is it in an acute phase, such as following a motor vehicle accident? Is it a chronic condition stemming from a postural disorder? The pressure/duration applied with IASTM will affect the way the body reacts to it. The heavier the pressure, the greater the fibroblastic proliferation and the greater the inflammatory response. The lighter the pressure, the more the treatment orients to a neurologic response and superficial vascular changes.

In this chapter, different cervical impairments associated with neck pain will be presented using a standardized approach. First, a provocation technique is applied to elicit symptoms before treatment, which is repeated after treatment to measure effectiveness. Next, the treatment region is identified. The treatment is then described, often involving active or resisted movement, along with the types of IASTM stroke, pressure, and duration. Finally, the goals of the treatment are established. Common impairments include acute pain, myofascial pain, cervicogenic headaches, upper crossed syndrome, and facet disorders.

Acute Pain

In the acute phase, particularly after whiplash, this is an inflammatory state and should be treated with much lighter pressure. Anterior cervical structures including the sternocleidomastoid and scalene muscles, the suboccipital musculature, upper trapezius, levator scapulae, the facet ligaments, and intersegmental muscles may be treated. Compared to impairments discussed later in this chapter, the major difference in the acute state is the amount of pressure used. An anti-inflammatory treatment should be performed with less than the weight of the instrument against the skin. To ensure this, the clinician should not hold the instrument with a full grip. The instrument should be held with just enough grip to make sure that it can be controlled by the clinician and treatment rendered with accuracy (Box 21.1; Figure 21.1).

Box 21.1

IASTM treatment protocol for acute neck pain

Provocation assessment: The position, motion, or activity that reproduces the pain

Treatment: Use the position or motions that provoke symptoms initially

Region: Tissues associated with whiplash (upper trapezius, levator scapulae, sternocleidomastoid, scalene muscles, cervical erector/paraspinal musculature, suboccipital musculature)

Type of stroke: Broad, longer strokes about 10 cm (4 inches) in length with overlapping motions

---

over the larger muscles (upper trapezius, levator scapulae, sternocleidomastoid, cervical erector/paraspinal musculature, suboccipital musculature) at a 30–60-degree angle. Smaller strokes about 1.25–5 cm (½–1 inch) over the focal lesions maintain a 30–60-degree angle to keep the pressure light, but progress to 90 degrees in more chronic situations

Application/pressure: Anti-inflammatory/neurosensory/weight of instrument to slightly deeper on less sensitive tissue (neurosensory) and not even the weight of the instrument over the acute highly sensitive tissue (anti-inflammatory). For smaller strokes, use the non-instrument hand to achieve a depth of penetration and skin pull; then place the instrument to that depth and see treatment strokes above

Duration: Until a very light hyperemia is created then reassess. No more than three reassessments in a treatment

Goal: Always start initial treatment assessment by having the patient note their pain level during provocation as "10" before treatment. The clinician should hope to reduce symptoms to 5 or below by post-assessment.

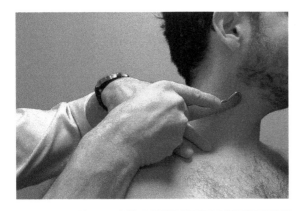

Figure 21.1 IASTM to the anterior cervical musculature during rotation with anti-inflammatory application of very light pressure

Myofascial Pain

In the case of myofascial pain, most of the treatment is aimed at resetting the firing pattern of the involved muscles. For this situation, the goal is to stimulate as many of the afferent sensory receptors as possible to neurologically reset the tone of tissue. In these situations, the clinician can increase the neurologic stimulation to the tissue by stimulating more than the nerve receptors in the skin, and may introduce stimulation to mechanoreceptors and nerve receptors in the muscles/fascia through movement. First, the clinician should determine the motions of restriction or pain. In most situations, a lighter pressure, about the weight of the instrument or slightly more, should be applied to the soft tissue while the patient reproduces the restricted or painful motions. Once a hyperemia has developed on the affected region, the clinician should reassess the patient's progress. As symptoms dissipate, the clinician may need to look at secondary sites or more focal lesions (Box 21.2; Figure 21.2).

Box 21.2

IASTM treatment protocol for myofascial pain

Provocation assessment: The position, motion, or activity that reproduces the pain/restriction

Treatment: In the position, motion, or activity that reproduces the pain/restriction

Region: Tissues associated with the myofascial pain

Type of stroke: Broad, longer strokes about 10 cm (4 inches) in length with overlapping strokes at a 30–60-degree angle

Application/pressure: Neurosensory/weight of instrument to slightly deeper

Duration: Until a hyperemia is created; then reassess. No more than three reassessments in a treatment

Goal: Always start initial treatment assessment as 10 on provocation. The clinician should hope to reduce symptoms to 5 or below by last assessment

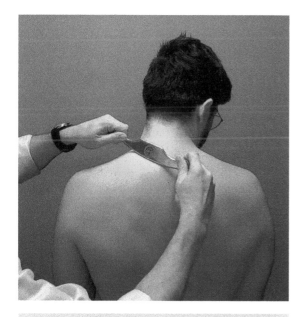

Figure 21.2 IASTM for myofascial pain over the upper trapezius and levator scapulae region in a position of provocation

Cervicogenic Headaches

With cervicogenic headaches, many of the same tissues and applications of myofascial pain should be addressed; however, it is important to understand the muscles that frequently refer pain to the head. The temporomandibular joint, sternocleidomastoid, and suboccipital muscles will very commonly refer pain to the head on palpation. The most common referral patterns include "headband," "question mark," and temporal distributions. Many of these muscles are best treated by adding movement to the cervical spine. Rotation is the best oriented

movement to stimulate the neurology associated with these muscles. Treatment should be targeted to the referring muscles, which can usually be discovered to cause referral patterns through simple palpation. Once the muscles creating the referral patterns have been discovered, start using IASTM with motion over the affected areas. Pressure should be consistent with the weight of the instrument or lighter while the patient moves slowly through restricted or painful patterns (Box 21.3; Figure 21.3).

Box 21.3

IASTM treatment protocol for cervicogenic headache

Provocation assessment: The position, motion, or activity that reproduces the pain

Treatment: In the position, motion, or activity that reproduces the pain

Region: Tissues associated with referral patterns of the headache

Type of stroke: Broad, longer strokes about 10 cm (4 inches) in length with overlapping strokes over the larger muscles (upper trapezius, levator scapulae, sternocleidomastoid, cervical erector/paraspinal musculature) at a 30–60-degree angle. Smaller strokes about 1.25–2.5 cm (½-1 inch) over the focal suboccipital musculature closer to a 90-degree angle

Application/pressure: Neurosensory/weight of instrument to slightly deeper. For smaller strokes, use the non-instrument hand to achieve a depth of penetration and skin pull; then place the instrument to that depth and see treatment strokes above

Duration: Until a hyperemia is created; then reassess. No more than three reassessments in a treatment

Goal: Always start initial treatment assessment as 10 on provocation. The clinician should hope to reduce symptoms to 5 or below by last assessment

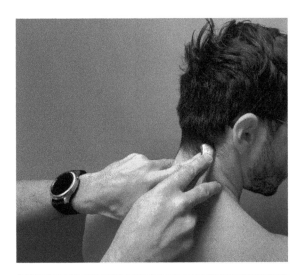

Figure 21.3 IASTM for suboccipital muscles using rotation movement, with the non-treatment hand finding depth and skin pull

Upper Crossed Syndrome

With upper crossed syndrome patterns, other muscles are to be considered. In an upper crossed posture, several muscles are hypertonic, including the upper trapezius, levator scapulae, suboccipitals, sternocleidomastoid, scalenes, anterior deltoid, teres major, latissimus dorsi, and pectoralis. In short, the clinician will address the muscles that are chronically shortened by neurologically normalizing the tone of these tissues with soft tissue treatments while simultaneously strengthening the weaker postural muscles, including the deep neck flexors, posterior medial and lower scapular stabilizers, and serratus anterior. By strengthening the weaker tissue at the same time as performing soft tissue treatments to the tighter tissues, the clinician can balance the "see-saws" associated with an upper crossed syndrome (Box 21.4; Figure 21.4).

Box 21.4

IASTM treatment protocol for upper crossed syndrome

Provocation assessment: The position, motion, or activity that reproduces the pain

Treatment: Use activities that stimulate postural muscles (medial and lower scapular stabilizers, deep neck flexors) of the cervical spine while treating the chronically tightened tissues described above

Region: Tissues associated with upper crossed syndrome (upper trapezius, levator scapulae, sternocleidomastoid, cervical erector/paraspinal musculature, pectoralis musculature, latissimus dorsi, suboccipital musculature)

Type of stroke: Broad, longer strokes about 10 cm (4 inches) in length with overlapping motions over the larger muscles (upper trapezius, levator scapulae, sternocleidomastoid, cervical erector/paraspinal musculature, pectoralis musculature, latissimus dorsi) at a 30–60-degree angle. Smaller strokes about 1.25–2.5 cm (½–1 inch) over the focal lesions closer to a 90-degree angle

Application/pressure: Neurosensory/weight of instrument to slightly deeper. For smaller strokes, use the non-instrument hand to achieve a depth of penetration and skin pull; then place the instrument to that depth and see treatment strokes above

Duration: Until a hyperemia is created; then reassess. No more than three reassessments in a treatment

Goal: Always start initial treatment assessment as 10 on provocation. The clinician should hope to reduce symptoms to 5 or below by last assessment. If there is no true provocation of pain or lost ROM, it may be difficult to achieve a 50 percent reduction during treatment but the patient should be able to notice the reduction of pain on return to the provoking activity.

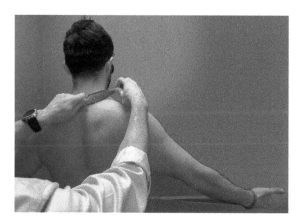

Figure 21.4 IASTM for upper trapezius/levator musculature during resisted abduction/external rotation with an elastic band

Facet Disorders

While facet disorders are primarily a joint issue, the clinician should not forget the small intersegmental muscles and capsule/ligaments associated with the involved facet. It is also important to understand that, in many necks, it may be very difficult to achieve a depth that addresses these specific deep tissues. However, if the clinician remembers that most soft tissue treatments aim for a neurologic effect, they will attempt to reach the necessary depth of the tissue with the non-treatment hand, then, with minimal added pressure, treat at the pinpoint region associated with facet injuries. This is not to say that more global treatments of the surrounding area are not necessary, but they have been described in other sections and can be added to the specific focal region discussed here. As most facet injuries are connected with movement-associated pain, finding the motion or position of pain should be the starting point. If extension is the primary position or motion, it may need to be limited to allow for the instrument to treat the involved region. That

being stated, side flexion and rotation used in conjunction with IASTM usually resolve the issue (Box 21.5; Figure 21.5).

Box 21.5

IASTM treatment protocol for facet disorders

Provocation assessment: The position, motion, or activity that reproduces the pain (usually easy to find with a position of provocation using either individual or a combination of lateral flexion, rotation and/or extension)

Treatment: Use positions or motions that provoke symptoms

Region: Tissues associated with the facet injury should be treated bilaterally with larger treatment strokes (upper trapezius, levator scapulae, sternocleidomastoid, cervical erector/paraspinal musculature, suboccipital musculature), and focal injured regions should be treated unilaterally with smaller strokes

Type of stroke: Broad, longer strokes about 10 cm (4 inches) in length with overlapping strokes over the larger muscle groups at a 30–60-degree angle. Smaller strokes about 1.25–2.5 cm (½–1 inch) over the focal lesions (smaller intersegmental muscles or facet capsule) closer to a 90-degree angle

Application/pressure: Neurosensory/weight of instrument to slightly deeper. For smaller strokes, use the non-instrument hand to get a depth of penetration and skin pull; then place the instrument to that depth and see treatment strokes above

Duration: Until a hyperemia is created; then reassess. No more than three reassessments in a treatment.

Goal: Always start initial treatment assessment as 10 on provocation. The clinician should hope to reduce symptoms to 5 or below by last assessment

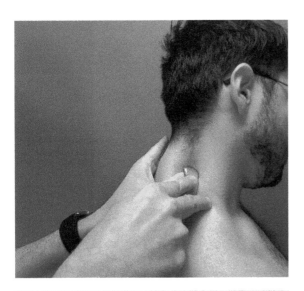

Figure 21.5 IASTM for facet treatment with the non-contact hand achieving depth and skin pull

Diagnosis: Chronic Low Back Pain

This chapter describes the treatment of a 45-year-old female patient with an acute episode of low back pain.

The following Functional Evaluation (FE) measures were used:

- finger–floor distance measured in centimeters from the fingertip of the middle finger to the floor
- Numeric Pain Rating (NRS) scale with classification from 0 to 10
- attempt to reach the foot with both hands, as if the patient were trying to soap her foot.

Due to the reported pain and functional limitations, with their corresponding effects on participation in daily life, the author decided to deviate from the standard protocol and carry out the analgesia technique first.

Assessment

After history taking, review of medical findings, and exclusion of red flags, FE was performed:

- finger–floor distance: 38 cm
- NRS: 7 in the lumbar region
- attempt to reach the right foot with both hands: foot not reachable, NRS 5 in the gluteal area.

Box 22.1

Case example

Starting position: Since I do not want the patient to change position unnecessarily because of the severe pain, the treatment begins in a standing position (Figure 22.1). The patient supports herself with both hands on the treatment couch.

Pain Relief Technique: The first technique is the so-called Pain Relief Technique, applied with a curved instrument. A little gel is used as lubricant in order to protect the patient's skin. The right lumbar region and the upper gluteal zone are treated. The treatment lasts about 45 seconds. The main focus is on the lumbar region, as this is where the patient has expressed her pain to be strongest.

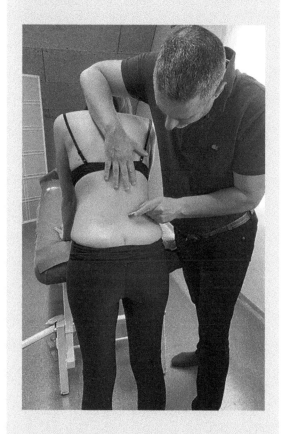

Figure 22.1 Pain Relief Technique in the standing position

Functional evaluation: After this treatment step, another FE is performed with the following results:

- finger–floor distance: 26 cm
- NRS: 4 in the lumbar region
- attempt to reach the right foot with both hands: foot reachable, NRS 5 in the gluteal area.

Rehydration Technique: The next treatment step is the Rehydration Technique. This is performed in the same position (standing). Furthermore, the targeted treatment areas are the right lumbar region and the upper right gluteal zone (Figure 22.2). Three slow and deep thrusts are performed for

each region. The direction of thrust in each case is from craniomedial to caudolateral, and is based on the fiber directions of the thoracolumbar fascia and the gluteal fascia. During this treatment step, the patient expresses mild pain at two points in the gluteal region. Palpation reveals a point of tension at each of these areas, indicating a local increase in tone.

Functional evaluation: Again, after this treatment step, FE is performed with the following results:

- finger–floor distance: 26 cm
- NRS: 2 in the lumbar region and hamstring stretch that is stiffer on the right than the left

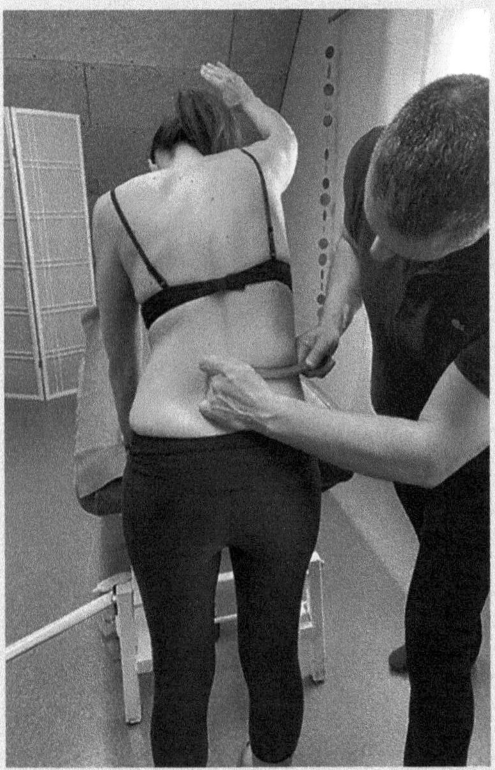

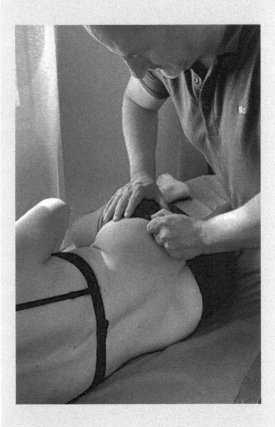

Figure 22.2 Rehydration Technique in the standing position

Figure 22.3 Regulation of Tone Technique in the left lateral position

- attempt to reach the right foot with both hands: foot reachable, NRS 5 in the gluteal region.

Regulation of Tone Technique: The next treatment step is Regulation of Tone, using an instrument which has a rounded tip (straight short instrument). The patient is now in the left lateral position. The lower leg is extended; the upper leg is bent. The points to be treated are determined by palpation and treated one after the other with the instrument (Figure 22.3). In this Regulation of Tone Technique, the patient is initially passive but helps

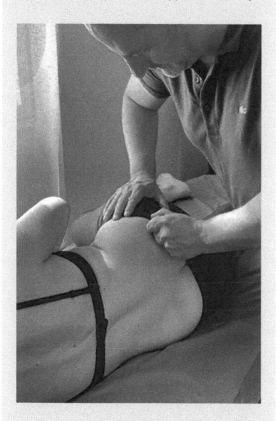

Figure 22.4 Regulation of Tone Technique: small-angle variations in the pressure vector and a high but still comfortable pressure intensity

by giving verbal feedback regarding the pressure intensity and angle, this exchange between practitioner and person being treated being very useful. The author's experience shows that small-angle variations in the pressure vector and a high but still comfortable pressure intensity produce good results (Figure 22.4). Both points are treated until a release sets in. To support the treatment, the patient can activate the right gluteus maximus muscle by very gently making an extension movement in the hip.

Progression: As a progression step, an elastic band can be wrapped around the right foot and a hip extension performed against resistance.

Functional evaluation: After Regulation of Tone, an FE is again performed:

- finger–floor distance: 22 cm
- NRS: 2 in the lumbar region and hamstring stretch ischiocrural resolved
- attempt to reach the right foot with both hands: no findings – that is, in the normal range, NRS 2.

With this result, the first treatment session is completed.

Planning a Further Course of Treatment

The interval for the second treatment is set at 3–5 days. As homework (self-treatment), the patient receives gentle daily rollouts of the region with a fascial roller and analgesic treatment with a towel as needed.

If the results of the FE persist, progressions are expanded and more emphasis is placed on exercise in subsequent treatments. Among the most important aspects of low back pain is the promotion of physical activity and the avoidance of fear of movement. In this way, a chronic form of symptom progression can be avoided.

The homework gives the patient a sense of self-efficacy, which is also extremely beneficial for the healing process. The intervals between further treatments are extended to up to 4 weeks. As soon as the patient can participate fully in everyday life again and has reached her old activity level, the treatment is considered complete.

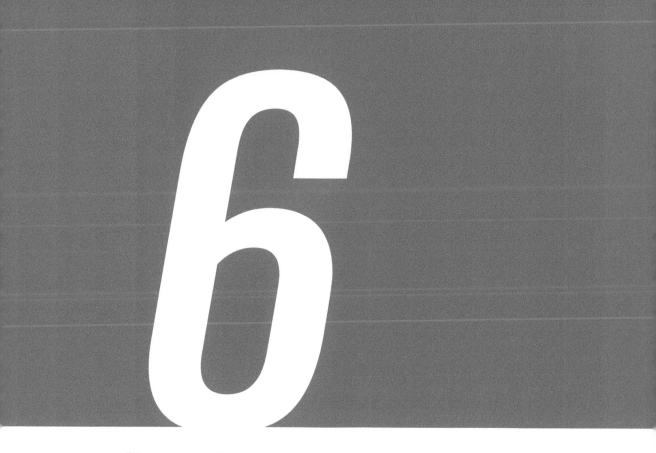

6

Therapeutic Integration

This final part of the book can certainly be described as a highlight, at least in the authors' view. Experienced therapists report on their specialty or on the opportunities for integrating IAMT into certain clinical scenarios along with other therapeutic modalities or into the treatment of special patient groups (such as children). Eminent colleagues have agreed to share their knowledge and skills with our readers here. These illustrated chapters are intended to tempt the reader to combine different therapy options for the benefit of patients. Our experts, who are based in different regions of the world (USA, Germany, and Norway), share their own experience with therapy techniques such as cupping and kinesiology taping, as well as active fascial training and the special field of the treatment of children. The authors are sure that every reader can personally benefit from this, be it in discovering new integration possibilities or getting to know other treatment options and wanting to try them out. Of course, in this case, participation in appropriate further training is an option. It is not possible here to illuminate the treatments shown in their entirety; we can only present connection and treatment possibilities in the hope of arousing readers' curiosity.

Therapeutic Integration

Introduction

Cupping, or vacuum therapy, is a long-used modality that has seen a recent resurgence in manual therapy and sports medicine. It is a traditional Chinese therapy that has been used for treatment of all types of ailments and dates back at least 2,000 years (Chirali 2014). Several review articles have looked into the effectiveness of cupping therapy (Tham et al. 2006; Gao et al. 2019; Rozenfeld and Kalichman 2016; Li et al. 2017; Chi et al. 2016; Zhang et al. 2017). Conclusions from the accumulation of these reviews were that most studies on cupping therapy were generally of low methodological quality, adding to the difficulty of drawing conclusions about the therapeutic value of cupping. However, the conditions for which cupping therapy was most commonly applied were herpes zoster, facial paralysis or Bell's palsy, musculoskeletal conditions, and spinal conditions like disk herniations and spondylosis.

Cupping Therapy and Microcirculation/Blood Flow

Effects

When a cup is applied, centrally localized negative pressure produces compression of the skin at the rim of the cup and distraction of the skin and underlying tissue that is maximal at the center of the cup (Tham et al. 2006). The pressure differential between the outer rim and center of the cup creates an immediate and visible vasodilation, even with low pressure, and can rupture capillaries, resulting in bruising under the cup (Tham et al. 2006; Gao et al. 2019). It is this capillary rupture that provides the classic red circles and petechiae described by so many in the literature (Rozenfeld and Kalichman 2016). It is commonly demonstrated that cupping therapy and negative pressure have demonstrated an association with

circulatory changes, pain decreases, tissue changes in fascial fibrosis/densifications, and increases in function or range of motion (Gao et al. 2019; Li et al. 2017; Chi et al. 2016; Zhang et al. 2017; DaPrato et al. 2018; Schafer 2018; Lacross 2011; Yim et al. 2017). In this way, cupping can be used to stimulate angiogenesis in chronically ill tissues.

Healthy tissue, with less capillary fragility and inflammation, will become red from erythema but will not bruise as substantially (Lowe 2017; Pober and Sessa 2015). In most cases, bruises caused by cupping are relatively painless, will not impair patient function, and will disappear within 3–4 days without additional treatment. Note that cupping bruises can last longer on some individuals as the circulatory system adapts. As better circulation is returned to the tissues, the bruises resolve faster with each successive treatment (Lowe 2017). If the marks do not fade or become symptomatic within that time period, a medical doctor should be consulted for professional advice.

Technique

Nomenclature for the techniques presented in this chapter are for "cup on body." So, a "static/static technique" is a static cup on a static body. This means that the patient is in a static position; once the cups are applied, they remain in situ until they are removed (Boxes 23.1 and 23.2; Figure 23.1).

Box 23.1

Keys to performance for all techniques

- Position the patient in a comfortable position that allows maximal exposure of the treatment area.
- Identify the treatment area where you want to have an effect. Determine where on the body to place the cups.

- Consider removing any body hair from the treatment site or apply ointment to the skin, if needed, to keep the cups in place. This step is optional only for static cupping and may be omitted if desired. Following this step can reduce irritation and may make it easier for the cups to stay in place during treatment.

- Use an appropriate cup size for the treatment area. The size of the treatment area dictates the size of cup.

- Apply the cup to the skin and create suction via the cup over the target area. This will draw the tissue up into the cup.

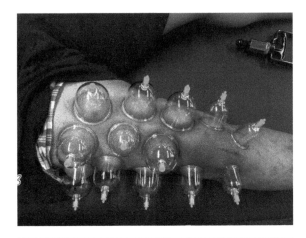

Figure 23.1 Cupping therapy and microcirculation/blood flow

Copyright Falsone S (2018) *Bridging the Gap from Rehab to Performance*. Aptos, CA: On Target Publications.

Box 23.2

Keys to performance for a static/static technique

- Leave the cups in place until you achieve an erythematic appearance. Petechiae (tiny red spots on the skin) may begin to appear within a few minutes. These pinpoint spots are caused by bleeding under the skin and are a sign indicating that the treatment should be concluded.

- Remove the cups by simply lifting them off with your hands or pulling the tab on top of the cup.

- If the suctioning is too painful, remove the cups and draw less suction to the area.

Cupping Therapy and Fascial Fibrosis/Densification

Effects

Cupping can theoretically be used to address myofascial fibrosis and densification. Recent research has provided new and growing information on the role of superficial and deep fascia in myofascial pain syndromes and movement dysfunctions

(Stecco and Day 2010). The terms "fibrosis" and "densification" are often used to indicate such fascial alterations (Stecco and Day 2010; Stecco and Hammer 2014). Fibrosis is similar to the process of scarring, with the deposition of excessive amounts of fibrous connective tissue, reflective of an inflammatory and/or repair process. Fibroses can change the architecture and function of the involved tissue. On the other hand, densification indicates an alteration of the viscosity of hyaluronan molecules within the layers of the deep fascia (Pavan et al. 2014). These densifications are able to modify the stress/strain properties of fascia without altering its general structure (Pavan et al. 2014). Thus, use of a moving cup can alter the tensile stress from rim to center, and gliding that cup longitudinally along the lines of pull of a myofascial structure should allow for disruption of these irregular type III collagen fibers in the tissue. Improving the viscosity of hyaluronan within the deep fascial layers has been shown to improve sliding and gliding of one tissue on an adjacent tissue (Tham et al. 2006; Pavan et al. 2014). To date, there is little evidence to demonstrate these decompressive changes in densification with cupping (DaPrato et al. 2018; Cage et al. 2017).

Technique

This is a dynamic/static technique, meaning that the patient is in a static position and the cup is moved so it manipulates the tissues underneath the cup. By dragging the cup longitudinally along the skin parallel to the functional forces in the myofascial unit, the biomechanical properties of the cup (compression of tissue at the rim and decompression of tissue at the center) can be used to apply a tensile force to manipulate the myofascial unit. Remember that there may be some bruising. Again, bruises caused by cupping are relatively painless and will disappear within 3–4 days without additional treatment. This treatment should be followed with therapeutic exercise to the myofascial unit treated (Box 23.3; Figure 23.2).

Box 23.3

Keys to performance for a dynamic/static technique

- Consider removing any body hair from the treatment site and apply ointment to the skin. This step is necessary for this technique.

- Use an appropriate cup size for the treatment area. The cup should be medium in size, typically around 5 cm (2 inches) in diameter.

- Create suction via the cup on the skin over the target area. This will draw the tissue up into the cup. For this technique the draw should be sufficient to adhere the cup but not make it painful to move the cup on the skin.

- Apply a distraction force to the cup (but not enough force to remove the cup) and slide the cup longitudinally along the skin parallel to the

functional forces in the myofascial unit. This draws the tissue up into the cup and then out of the cup as you move the cup longitudinally, distracting and manipulating the tissue.

- Move the cup longitudinally along the tissue, back and forth, until the tissue has an erythematic appearance and you feel a decrease in tissue tension/compression.

- Remove the cups by simply lifting them off with your hands or pulling the tab on top of the cup.

- If the suctioning becomes too painful, remove the cup and draw less suction to the area. Remember, you want to be able to glide the cup over the tissue, but this should not be painful for the patient.

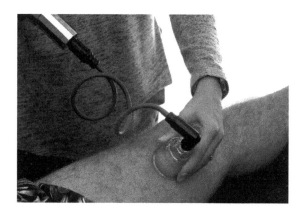

Figure 23.2 Cupping therapy and fascial fibrosis/densification

Copyright Falsone S (2018) *Bridging the Gap from Rehab to Performance.* Aptos, CA: On Target Publications.

Cupping Therapy and Range of Motion

Effects

This technique is similar in philosophy to many traditional manual therapy techniques. Whatever their various commercial names, the techniques all essentially use "pin and stretch" or "anchor and stretch" of the soft tissue structures. This is a static/dynamic technique, where the cup does not move but the patient moves the body part through a range of motion. The cup is used to distract and "hold" and/or "pin" tissues while the patient is instructed to move a body part. The practitioner monitors pressure and the region under the cup. The capture of the tissue can clearly be seen via MRI evidence provided by DaPrato et al. (2018). This constitutes a longitudinal manipulation of soft tissues by using the active motion of the patient's body, thus placing a higher demand on the "free" tissues to accomplish the task. This boosts tensile stretching of those tissues, increasing the total elasticity of the myofascial unit. There is evidence for increased ROM through the theoretic "pinning" of myofascial tissues and active range of motion in its various forms (DaPrato et al. 2018; Schafer 2018; Yim et al. 2017). While only a few authors have demonstrated evidence of the use of cupping for this purpose, clinically the authors have seen dramatic changes in ROM using this technique.

Technique

This is a static/dynamic technique, meaning the cup "pins" the tissue in a static position and the patient engages in active range of motion exercises while the cup is monitored for signs of erythema/petechiae. This provides a manipulation of soft tissues by use of active motion, thus placing a higher demand on the "free" tissues to accomplish the task. This increases tensile stretching on those tissues, boosting the total elasticity of the myofascial unit (Box 23.4; Figure 23.3).

Box 23.4

Keys to performance of a static/dynamic technique:

- The cups should be applied with the muscle in a relaxed position, typically around the mid-range of available ROM.

- Consider removing any body hair from the treatment site or apply ointment to the skin, if needed, to keep cups in place. This step helps prevent the cups from falling off during active ROM for this technique.

- Use an appropriate cup size for the treatment area. The cup should be medium in size, typically around 5 cm (2 inches) in diameter, depending on the treatment area.

- Apply the cup to the skin by creating suction via the cup over the targeted area. This will draw the tissue up into the cup. For this technique, the draw should be sufficient to adhere the cup but not so much to overly restrict ROM. The patient should be able to move through an extended ROM.

- Monitor the cups in place until you achieve an erythematic appearance. When the skin beneath the cup begins to progress to petechiae, this is the sign indicating that treatment should be concluded. This typically occurs quite quickly, as you are moving the body part and increasing circulation to the extremity.

- Remove the cups by simply lifting them off with your hands or pulling the tab on top of the cup.

- If the suctioning becomes too painful, remove the cups to draw less suction to the area and repeat the ROM.

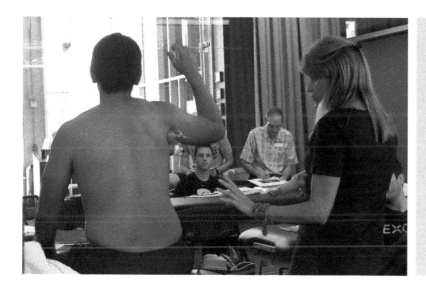

Figure 23.3 Cupping therapy and range of motion

Copyright Falsone S (2018)
Bridging the Gap from Rehab to Performance. Aptos, CA: On Target Publications

Summary

The majority of the available evidence around cupping is rooted in pain modulation. There appears to be moderate evidence for the use of various cupping techniques to improve patient-reported outcome measures related to pain. Emerging cupping techniques, such as improving fascial extensibility and joint range of motion, may also be effective, although more research is needed.

References

Cage SA, Gallegos DM, Warner BJ (2017) Utilization of cupping therapy in the treatment of vascular thoracic outlet syndrome in a collegiate pitcher: a case study. J Sports Med Allied Health Sci Off J Ohio Athl Train Assoc 3(2).

Chi L-M, Lin L-M, Chen C-L et al. (2016) The effectiveness of cupping therapy on relieving chronic neck and shoulder pain: a randomized controlled trial. Evid Based Complement Alternat Med 2016(7358918):1–7.

Chirali IZ (2014) History of cupping therapy. In: Chirali IZ, ed. Traditional Chinese Medicine Cupping Therapy, 3rd edn. Edinburgh: Churchill Livingstone.

DaPrato C, Krug R, Souza R et al. (2018) The immediate and long-term effects of negative pressure soft tissue mobilization on the iliotibial bands of runners using magnetic resonance imaging. J Bodyw Mov Ther 22(4):863.

Gao C, Wang M, He L et al. (2019) Alternations of hemodynamic parameters during Chinese cupping therapy assessed by an embedded near-infrared spectroscopy monitor. Biomed Opt Express 10(1):196.

Lacross Z (2011) Treatment Outcomes of Myofascial Decompression on Hamstring Pathology [MS Thesis]. Ypsilanti, MI: Eastern Michigan.

Li T, Li Y, Lin Y et al. (2017) Significant and sustaining elevation of blood oxygen induced by Chinese cupping therapy as assessed by near-infrared spectroscopy. Biomed Opt Express 8(1):223.

Lowe DT (2017) Cupping therapy: an analysis of the effects of suction on skin and the possible influence on human health. Complement Ther Clin Pract 29:162–168.

Pavan PG, Stecco A, Stern R et al. (2014) Painful connections: densification versus fibrosis of fascia. Curr Pain Headache Rep 18(8):441.

Pober JS, Sessa WC (2015) Inflammation and the blood microvascular system. Cold Spring Harb Perspect Biol 7(1).

Rozenfeld E, Kalichman L (2016) New is the well-forgotten old: the use of dry cupping in musculoskeletal medicine. J Bodyw Mov Ther 20(1):173–178.

Schafer M (2018) The Acute Effects of Cupping Therapy on Hamstring Range of Motion Compared to Sham [PhD Thesis]. Las Vegas: UNLV Theses, Dissertations, Professional Papers, and Capstones.

Stecco C, Day JA (2010) The fascial manipulation technique and its biomechanical model: a guide to the human fascial system. Int J Ther Massage Bodyw 3(1):38–40.

Stecco C, Hammer WI (2014) Functional Atlas of the Human Fascial System. Edinburgh: Churchill Livingstone.

Tham LM, Lee HP, Lu C (2006) Cupping: from a biomechanical perspective. J Biomech 39(12):2183–2193.

Yim J, Park J, Kim H et al. (2017) Comparison of the effects of muscle stretching exercises and cupping therapy on pain thresholds, cervical range of motion and angle: a cross-over study. Phys Ther Rehabil Sci 6(2):7.

Zhang Y-J, Cao H-J, Li X-L et al. (2017) Cupping therapy versus acupuncture for pain-related conditions: a systematic review of randomized controlled trials and trial sequential analysis. Chin Med 12(1):21.

Introduction

If we use instruments for myofascial therapy, elastic taping may and must be called an instrument. As with IAMT, the mechanical stimulus through the skin is the basis for the mode of action of this therapy.

We owe the origin of this method to Dr Kenzo Kase (a Japanese chiropractor), who made the technique possible with the invention of elastic tape material in the late 1970s. At the beginning of the 2000s, this tape method became popular in Europe through professional sports and is now used in almost every practice.

To date, according to the current state of research, it is not possible to speak of an evidence-based treatment technique, as nearly all studies write only of "non-significant positive effects." However, the feedback from athletes and patients is quite positive and the technique should therefore not be dismissed as "useless," even if it only produces a feeling. That we can achieve an effect on hematomas is shown by the figures in this chapter, which at least suggest that metabolic processes are accelerated.

As contraindications, skin diseases and injuries of the skin must be taken into account. Sunburn and plaster allergies must be excluded in advance.

Before the tapes are applied, the skin should be free of hair and grease (body lotion/cream). During application of the tapes, the adhesive surface should not be touched with the fingers and the position of the tape should not be corrected after contact with the skin; otherwise, skin particles already adhering will negatively influence the adhesive quality.

Principles

Due to the stretchable material that constitutes the elastic tapes, stimuli of different strengths can be given to the skin and the underlying layers. We can influence the superficial lymphatic system (improved lymphatic drainage) and also reach fascia layers such as the superficial fascia or the deeper muscle fascia by pulling the tape more strongly. Proprioception and nociception additionally play a crucial role.

The basic idea, in contrast to most fascia techniques, is not pressure and the resulting displacement of tissue, but rather lifting of the tissue and fascial layers and the resulting pressure reduction.

The elastic taping method should not be seen as a stand-alone treatment technique. In connection with IAMT, however, we can speak of a temporal extension of the therapy stimulus. Therefore, the techniques fit well together in the appropriate sequence. The previously treated tissue is kept in motion by the lifting function of the tape, and the gliding ability of the fascia layers continues to be maintained over the wearing time of the elastic tapes (up to 4–5 days is possible).

Using two different basic techniques for the elastic taping method, we can easily demonstrate how the mechanical stimulus acts on the skin. The difference is in the application technique and timing (before or after IAMT). The skin surface can be pre-stretched via movement of the joint, or the elastic tape material is pre-stretched with traction and glued on. The effect differs visually and in sensitivity.

In the lymphatic technique we have a visible lifting of the skin and thus a drainage effect whereby the lymphatic system is stimulated. The tape can be applied before the lymphatic drainage, thus increasing the area treated during manual lymphatic drainage.

The removal of a hematoma is also clearly visible after 2 days (Figures 24.1 and 24.2). Especially in the case of hematomas, we do not have many options with IAMT, as these are often a

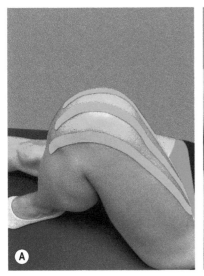

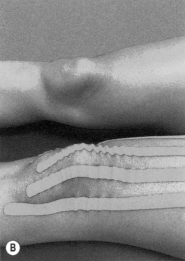

Figure 24.1 Convolutions (rippling) are clearly visible, lifting the skin and thus reducing pressure in the underlying fascial tissue (nociception/analgesia)

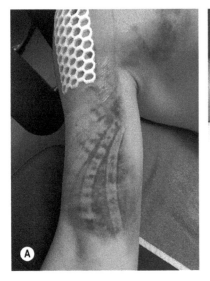

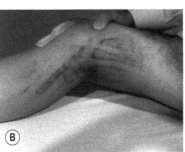

Figure 24.2 (A) After removal of a lymph tape applied postoperatively after a humeral head fracture for 2 days. (B) After removal of a lymph tape, which was applied postoperatively after anterior cruciate ligament surgery for 2 days.

contraindication. Using elastic taping as an instrument, we can also work in the early phase after an injury.

In the fascia technique, we pull the well-fixed base (base glued on without traction) of the elastic tape flat over the surface of the body to achieve a displacement transversely and longitudinally to the fiber course of the superficial fascia layer to deeper fascia. In this case, IAMT is performed before application of the elastic taping fascia technique (Figure 24.3). The structures to be treated are worked on with the instruments and their different techniques (Rehydration, Pain Relief, Mobilization, Regulation of Tone, Metabolization). Immediately afterwards, the tape is applied. However, no gel should be used in the IAMT because

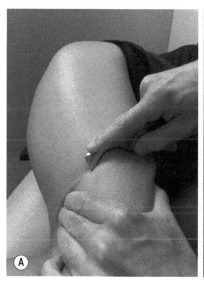
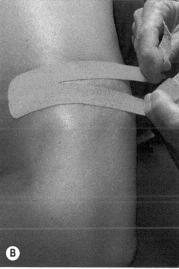

Figure 24.3 (A) First the IAMT treatment is performed. (B) Then the tape is applied.

the adhesive ability of the tape would be reduced or it would even be impossible to apply.

Since the elastic tapes remain in place for several days, the mechanical stimulus on the skin is also maintained and is further enhanced by movements of the patient. The goal, in addition to improving mobility, is hyperemia (metabolization) in the various tissue layers.

The sensation of wearing the tape is usually very pleasant and is often described as stabilizing, although this is only a proprioceptive input and not real, passive stability (compared with classical tape application). A sensation of warmth and pain relief is also frequently reported, which can be explained by hyperemia. This can be detected by a thermal imaging camera. Again, we have the same goal with the tapes as with IAMT.

Movement of the taped area is important for the effectiveness of the elastic tapes. The tapes are not intended for immobilization because only with movement can the mechanical stimulus on the skin achieve its effect. The movements are ideally active, but they can also be implemented, for example, post-operatively, through a movement

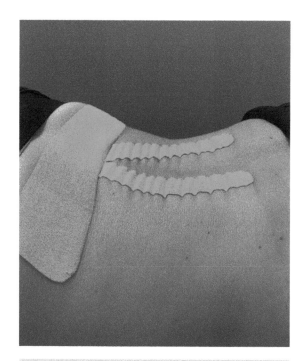

Figure 24.4 Two techniques in combination: with convolutions (applied without tension) and the fascia technique (applied with tension)

splint. Since this taping method should not restrict movements, it is often used by athletes.

As with sports bandages, taped joints provide improved proprioception, which optimizes the perception of movement (Pain Relief, Regulation of Tone).

In summary, the elastic taping method is a useful complement to IAMT. Both treatment techniques performed in the right order in a therapy plan are a good combination with the same objective (Figure 24.4).

A basic assumption of fascia training is that a physiotherapeutic treatment will be more effective and, above all, more sustainable if the patient moves actively in a targeted manner and adjusts their posture. If they do this, permanent structural changes are brought about, in line with the well-known dictum "Form follows function." These changes should, in turn, promote a natural strain on the structures. The functionality of the body is dependent not only on the muscles, but also on the fasciae. The (myo)fascial system is a "global player"; in training, muscles and fasciae cannot be separated, but it is possible to put the emphasis on muscular training or fascial training. The latter is presented in this chapter. The combination of IAMT and meaningful fascial movements seems to increase treatment success significantly and could lead to better sustainability of the treatment outcome. The fact that the (myo)fascial system connects everything to everything in our body and that unhealthy fasciae have poor characteristics are the reasons for this.

The (myo)fascial system is a continuum, and in order to maintain the positive change induced by IAMT, the treated structure must be functionally and regularly stimulated. The change must be integrated into the body perception and the movement behavior must be changed on a permanent basis (Figure 25.1).

Unhealthy fasciae have two bad characteristics:

- They develop hypomobilities: that is, a reduction in their ability to be made more flexible.
- They lose the ability to store kinetic energy.

Healthy components of fascial structures (the parallel parts of the so-called "loose connective tissue")

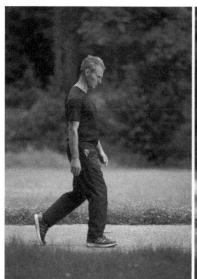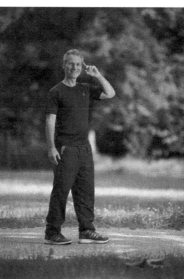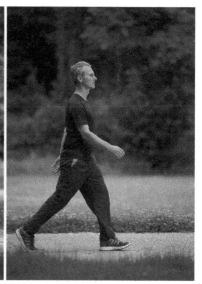

Figure 25.1 From a poor posture to an upright, healthy posture

store 30 percent of kinetic energy and transmit it to adjacent body structures during movement (Hujing and Baan 2003). Sticky ones do not! These hypomobilities can be resolved very efficiently with IAMT. Specific training, however, optimizes the mechanical properties of the fasciae. The optimal stimuli for the (myo)fascial system are maximum stretching over the longest possible chains (tensegrity mode); activation of the musculature in a lengthened position; and bouncing (or rocking) in the final pre-stretched area and an important variety of movements.

Maximum Stretching over Long Chains (Tensegrity Mode)

Fascia loves to be stretched maximally. It releases fascial hypomobilities, and moves and distributes fluids whose optimal consistency is thus maintained. Since everything is connected to everything else, it makes absolute sense to operate fascial chains that are as long as possible. Stretching should be done according to the "tensegrity mode" (Figure 25.2): it all depends on the detail. Every structure in the chain should be stretched according to an individual's possibilities – from the toes to the fingertips!

Activation of the Musculature in Lengthened Position

Kurt Mosetter has shown us with his KID method (Kraft in der Dehnung – strengthening in lengthened position; Mosetter and Mosetter 2012) how effective activating the muscles in a lengthened position is (Figure 25.3). The fact is that the length of muscles or muscle fibers cannot be increased by stretching and cannot be shortened by strength training (studies have never been able to show the opposite). Rather, it is the fascial system around the muscles that gives us the feeling of stiffness and shortened muscles. A study

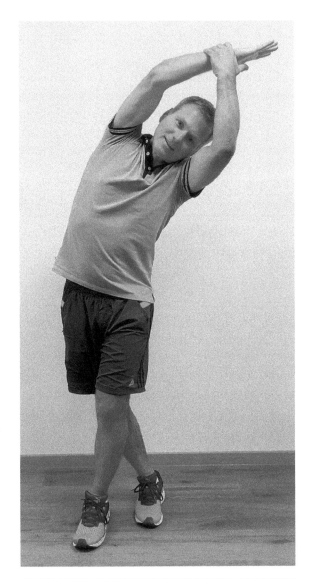

Figure 25.2 An exercise in "tensegrity mode"

from Brazil (Aquino et al. 2009) concludes that the exercise technique of "activating the muscles lengthwise" causes the surrounding fascial structures of the muscles to slacken; passive stretching does not do this. Thus, this technique would be the best method to improve flexibility. If we summarize all the elements of this technique, we inevitably come to the conclusion that these exercises are the most efficient and time-saving ones for health. You kill three birds with one stone! With one exercise you train strength, flexibility, and upright posture.

Bouncing (Rocking) in the Final Pre-stretched Area

As explained before, fascia training is not only about loosening and reorganizing the fascia, but also about the ability to store kinetic energy for a short time and to transport it further. Optimal

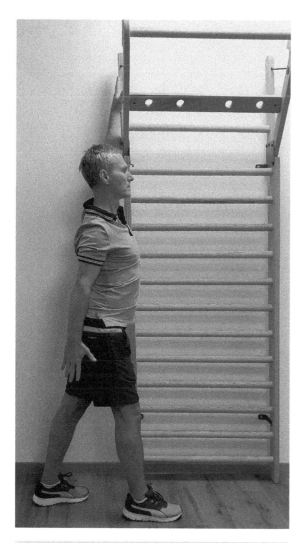

Figure 25.3 Activation of the musculature in a lengthened position

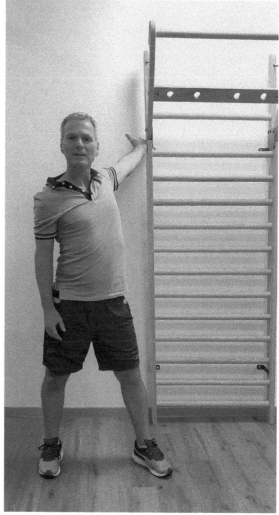

Figure 25.4 Bouncing (rocking) in the final pre-stretched area

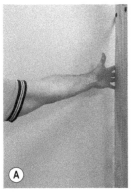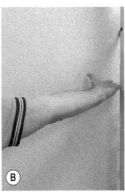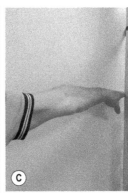

(A) (B) (C)

Figure 25.5 (A–C) Varieties of movement

stimuli for this are bouncing (rocking) movements in a maximally pre-stretched state (Figure 25.4). This applies to the parallel fibers of the "loose connective tissue," as well as to ligaments/tendons and joint capsules. For the latter structures, there are two components to consider during training: the production of collagen fibers and the building and breaking down of so-called cross-links. Both are promoted by these exercises – breakdown of cross-links more so than the building of collagen.

An Important Variety of Movement

If everything in our body is connected to everything else by millions of collagenous, elastic fibers, and if these fibers are criss-crossed and completely disorganized, then movement variety has to be introduced in order to really offer all fibers an optimal stimulus (Figure 25.5). If stretching occurs along the axis only, then only some of the fibers receive the movement impulse they need to remain elastic and flexible. The result: disbalances in the fascial system – structures that are too firm collide with structures that are too soft. During movement, this inevitably leads to incorrect and excessive strain and thus to injuries.

Summary

Of course, a combination of these four movement stimuli is interesting for training the myofascial system and leading it to sustainable health. So-called "all-in-one exercises" stimulate all the important components of the myofascial system in the best possible way. This sounds like a very time-consuming workout – but it is not!

References

Aquino CF, Fonseca ST, Gonçalves GGP et al (2009) Stretching versus strength training in lengthened position in subjects with tight hamstring muscles: a randomized controlled trial. J Man Ther (1-6). doi:10.1016/j.math.2009.05.006.

Hujing PA, Baan GC (2003) Myofascial force transmission: muscle relative position and length determine agonist and synergist muscle force. J Appl Physiol 94:1092–1107.

Mosetter K, Mosetter R (2012) Strength in Stretching: A Practical Book for Stress, Permanent Load and Trauma. Düsseldorf: Patmos.

In physiotherapy, children are not treated like adults in miniature, but as people in a high-paced developmental process. The younger the child, the faster the development. This is true on all levels: motor, cognitive, and emotional. An effective and targeted therapy is the best prerequisite for optimal promotion of the existing developmental potential.

Common problems in pediatric physiotherapy, which allow meaningful use of IAMT as a support, include the therapy of children with neurological challenges, such as cerebral palsy, but in my experience supportive IAMT is often very useful in rehabilitation after brain and spinal surgeries also. The improvement in tissue quality is directly reflected in improved sensory function and thus in motor function also. The maintenance of mobility in these children is a relevant physiotherapeutic objective due to the disease-related tendency to contractures. IAMT is an important method to achieve this goal, especially as experience shows that the children usually require lifelong treatment. In the field of orthopedic diseases IAMT can also be used profitably. Typical diagnoses include clubfoot, Perthes' disease, scoliosis, developmental asymmetries, and postural deficits. There are more and more children who develop asymmetrically and are motorically conspicuous, and not infrequently show a postural deficit too. In the anamnesis interview it often turns out that there were already problems with motor skills and symmetry in babyhood. Nowadays, many children are delivered by suction cup and cesarean section. These birth mechanisms are a great challenge for the fascia system. Often this is a traumatic event that can additionally affect fascia quality. In recent years, the number of babies with a torticollis/CISS (upper cervical joint-induced symmetry disorder) has increased significantly. Disorders of the fascia from birth can affect motor development in a negative direction. Many babies are treated for this. Asymmetry and coordination problems can reappear in infancy and childhood, especially during growth spurts.

IAMT is an effective method to rebalance the fascia and thus achieve an optimization of posture and symmetry. Many children describe after IAMT how they feel lighter and movement is more fun. The effect of IAMT on children is prompt and spontaneous. Targeted therapeutic exercises, such as in Vojta therapy, are easier to perform, and the treatment effect is more marked. Also the application of kinesiotape (see Chapter 24) has a greater effect after treatment with instruments. To illustrate these statements, here are two case studies from my practice.

Box 26.1

Case report 1: Carolin

Carolin is 8 years old. Her diagnosis is brachial plexus damage in the form of Erb's palsy, right side.

Typical in such a brachial plexus paresis are the clearly weaker shoulder joint external rotators in relation to the internal rotators. Here, there is a risk of internal rotation contracture, and in the worst case, (sub)dislocation of the shoulder. Similarly, shoulder joint abduction and adduction, as well as flexion and pronation–supination in the forearm, are affected. The wrist is limited in palmar flexion, as are finger flexion–extension and thumb opposition. The body schema is disrupted and the arm is in "learned-non-use" mode. This often leads to growth disturbances and is manifested by poor shoulder joint centering and arm length discrepancy. This in turn can lead to asymmetries and scoliosis development.

Carolin's right-sided Erb's palsy was caused by a traumatic birth. No nerve grafting was performed. From the 10th day of life, Carolin received regular physiotherapy in the form of Vojta therapy, and IAMT in addition since the age of 4. Vojta therapy has been performed in intervals since the 4th year of life, and IAMT about once a week, at intervals of 2–3 weeks, depending on growth spurt and development. In addition, daily passive stretching is performed. If arm function worsens, IAMT and Vojta therapy are resumed.

It has been shown that deterioration can be quickly recovered, providing control over function and growth. The biggest challenge is bringing the internal rotation contracture under control. The subscapularis muscle and the external rotators of the shoulder must be treated regularly, as well as the internal rotation tendency in the forearm. Regular treatment of the fascia with IAMT, accompanied by passive stretching and Vojta therapy, which has been going on for years now, has resulted in sufficient shoulder stability. Shoulder surgery that is "normally" required is still considered unnecessary in Carolin's case. Arm length discrepancy is no longer seen. In daily life (activities of daily living) Carolin has almost no problems: she can brush her hair, go to the toilet without problems, put on her jacket and close the zipper, and tie her shoes. Carolin is right-handed and manages to use her right hand for writing. She needs only a few aids, such as table-top dry-erase board on an easel and a grip aid on the pen.

Box 26.2

Case report 2: Mathilde

Mathilde is 8 years old. Her diagnosis is 8p-inverted duplication/deletion syndrome.

Chromosome 8 deletion is a chromosome abnormality that affects many different parts of the body. People with this condition are missing genetic material located on the short arm (p) of chromosome 8 in each cell. The severity of the condition and the associated signs and symptoms vary based on the size and location of the deletion and which genes are involved. Most cases are not inherited, although affected people can pass the deletion on to their children. Treatment is based on the signs and symptoms present in each person. (NIH/GARD 2015)

Mathilde has an unsteady supine position and limited range of motion in all joints. She moves primarily in the sagittal plane. She has difficulty with rotation in the spine. She moves independently from supine to sitting. She sits with her legs crossed and can hold herself in the sitting position for a while. She sits behind the sitting bones with a kyphotic spine. She moves in homologous sliding.

After IAMT she is better able to use reciprocal leg movements; the focus is on regulating the tone in the entire spine, hip flexors, and adductors and buttocks, as well as hamstrings and calf muscles, including the Achilles tendon. Preparation with IAMT makes it possible for her to take up the initial position in Vojta exercises more easily and permits improved freedom of movement. Subsequent Vojta therapy consists mainly of reflex creeping in the prone position. The arm that the head is rotated towards (the facial arm) is flexed to 135 degrees with contact of the medial humeral epicondyle; the leg opposite the direction in which the head is rotated (the occipital leg) is flexed to 45 degrees with contact of the medial femoral epicondyle. Triggering of the zones is performed to activate the innate movement patterns of creeping. Matilde's mother reported after the first IAMT session that her daughter spontaneously showed more joy of movement and tried new movements. She had better blood circulation and warmer feet. Vojta therapy was clearly easier to perform.

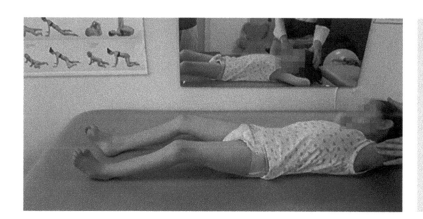

Figure 26.1 Before IAMT: marked knee and hip contraction, supinated feet, and poorly perfused tissues

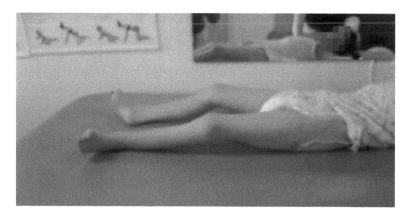

Figure 26.2 After IAMT, feet more in the middle position, much better knee extension, more relaxed hip rotation, and better perfused tissue

References

MIH/GARD (2015) Chromosome 8p deletion. Genetic and Rare Diseases Information Center. Available: https://rarediseases.info.nih.gov/diseases/3768/chromosome-8p-deletion [April 6, 2022].

INDEX

Note: Page numbers followed by italics denotes figures and bold denotes tables respectively.

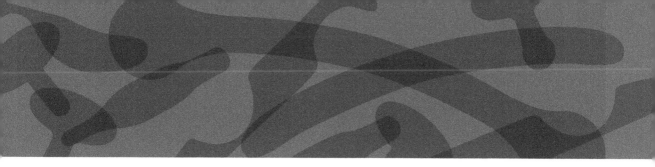

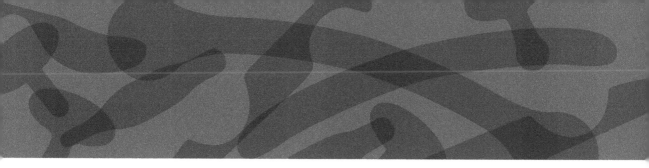

THE FASCIA

Recent research shows that connective tissue has many important functions:

1. Independent organ that supports and shapes the body.
2. Central organ of body perception (influence on immune system and psyche).
3. Protection of spinal cord and joints.
4. Transfer, provision and generation of force (strength).
5. Ability to store kinetic energy.

IASTM – INSTRUMENT-ASSISTED THERAPY WITH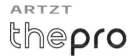

Based on these important functions, myofascial interventions play an increasingly important role in therapy. Functional devices can facilitate the therapist's work, spare their hands and provide an effective therapy supplement.

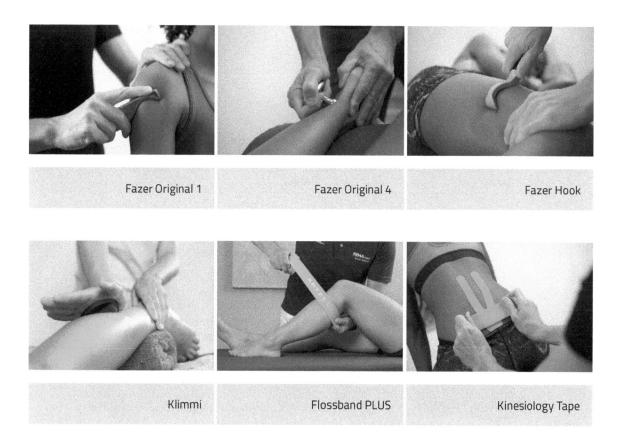

| Fazer Original 1 | Fazer Original 4 | Fazer Hook |
| Klimmi | Flossband PLUS | Kinesiology Tape |

With ARTZT thepro devices you are well equipped: expert knowledge from decades of research as well as first-class quality are combined to create an indispensable tool for daily professional use. This is what the name ARTZT has stood for for over 40 years.

The applied techniques and devices, with their unique shape and material are quick to apply, easy to grasp and produce incredible results in practice.

Leading experts from physiotherapy and medicine such as DFB physio Klaus Eder, fascia expert Dr Robert Schleip or soccer fitness coach Dr Andreas Schlumberger have contributed their expertise and experience to the product development. Each device was designed and forged for special treatment techniques or body regions.

This close contact with professionals makes ARTZT thepro so special and guarantees unparalleled quality and scientific expertise.

ARTZT
thepro

Trust the professionals. Trust ARTZT thepro.

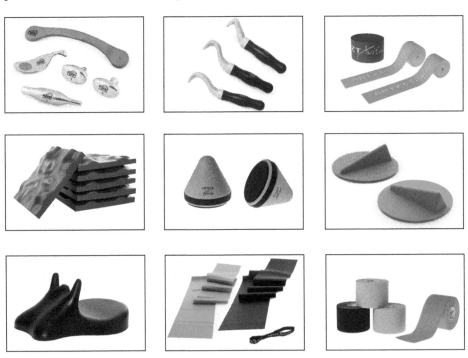

Visit us at **www.artzt.eu/thepro**